AF323012

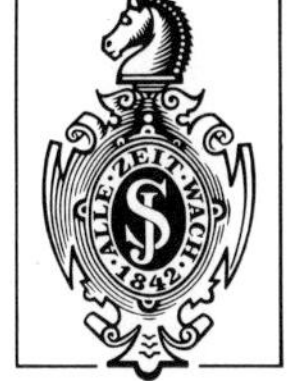

R. Erbel · B. K. Khandheria · R. Brennecke
J. Meyer · J. B. Seward · A. J. Tajik (Eds.)

Transesophageal Echocardiography

A New Window to the Heart

With 176 Figures, Some in Color

Springer-Verlag Berlin Heidelberg New York
London Paris Tokyo Hong Kong

RAIMUND ERBEL, M. D.
II. Medical Clinic
Johannes Gutenberg-University
Mainz
Langenbeckstr. 1
6500 Mainz 1, FRG

BIJOY K. KHANDHERIA, M. D.
Cardiovascular Diseases and
Internal Medicine
Mayo Clinic
Rochester, MN 55905, USA

RÜDIGER BRENNECKE, Ph. D.
II. Medical Clinic
Johannes Gutenberg-University
Mainz
Langenbeckstr. 1
6500 Mainz 1, FRG

JÜRGEN MEYER, M. D.
II. Medical Clinic
Johannes Gutenberg-University
Mainz
Langenbeckstr. 1
6500 Mainz 1, FRG

JAMES B. SEWARD, M. D.
Cardiovascular Diseases and
Pediatric Cardiology
Echocardiographic Laboratory
Mayo Clinic
Mayo Medical School
Rochester, MN 55902, USA

A. JAMIL TAJIK, M. D.
Cardiovascular Diseases and
Pediatric Cardiology
Echocardiographic Laboratory
Mayo Clinic
Mayo Medical School
Rochester, MN 55902, USA

ISBN 3-540-50507-5 Springer-Verlag Berlin Heidelberg New York
ISBN 0-387-50507-5 Springer-Verlag New York Berlin Heidelberg

Typesetting, printing and bookbinding: Druckerei Parzeller, Fulda
2121/3130-543210 − Printed on acid-free paper

Preface

Echocardiography has been one of the most significant advances in cardiology in the past two decades. It can provide anatomic, functional hemodynamic, and blood flow information. Conventional transthoracic echocardiography has limitations, particularly in certain patients such as those with obesity, chronic lung disease, or chest wall deformity, or in those where a transthoracic approach is difficult for reasons including trauma, life support apparat uses, and surgical dressings. There are also certain disease states or conditions in which transthoracic echocardiography expectedly gives incomplete or inadequate information.

Transesophageal echocardiography has opened a unique "new window to the heart." The immediate proximity of the esophagus and the posterior heart permits exceptionally high resolution images, particularly of the left atrium, mitral valve, and intraatrial septum. Additionally, from the stomach (transgastric views), the ventricles can be dependably imaged.

Transesophageal echocardiography presently is utilized in two environments: intraoperatively and for outpatient examinations. Intraoperatively, TEE is utilized to monitor cardiac function and detect intracardiac air or debris, to diagnose or quantitate cardiac pathology, and to access operative results.

Applications of TEE out of the operating room continue to be defined. Clinical diseases or circumstances which appear to be particularly suited for TEE include: (1) assessment of prosthetic heart valves to better define malfunction and important pathologic associations; (2) native valve disease, particularly mitral valve regurgitation and chordal/papillary muscle rupture; (3) detection of thrombus and tumors including atrial and atrial appendage thrombus and atypical or otherwise poorly imaged tumors; (4) endocarditis and detection of vegetations and complications such as abscess formation; (5) thoracic aortic pathology including dissection, aneurysm, and atherosclerosis; (6) congenital heart disease, particularly atrial septal defect; and (7) critically ill patients on life-support who cannot be easily moved or imaged by other modalities, including transthoracic echocardiography. In these circumstances, TEE is often a superior examination or adds unique anatomic or hemodynamic information.

TEE has indeed opened a new and exciting window to the heart. This book of the symposium proceedings presents an overview of current and promising applications of TEE. Methods, technique, anatomic correlation, and future applications are all discussed by recognized experts. Technical aspects of probe design, safety, and current applications are also dealt with.

The editors are particularly grateful to the contributors for their cooperation in preparing manuscripts of their presentations. We are confident that readers will find the contents of the book complete and extremely helpful in understanding the basics as well as the more intricate applications of this new ultrasound technology.

RAIMUND ERBEL, M. D.   BIJOY KHANDHERIA, M. D.
RÜDIGER BRENNECKE, Ph. D.   JAMES SEWARD, M. D.
A. JAMIL TAJIK, M. D.   JÜRGEN MEYER, M. D.

Contents

Masses and Vegetation

Aortic Dissection

Prosthetic Valve Function

**Transesophageal Echocardiography in Critically Ill Patients,
Monitoring by Transesophageal Echocardiography**

Transesophageal Echocardiography in the Operating Room

Transesophageal Echocardiography Versus Epicardial Echo

Perspectives on Transesophageal Echocardiography

Contributors

ABEL M. D., M. D., Departments of Anesthesiology and Internal Medicine, Division of Cardiovascular Diseases and Internal Medicine, Mayo Clinic, Rochester, MN 55905, USA

ADACHI H., M. D., Department of Surgery, Saitama Medical School, 38 Morohongo, Moroyama, 350−04 Saitama, Japan

AFFELD K., M. D., Klinikum Rudolf-Virchow, Spandauer Damm 130, 1000 Berlin 19, Standort Charlottenburg, FRG

ANGELSEN B. A. J., Ph. D., Department of Biomedical Engineering, University of Trondheim, Eirik Jarls gt. 10, 7006 Trondheim-Rit, Norway

ANGERMANN C. E., M. D., Department of Cardiology, Medical Clinic, University of Munich, Ziemsenstr. 1, 8000 München, FRG

BASART D. C. G., M. D., Academic Medical Center Amsterdam, Radboud Hospital Nijmegen, Interuniversity Cardiological Institute Utrecht, Meibergdreef 9, 1105 AZ Amsterdam Zuidoost, The Netherlands

BIAS H., M. D., Klinikum Rudolf-Virchow, Spandauer Damm 130, 1000 Berlin 19, Standort Charlottenburg, FRG

BOM N., M. D., Interuniversity Cardiology Institute of the Netherlands (ICIN)

BOSCH H. G., M. D., Erasmus University Rotterdam, Postbus 1738, 3000 DR Rotterdam, The Netherlands

BRENNECKE R., P. D., Ph. D., II. Medical Clinic, Johannes Gutenberg-University Mainz, Langenbeckstr. 1, 6500 Mainz, FRG

BROMMERSMA P., M. D., Thoraxcenter, Erasmus University Rotterdam and Academic Rotterdam-Dijkzigt, Postbus 1738, 3000 DR Rotterdam, The Netherlands

BRUGADA P., M. D., Academic Hospital, University of Limburg, P.O. Box 1918, 6201 BX Maastricht, The Netherlands

BURG B. V.D., M. D., Academic Medical Center Amsterdam, Radboud Hospital Nijmegen, Interuniversity Cardiological Institute Utrecht, Meibergdreef 9, 1105 AZ Amsterdam Zuidoost, The Netherlands

CAHALAN M. K., M. D., University of California, San Francisco, Department of Anesthesia, San Francisco, CA 94143−0648, USA

CATTELAENS N., M. D., Medical Clinic, Cardiology, Hospital Siegburg, Ringstr. 48, 5200 Siegburg, FRG

CHAPMAN J., Department of Biomedical Engineering, University of Trondheim, Eirik Jarls gt. 10,7006 Trondheim-Rit, Norway

CHERIEX E. C., M. D., Academic Hospital, University of Limburg, P.O. Box 1918, 6201 BX Maastricht, The Netherlands

CLEMENTS F. M., M. D., Duke University Medical Center, Durham NC 27710, USA

CURTIUS J. M., M. D., Medical Clinic III, University of Cologne, Joseph-Stelzmann-Str. 9, 5000 Köln 41, FRG

DANIEL W. G., M. D., Division of Cardiology and Thoracic Surgery, Hannover Medical School, Konstanty-Gutschow-Str. 8, 3000 Hannover 61, FRG

DANIELS O., M. D., Academic Medical Center Amsterdam, Radboud Hospital Nijmegen, Interuniversity Cardiological Institute Utrecht, Meibergdreef 9, 1105 AZ Amsterdam Zuidoost, The Netherlands

DAVID G. K., M. D., Department of Cardiology of the Academic Medical Center, Amsterdam, and the Interuniversity Cardiology Institute Utrecht, Meibergdreef 9, 1105 AZ Amsterdam Zuidoost, The Netherlands

DE BRUIJN N. P., M. D., Duke University Medical Center, Durham NC 27710, USA

DE JONG N., M. D., Thoraxcenter, Erasmus University Rotterdam and Academic Rotterdam-Dijkzigt, P.O. Box 1738, 3000 DR Rotterdam, The Netherlands

DE MARTINO G., M. D., Division of Cardiology, University of Bari, Piazza Giulio Cesare, 70124 Bari, Italy

DESIDERI A., M. D., Klinikum Rudolf-Virchow, Spandauer Damm 130, 1000 Berlin 19, Standort Charlottenburg, FRG

DØRUM S., M. D., Department of Biomedical Engineering, University of Trondheim, Eirik Jarls gt. 10, 7006 Trondheim-Rit, Norway

DREXLER M., M. D., II. Medical Clinic, Johannes Gutenberg-University, Langenbeckstr. 1, 6500 Mainz, FRG

DREYSE S., M. D., Klinikum Rudolf-Virchow, Spandauer Damm 130, 1000 Berlin 19, Standort Charlottenburg, FRG

DUNNING A. J., M. D., Department of Cardiology of the Academic Medical Center, Amsterdam, and the Interuniversity Cardiology

Institute Utrecht, Meibergdreef 9, 1105 AZ Amsterdam Zuidoost, The Netherlands

EFFERT S., M. D., Medical Clinic I RWTH, Pauwelsstraße, 5100 Aachen, FRG

ENGBERDING R., M. D., Medical Clinic, Department of Internal Medicine C, University Münster, Albert-Schweitzer-Str. 33, 4400 Münster, FRG

ERBEL R., M. D., II. Medical Clinic, Johannes Gutenberg-University Mainz, Langenbeckstr. 1, 6500 Mainz, FRG

ERNST S. M. P. G., M. D., Departments of Cardiology of the Academic Medical Center Amsterdam and the Sint Antonius Hospital Nieuwegein and the Interuniversity, Cardiology Institute Utrecht, Meibergdreef 9, 1105 AZ Amsterdam Zuidoost, The Netherlands

ERTL G., M. D., University Hospital of Internal Medicine, Josef-Schneider-Str. 2, 8700 Würzburg, FRG

ESCHENBRUCH C., M. D., Division of Cardiology and Thoracic Surgery, Hannover Medical School, Konstanty-Gutschow-Str. 8, 3000 Hannover 61, FRG

FLACHSKAMPF F. A., M. D., Klinikum RWTH, Pauwelsstraße, 5100 Aachen, FRG

FRANK G., M. D., Division of Cardiology and Thoracic Surgery, Hannover Medical School, Konstanty-Gutschow-Str. 8, 3000 Hannover 61, FRG

GEIBEL A., M. D., Internal Medicine and Cardiovascular Surgery, Albert-Ludwig University of Freiburg, Hugstetter Str. 55, 7800 Freiburg, FRG

GERBER TH., cand. med., II. Medical Clinic, Johannes Gutenberg-University Mainz, Langenbeckstr. 1, 6500 Mainz, FRG

GERBRANDS J. J., M. D., Erasmus University Rotterdam, P.O. Box 1738, 3000 DR Rotterdam, The Netherlands

GERCKENS U., M. D., Department of Cardiology, University Hospital Siegburg, Ringstr. 49, 5200 Siegburg, FRG

GROTE J., M. D., Division of Cardiology and Thoracic Surgery, Hannover Medical School, Konstanty-Gutschow-Str. 8, 3000 Hannover 61, FRG

GRUBE E., M. D., Department of Cardiology, University Hospital Siegburg, Ringstr. 49, 5200 Siegburg, FRG

GUSSENHOVEN W. J., M. D., Interuniversity, Cardiology Institute Utrecht, Meibergdreef 9, 1105 AZ Amsterdam Zuidoost, The Netherlands

HAAGEN F. D. H., M. D., Departments of Cardiology of the Academic Medical Center Amsterdam and the Sint Antonius Hospital Nieuwegein and the Interuniversity, Cardiology Institute Utrecht, Meibergdreef 9, 1105 AZ Amsterdam Zuidoost, The Netherlands

HAKE U., M. D., II. Medical Clinic, Johannes Gutenberg-University Mainz, Langenbeckstr. 1, 6500 Mainz, FRG

HANDT S., M. D., Klinikum RWTH, Pauwelsstraße, 5100 Aachen, FRG

HANRATH P., M. D., Medical Clinic I RWTH, Pauwelsstraße, 5100 Aachen, FRG

HAUDE M., M. D., II. Medical Clinic, Johannes Gutenberg-University Mainz, Langenbeckstr. 1, 6500 Mainz, FRG

HEINRICH H., M. D., University Clinic of Anesthesia, Steinhövelstr. 9, 7900 Ulm, FRG

HENRICHS K. J., M. D., II. Medical Clinic, Johannes Gutenberg-University Mainz, Langenbeckstr. 1, 6500 Mainz, FRG

HEROLD M., M. D., Klinikum RWTH, Pauwelsstraße, 5100 Aachen, FRG

HESS J., M. D., Departments of Clinical Echocardiography, Pediatric Cardiology and Cardiac Surgery, Thoraxcenter, Erasmus University Rotterdam and the Sophia Kinderziekenhuis, Postbus 1738, 3000 DR Rotterdam, The Netherlands

HOEDEMAKER G., M. D., Department of Cardiology of the Academic Medical Center, Amsterdam, and the Interuniversity Cardiology Institute Utrecht, Meibergdreef 9, 1105 AZ Amsterdam Zuidoost, The Netherlands

HOEM J., M. D., Department of Biomedical Engineering, University of Trondheim, Eirik Jarls gt. 10, 7006 Trondheim-Rit, Norway

HOFMANN T., M. D., Internal Medicine and Cardiovascular Surgery, Albert-Ludwig University of Freiburg, Hugstetter Str. 55, 7800 Freiburg, FRG

HOJO H., M. D., Department of Cardiovascular Surgery, Showa General Hospital, 2−450, Tenjin-cho, Kodaira, Tokyo 187, Japan

ILICETO S., M. D., Division of Cardiology, University of Bari, Piazza Giulio Cesare, 70124, Bari, Italy

IVERSEN S., M. D., II. Medical Clinic, Johannes Gutenberg-University Mainz, Langenbeckstr. 1, 6500 Mainz, FRG

JAARSMA W., M. D., St. Antonius Ziekenhuis, Postbus 2500, 3430 EM Nieuwgein, Belgium

Jakob H., M. D., II. Medical Clinic, Johannes Gutenberg-University Mainz, Langenbeckstr. 1, 6500 Mainz, FRG

Johnson S. H., M. D., Duke University Medical Center, Department of Surgery, Durham, NC 27710, USA

Just H., M. D., Internal Medicine and Cardiovascular Surgery, Albert-Ludwig University of Freiburg, Hugstetter Str. 55, 7800 Freiburg, FRG

Kabas J. S., M. D., Duke University Medical Center, Department of Surgery, Durham, NC 27710, USA

Karnik R., M. D., II. Medizinische Abteilung, Krankenhaus Rudolfstiftung, Juchgasse 25, 1030 Wien, Austria

Kasper W., M. D., Internal Medicine and Cardiovascular Surgery, Albert-Ludwig University of Freiburg, Hugstetter Str. 55, 7800 Freiburg, FRG

Kemkes B. M., M. D., Department of Cardiac Surgery, Klinikum Großhadern, University of Munich, Marchioninistr. 15, 8000 München 70, FRG

Khandheria B. K., M. D., Cardiovascular Diseases and Internal Medicine, Mayo Clinic, Rochester, MN 55905, USA

Kisslo J., M. D., Duke University Medical Center, Department of Surgery, Durham, NC 27710, USA

Kleinert C., M. D., University Hospital of Internal Medicine, Josef-Schneider-Str. 2, 8700 Würzburg, FRG

Kochsiek K., M. D., University Hospital of Internal Medicine, Josef-Schneider-Str. 2, 8700 Würzburg, FRG

Koolen J. J., M. D., Department of Cardiology of the Academic Medical Center Amsterdam, Meibergdreef 9, 1105 AZ Amsterdam Zuidoost, The Netherlands

Küpper W., M. D., Klinikum RWTH, Pauwelsstraße, 5100 Aachen, FRG

Kreis A., M. D., Medical Clinic I, RWTH Aachen, Pauwelsstraße, 5100 Aachen, FRG

Krüger W., M. D., II. Medical Clinic, AK St. Georg, 2000 Hamburg, FRG

Kupferwasser I., cand. med., II. Medical Clinic, Johannes Gutenberg-University Mainz, Langenbeckstr. 1, 6500 Mainz, FRG

Kyo S., M. D., Department of Surgery, Saitama Medical School, 38 Morohongo, Moroyama, Saitama 350−04, Japan

LAM J., M. D., Academic Medical Center Amsterdam, Radboud Hospital Nijmegen, Interuniversity Cardiological Institute Utrecht, Meibergdreef 9, 1105 AZ Amsterdam Zuidoost, The Netherlands

LAMBERTZ H., M. D., Klinikum RWTH, Pauwelsstraße, 5100 Aachen, FRG

LAMBREGTS H., M. D., Academic Hospital, University of Limburg, P.O. Box 1918, 6201 BX Maastricht, The Netherlands

LANCÉE C. T., Ph. D., Thoraxcenter, Erasmus University Rotterdam and Academic Rotterdam-Dijkzigt, P.O. Box 1738, 3000 DR Rotterdam, The Netherlands

LANGENSTEIN B., M. D., II. Medical Clinic, AK St. Georg, 2000 Hamburg, FRG

LICHTLEN P. R., M. D., Division of Cardiology and Thoracic Surgery, Hannover Medical School, Konstanty-Gutschow-Str. 8, 3000 Hannover 61, FRG

LO H. B., M. D., Klinikum RWTH, Pauwelsstraße, 5100 Aachen, FRG

LOOS D., M. D., Klinikum Rudolf-Virchow, Spandauer Damm 130, 1000 Berlin 19, Standort Charlottenburg, FRG

LU W., M. D., II. Medical Clinic, Johannes Gutenberg-University Mainz, Langenbeckstr. 1, 6500 Mainz, FRG

MAISCH B., M. D., Department of Internal Medicine and Cardiology, Philipps University Marburg, Baldingerstraße, 3550 Marburg, FRG

MATSUMURA M., M. D., Department of Surgery, Saitama Medical School, 38 Morohongo, Moroyama, Saitama 350−04, Japan

MATSUNAKA T., Medical Ultrasound, Department, Aloka Co. Ltd, Mure-6-22-1, Mitaka-shi, Tokyo, 181, Japan

MAYER E., M. D., Clinic for Cardiothoracic and Vascular Surgery, Johannes Gutenberg-University Mainz, Langenbeckstr. 1, 6500 Mainz, FRG

MEMMOLA C., M. D., Division of Cardiology, University of Bari, Piazza Giulio Cesare, 70124 Bari, Italy

MESSMER B. J., M. D., Klinikum RWTH, Pauwelsstraße, 5100 Aachen, FRG

MEYER J., M. D., II. Medical Clinic, Johannes Gutenberg-University Mainz, Langenbeckstr. 1, 6500 Mainz, FRG

MOHR-KAHALY S., M. D., II. Medical Clinic, Johannes Gutenberg-University Mainz, Langenbeckstr. 1, 6500 Mainz, FRG

MÜGGE A., M. D., Division of Cardiology and Thoracic Surgery, Hannover Medical School, Konstanty-Gutschow-Str. 8, 3000 Hannover 61, FRG

NEYA K., M. D., Department of Surgery, Saitama Medical School, 38 Morohongo, Moroyama, Saitama 350−04, Japan

NIJVELD A., M. D., Academic Medical Center Amsterdam, Radboud Hospital Nijmegen, Interuniversity Cardiological Institute Utrecht, Meibergdreef 9, 1105 AZ Amsterdam Zuidoost, The Netherlands

NISHIMURA R. A., M. D., Departments of Anesthesiology and Internal Medicine, Division of Cardiovascular Diseases and Internal Medicine, Mayo Clinic, Rochester, MN 55905, USA

OELERT H., M. D., Division of Cardiothoracic and Vascular Surgery, Johannes Gutenberg-University Mainz, Langenbeckstr. 1, 6500 Mainz, FRG

OH J. K., M. D., Department of Cardiovascular Diseases and Internal Medicine, Mayo Clinic, Rochester, MN 55905, USA

OMOTO R., M. D., Department of Surgery, Saitama Medical School, 38 Morohongo, Moroyama, 350−04 Saitama, Japan

PICCINNI G., M. D., Division of Cardiology, University of Bari, Piazza Giulio Cesare, 70124 Bari, Italy

PIETERS F., M. D., Academic Hospital, University of Limburg, P.O. Box 1918, 6201 BX Maastricht, The Netherlands

QUAEGEBEUR J., M. D., Departments of Clinical Echocardiography, Pediatric Cardiology and Cardiac Surgery, Thoraxcenter, Erasmus University Rotterdam and the Sophia Kinderziekenhuis, P.O. Box 1738, 3000 DR Rotterdam, The Netherlands

RANKIN J. S., Duke University Medical Center, Durham NC 27710, USA

RAU G., Ph. D., Klinikum RWTH, Pauwelsstraße, 5100 Aachen, FRG

REIBER J. H. C., Ph. D., Erasmus University Rotterdam, P.O. Box 1738, 3000 DR Rotterdam, The Netherlands

RENNOLLET H., cand. med., II. Medical Clinic, Johannes Gutenberg-University Mainz, Langenbeckstr. 1, 6500 Mainz, FRG

REUL H., Klinikum RWTH, Pauwelsstraße, 5100 Aachen, FRG

RITTER G., M. D., Klinik für Unfallchirurgie, Johannes Gutenberg-University Mainz, Langenbeckstr. 1, 6500 Mainz, FRG

RIZZON P., M. D., Division of Cardiology, University of Bari, Piazza Giulio Cesare, 70124 Bari, Italy

ROELANDT J. R. T. C., M. D., Thoraxcenter, Erasmus University Rotterdam and Academic Rotterdam-Dijkzigt, P.O. Box 1738, 3000 DR Rotterdam, The Netherlands

SACK S., cand. med., II. Medical Clinic, Johannes Gutenberg-University Mainz, Langenbeckstr. 1, 6500 Mainz, FRG

SCHARTL M., M. D., Klinikum Rudolf-Virchow, Spandauer Damm 130, 1000 Berlin 19, Standort Charlottenburg, FRG

SCHLOSSER V., M. D., Internal Medicine and Cardiovascular Surgery, Albert-Ludwig University of Freiburg, Hugstetter Str. 55, 7800 Freiburg, FRG

SCHMIEDT W., M. D., II. Medical Clinic, Johannes Gutenberg-University Mainz, Langenbeckstr. 1, 6500 Mainz, FRG

SCHNEIDER B., M. D., II. Medical Clinic, AK St. Georg, 2000 Hamburg, FRG

SCHÜTZ A., M. D., Department of Cardiac Surgery, Klinikum Großhadern, Marchioninistr. 15, 8000 München 40, FRG

SCHULLER J. L., M. D., Academic Medical Center Amsterdam, Radboud Hospital Nijmegen, Interuniversity Cardiological Institute Utrecht, Meibergdreef 9, 1105 AZ Amsterdam Zuidoost, The Netherlands

SCHUSTER S., M. D., II. Medical Clinic, Johannes Gutenberg-University Mainz, Langenbeckstr. 1, 6500 Mainz, FRG

SEHNAL E., M. D., II. Medizinische Abteilung, Krankenhaus Rudolf-stiftung, Juchgasse 25, 1030 Wien, Austria

SEWARD J. B., M. D., Cardiovascular Diseases and Pediatric Cardiology, Echocardiographic Laboratory, Mayo Clinic, Mayo Medical School, Rochester, MN 55902, USA

SHAH P., M. D., Assistant of Anesthesiology, University Rochester, NY 14642, USA

SHEIKH K. H., M. D., Duke University Medical Center, Durham NC 27710, USA

SLANY J., M. D., II. Medizinische Abteilung, Krankenhaus Rudolf-stiftung, Juchgasse 25, 1030 Wien, Austria

SMITH P. K., M. D., Duke University Medical Center, Department of Surgery, Durham, NC 27710, USA

SPES C. H., M. D., Department of Cardiology, Medical Clinic, University of Munich, Ziemsenstr. 1, 8000 München, FRG

SPILLNER G., M. D., Internal Medicine and Cardiovascular Surgery, Albert-Ludwig University of Freiburg, Hugstetter Str. 55, 7800 Freiburg, FRG

STANLEY T., M. D., Duke University Medical Center, Durham NC 27710, USA

STEMPFLE H.-U., M. D., Department of Cardiology, Medical Clinic, University of Munich, Ziemsenstr. 1, 8000 München, FRG

STÖLLBERGER C., M. D., II. Medizinische Abteilung, Krankenhaus Rudolfstiftung, Juchgasse 25, 1030 Wien, Austria

STUMPER O. F. W., M. D., Departments of Clinical Echocardiography, Pediatric Cardiology and Cardiac Surgery, Thoraxcenter, Erasmus University Rotterdam and the Sophia Kinderziekenhuis, P.O. Box 1738, 3000 DR Rotterdam, The Netherlands

SUTHERLAND G. R., M. D., Adolescent/Adult Congenital Heart Disease Clinic, Department of Echocardiography, Thoraxcenter, Academisch Ziekenhuis Dijkzigt, Erasmus University Rotterdam, P.O. Box 1738, 3000 DR Rotterdam, The Netherlands

TAAMS M., M. D., Thoraxcenter, Erasmus University Rotterdam and Academic Rotterdam-Dijkzigt, P.O. Box 1738, 3000 DR Rotterdam, The Netherlands

TACHIKAWA K., Aloka Co Ltd., Mure 6-221, Mitaka-shi, Tokyo 181, Japan

TAJIK A. J., M. D., Cardiovascular Diseases and Pediatric Cardiology, Echocardiographic Laboratory, Mayo Clinic, Mayo Medical School, Rochester, MN 55902, USA

TAKAMOTO S., M. D., Department of Cardiovascular Surgery, Showa General Hospital, 2−450, Tenjin-cho Kodaira, Tokyo 187, Japan

TAMMEN A. R., M. D., Department of Cardiology, Medical Clinic University of Munich, Ziemsenstr. 1, 8000 München, FRG

THEISEN K., M. D., Department of Cardiology, Medical Clinic University of Munich, Ziemsenstr. 1, 8000 München, FRG

TIEDE N., M. D., Internal Medicine and Cardiovascular Surgery, Albert-Ludwig University of Freiburg, FRG

TODT M., M. D., II. Medical Clinic, Johannes Gutenberg-University Mainz, Langenbeckstr. 1, 6500 Mainz, FRG

VAN BURKEN G., M. D, Erasmus University Rotterdam, Postbus 1738, 3000 DR Rotterdam, The Netherlands

VAN DAELE M. E. R. M., M. D., Thoraxcenter, University Hospital Rotterdam-Dijkzigt, Dr. Molewaterplein 40, 3015 GD Rotterdam, The Netherlands

VANDENBOGAERDE J., M. D., Department of Intensive Care, University Hospital, Gent, Belgium

VAN WEZEL H. J., M. D., Department of Cardiology of the Academic Medical Center, Amsterdam, and the Interuniversity Cardiology Institute Utrecht, Meibergdreef 9, 1105 AZ Amsterdam Zuidoost, The Netherlands

VISSER C. A., M. D., Department of Cardiology of the Academic Medical Center Amsterdam, Meibergdreef 9, 1105 AZ Amsterdam Zuidoost, The Netherlands

WALKER P., M. D., Klinikum Rudolf-Virchow, Spandauer Damm 130, 1000 Berlin 19, Standort Charlottenburg, FRG

WEILEMANN L. S., M. D., II. Medical Clinic, Johannes Gutenberg-University Mainz, Langenbeckstr. 1, 6500 Mainz, FRG

WEIMANN E., M. D., Klinikum Rudolf-Virchow, Spandauer Damm 130, 1000 Berlin 19, Standort Charlottenburg, FRG

WELLEK S., II. Medical Clinic, Johannes Gutenberg-University Mainz, Langenbeckstr. 1, 6500 Mainz, FRG

WENDA K., M. D., Klinik für Unfallchirurgie, Johannes Gutenberg-University Mainz, Langenbeckstr. 1, 6500 Mainz, FRG

WITTLICH N., M. D., II. Medical Clinic, Johannes Gutenberg-University Mainz, Langenbeckstr. 1, 6500 Mainz, FRG

YOKOTE Y., M. D., Department of Surgery, Saitama Medical School, 38 Morohongo, Moroyama, Saitama 350−04, Japan

Technology, Normal Examination, Development, Anatomy

Technological Developments of Transesophageal Echocardiography in a Historical Perspective*

C. T. Lancée, N. de Jong, W. J. Gussenhoven, M. Taams, N. Bom, P. Brommersma, and J. R. T. C. Roelandt

Introduction

After the introduction of echocardiography [10], it soon became apparent that scanning of the heart is sometimes hindered by inadequate penetration of ultrasound through the thoracic wall and ribcage. This stimulated many investigators to search for alternative approaches using cavities within the thorax, with the exception of the bronchial tree.

There are two types of cavities leading to the heart or its close vicinity: the blood vessels and the esophagus. Historically, the intravascular approach became the first to be examined, since the presence of blood around the transducer facilitates the direct coupling of ultrasonic energy.

The Intravascular Approach

As early as 1960 a single element mounted on a catheter was introduced into the jugular vein of dogs [5] to observe echoes from cardiac structures on an oscilloscope screen (A mode), while the transducer remained in a stationary position. Three years later, a similar, slowly rotating device which was also introduced in the jugular or femoral vein was described [19]. Using ECG triggering, this technique provided a static cross-sectional image on a memory oscilloscope. A device to monitor the dynamic behavior of intracardiac dimensions was reported in 1968 [4] using an omnidirectional single element at the tip of a catheter. The dimensions had to be reconstructed from minimal and maximal echo arrival times.

Eggleton et al. [11] constructed a catheter with four elements at the tip. Using slow rotation and ECG triggering, a cross-sectional image of intracardiac structures was reconstructed by computer. Two years later, at the Thoraxcenter of the Erasmus University a real-time intracardiac scanner was reported on [1], which used an electronically phased circular array of 32 elements at the tip of a 9-French catheter. Image quality, however, was below the clinically acceptable level. To conclude this historical survey of intravascular scanning

* This work has been supported by grants from the Netherlands Heart Foundation (NHS), the Netherlands Technology Foundation (STW), and ICIN. Sponsoring by Oldelft is acknowledged.

Transesophageal Echocardiography
Edited by R. Erbel et al.
© Springer-Verlag Berlin Heidelberg 1989

devices, another monitoring device [22] should be mentioned. A catheter with two elements was maneuvered in the left ventricle such that the elements were opposite to one another. Following motion of opposing walls and by measuring the transmission of ultrasound, a dynamic recording of the ventricular short axis could be obtained.

But history repeats itself, since our department and others are at this very moment working on an endovascular scanner again. The scope, however, is completely changed, since these scanners are intended to visualize the vessel anatomy in real-time [2, 3].

The Transesophageal Approach

In 1968 a new generation of gastroscopes with a steerable tip was launched. Now a direct contact, without the need for balloons, between the esophageal wall and a tip-mounted ultrasound transducer became possible.

The first cardiac investigation with ultrasound via the esophagus was reported by Side and Gosling [20]. They used a dual element construction mounted on a standard gastroscope to obtain continuous wave (CW) Doppler cordings of cardiac flow. The use of Doppler recording through the esophagus was further expanded with the use of pulsed Doppler with a single element [6]. M-mode tracings obtained via the esophagus were reported by Frazin et al. [12].

Imaging through the esophagus began when Hisanaga et al. [14] reported on a two-dimensional real-time scanning system. The scanning device consisted of a rotating single element in a liquid-filled balloon mounted at the tip of a gastroscope. One year later the same group of researchers also described a mechanical linear scanning device for transesophageal use [15].

The next and most important stage in the development of transesophageal transducers was the introduction of electronic scanners. DiMagno et al. [9] described a high-frequency (10 MHz) linear array for small parts scanning, mainly organs in the gastrointestinal tract. An electronic phased array transducer [21] was particularly useful for cardiac imaging. The frequency of this transducer was the same as that of the precordial transducer (2.25 MHz). From this moment on, phased array scanning via the esophagus evolved rapidly.

In our institution the first transesophageal phased array transducer was constructed [17]. The design featured a tilted 24-element 3.1-MHz array with a pitch (element to element distance) of 400 μm (Fig. 1). Clinical studies, however, showed no need for the 20° inclination of the scanning plane and subsequent designs left the array in line with the gastroscope's long axis. Improvements in microminiature cutting and bonding technology resulted in a series of transducers with progressively better image quality.

In 1983 a 32-element, 3.5-MHz array with a pitch of 300 μm was constructed and its successor − a 52-element, 4.7-MHz array with a pitch of 210 μm − was introduced for clinical use in 1984 [7, 8]. The carrier was a gas-

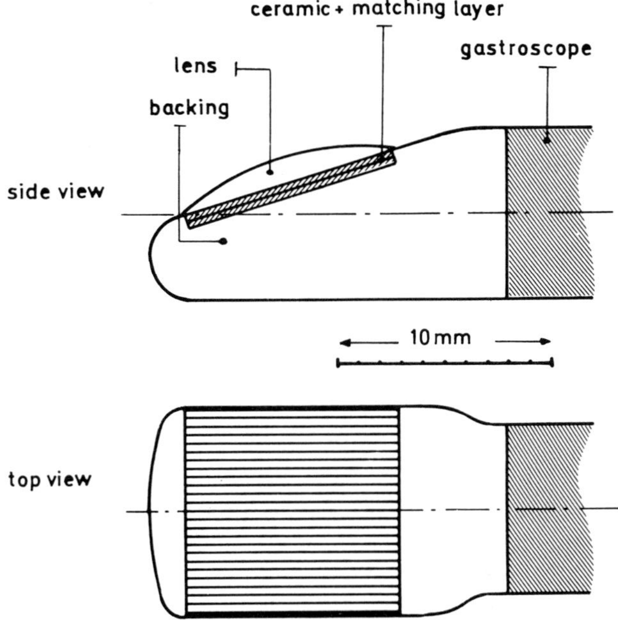

Fig. 1. Schematic drawing of the transesophageal transducer assembly

troscope of 9 mm diameter, while the scan head incorporated an active area of 10×10 mm^2. The final design was realized in 1985, featuring a 64-element, 5.6-MHz array with a pitch of only 160 µm. This design had an extremely low artifact level (grating lobes) combined with superior lateral and axial resolution [13, 18]. Experience with these transducers provided the clinical material presented at this meeting.

Design of Current Transesophageal Echocardiography Probes

The performance of the transducer is determined by its axial, transversal, and lateral resolution, assuming that the sensitivity is sufficient. For the whole system (including the electronics), it is important to have prior knowledge of the area to be imaged, i.e., the acoustic impedance of the different structures, attenuation of the different tissues, and the region of interest. As mentioned before, practical aspects limit the dimensions of the transducer.

The spatial resolution (the resolution cell) is determined by the axial, lateral, and transverse response of the transducer. These three responses are more or less mutually independent and will be discussed individually.

The Axial Resolution

The axial resolution is highly dependent on the ultrasound frequency and its impulse response. The frequency used depends on the attenuation in the medium. It was set to 5.6-MHz. With this setting, parameters for the matching and backing layers must be selected. The matching layer (quarter wave length or 1/4 λ layer) on the front of the ceramic adapts the mismatch in acoustic impedance between the ceramic and the tissue (30 MRayls and 1.5 MRayls, respectively). The backing must have a low impedance for high efficiency of the transducer and a high attenuation to avoid spurious echoes.

Using the Mason model it is possible to predict the impulse response theoretically. Optimal values of the density ϱ and the velocity c of the 1/4 λ layer can be calculated. The acoustic impedance, z_3, must be close to the optimal value given by Eq. (1):

$$z_3 = (2z_1^2 \, z_2)^{1/3} \tag{1}$$

(z_1 = acoustic impedance of the load medium, z_2 = acoustic impedance of the ceramic)

The optimal thickness and density of the 1/4 λ layer have to be determined experimentally because of the unpredictable change in velocity due to the necessary cutting of the material. With several combinations of density and thickness along an array these parameters can be evaluated in order to yield the shortest pulse response.

The Transverse Resolution (in the Elevation Plane)

In contrast to the beam width in the scanning plane, the transverse beam width cannot be controlled dynamically. The focusing in this direction is fixed and realized by a silicon rubber lens. The region of interest is between 2 and 12 cm of depth. In the majority of patients the most important structures (the valvular apparatus, left atrium and ventricle, the outflow tract, and the large vessels) are within 4–8 cm. Computer simulations predict an optimal beam with an aperture of 10 mm and a geometrical focus at 70 mm. Assuming a plane wave, the radius of curvature of the convex lens used is given by

$$R = F \, (1 - c_m/c_1) \tag{2}$$

where R = radius of the lens (m), F = geometrical focus (m), c_m = acoustic velocity in the load medium (m/s), and c_1 = acoustic velocity in the lens (m/s). When $c_1 = 1000$ m/s, then the radius of curvature of the lens will be 35 mm.

The Lateral Resolution (in the Azimuthal Plane)

In order to avoid ambiguity, the main beam should be narrow during transmission and reception, such as might be the case with dynamic focusing techniques. Any sensitivity outside the main beam direction may result in image artifacts. Lobes appearing outside the main beam direction are called side-lobes. A special side-lobe known as the grating lobe originates from the regular spacing of the transducer elements of the array.

The relationship between the angle of the grating lobe and the angle of the main lobe is given by the following equation:

$$\sin \varphi = \frac{\lambda}{p} - \sin \theta \tag{3}$$

where φ = angle of the grating lobe, θ = angle of the main lobe, λ = wavelength (m), and p = pitch (m).

The right-hand term of Eq. (3) will exhibit a range of λ/p to $\lambda/p - \sin \theta_{max}$ when the beam is steered from $\theta = 0$ to θ_{max}. There will be no grating lobe when $\lambda/p - \sin$ remains greater than 1. For $\theta_{max} = 45°$, it follows that $\lambda/p > 1.7$.

The requirement for the absence of grating lobes will be $p < 0.6\,\lambda$. When the array does not satisfy this for all wavelength there will be a grating lobe.

In general, the lateral directivity pattern depends on the total available aperture, the number of elements, and the bandwidth of the transducer. The total aperture determines the beamwidth, while the number of elements determines the occurrence of grating lobes. The bandwidth has a weak influence on the side-lobe level, but a strong influence on the grating lobe level.

Figure 2 shows the theoretical beam pattern for four steering angles with the following parameters: pitch 0.16 mm; number of elements 64; bandwidth of each element 50%. In this figure the patterns are calculated in the focal

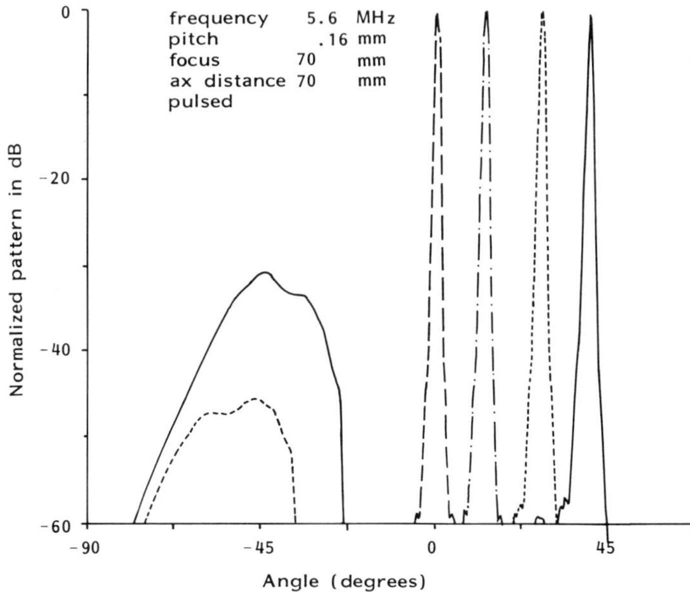

Fig. 2. Calculated beam patterns for steering angles of 0, 13, 27 and 40°, respectively. At large steering angles the grating lobe appears

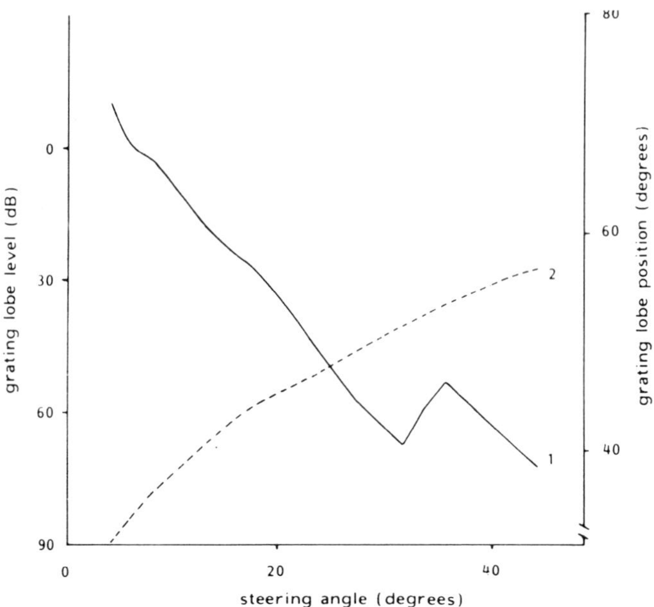

Fig. 3. Grating lobe position (*1, right*) and grating probe level (*2, left*) as function of the steering angle for the esophageal probe (0.16 mm, 5.6-MHz)

point 50 mm from the transducer. Tapering is applied in transmission. The 32 center elements have a factor of 1, the adjacent elements a factor of 0.75, and the outer elements a factor of 0.5. In the figure the beam patterns have been calculated for steering angles of 0°, 13°, 27°, and 40°. Only the last two steering angles have a grating lobe higher than −60 dB. The position and shape of the grating lobe change with the steering angle. The higher the steering angle, the smaller the angle of the grating lobe. In the grating lobe complex, the top moves to the left with an increase of the steering angle.

Figure 3 shows that there is no grating lobe at all at steering angles below 4°. At 4° the level is −90 dB and the position −73°. The grating lobe level increases gradually to −28 dB at the highest steering angle, with a position of −38°. Curve 1 (position of the top of the grating lobe) is not monotonously decreasing because of the change in shape of the grating lobe.

Results

For high performance, good lateral resolution is important. Figure 4 illustrates the measured and simulated beam profile of the esophageal probe at 40° steering angle. Focusing was at 50 mm and measurements were made with digitally phased electronics. As can be seen the measured and simulated data correspond well. Given the data measured in the other resolution planes, the overall resolution cell at the −6 dB level in the focal area was shown to be $1 \times 1 \times 0.3$ mm^3 (Fig. 5).

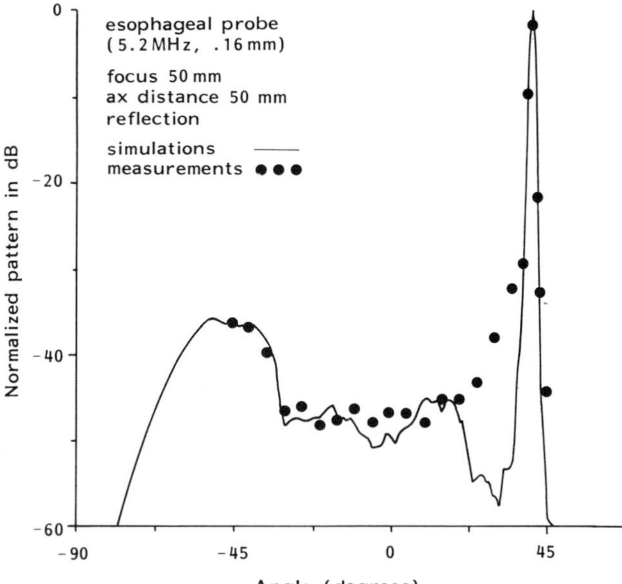

Fig. 4. Simulated (*line*) and measured beam profile (*filled circles*) of the esophageal probe (5.2-MHz, 0.16 mm) at 40° steering angle

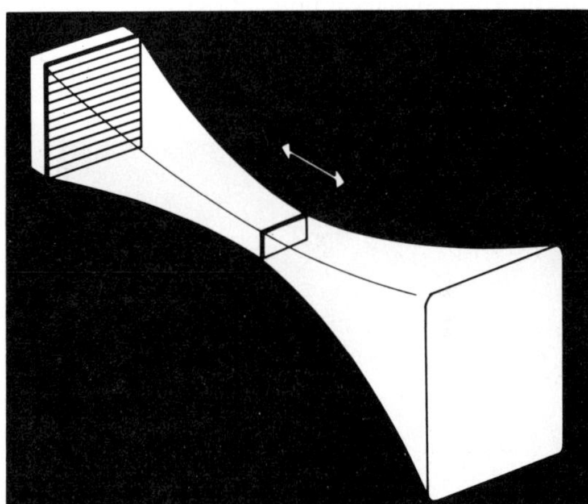

Fig. 5. The resolution of the esophageal probe. Axial resolution (−50 dB), 5 periods; lateral aperture angle (−20 dB), 50°; transverse aperture angle (−20 dB), 1.5°; resolution in focal area (−6 dB), $1 \times 1 \times 0.3$ mm³

The transesophageal probe is shown in Fig. 6. It turned out to perform excellently in clinical use. In patients in whom results of precordial investigation are inadequate, transesophageal scanning provides vital information. Based on a detailed study of the valve apparatus, corrective surgery has in some cases been performed without angiocardiography. The investigation takes less than 15 min and is well tolerated by the patients. The quality of left ventricular cross-sectional images made during surgery is excellent and allows for quantitative analysis. An example of the resulting image is shown in Fig. 7.

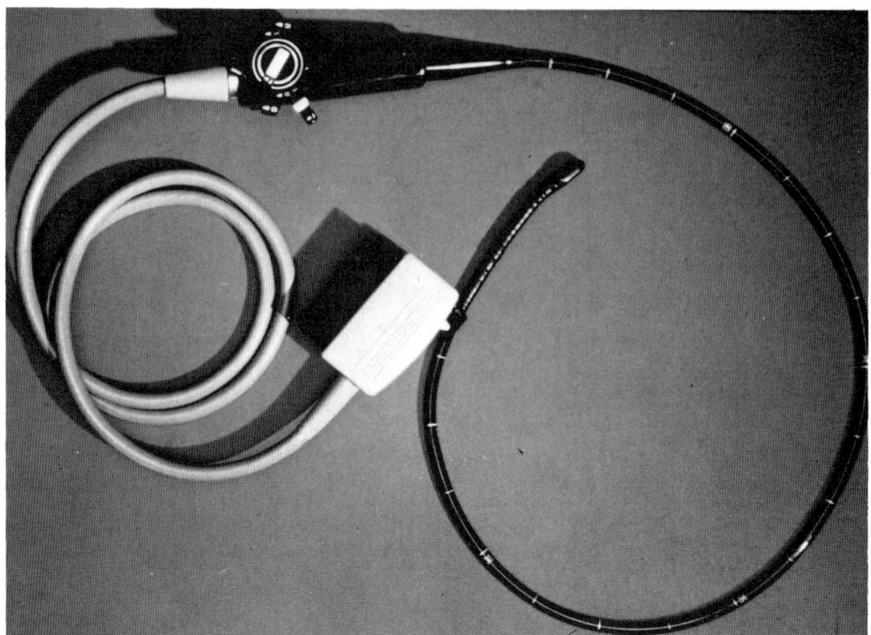

Fig. 6. The esophageal probe in its experimental stage

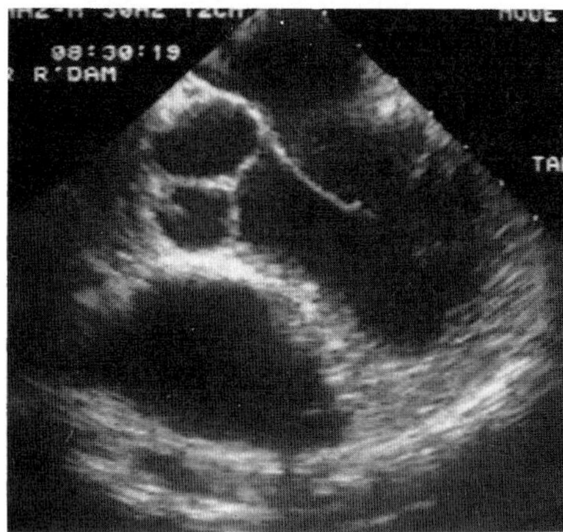

Fig. 7. Cardiac cross section obtained in diastole with the esophageal probe (the left atrium is at the *top* and the closed aortic valve cusps are seen in the *middle* of the image)

Future Developments

As a spin-off from the work on transesophageal transducers, research is currently being done in the field of miniaturized phased array transducers. These transducers are intended to be used as direct contact scanners during open-chest surgery and may operate at frequencies of 7.5-MHz or even higher. This new technology will also be of use for the design of pediatric transesophageal echocardiograpohy transducers, which will considerably increase the range of applications of the technique.

Acknowledgements. The authors are grateful for the enormous amount of work that has been done for our department at the Central Research Workshop of the Medical Faculty, in particular by Leo Bekkering.

References

1. Bom N, Lancée CT, van Egmond FC (1972) An ultrasonic intracardiac scanner. Ultrasonics 10:72–76
2. Bom N, Lancée CT, Slager CJ, de Jong N (1987) Ein Weg zur intraluminären Echoarteriographie. Ultraschall 8:233–236
3. Bom N, Slager CJ, van Egmond FC, Lancée CT, Serruys PW (1988) Intra-arterial ultrasonic imaging for recanalization by spark erosion. Ultrasound Med Biol 14:257–261
4. Carleton RA, Clark JG (1968) Measurement of left ventricular diameter in the dog by cardiac catheterization. Validation and physiologic meaningfulness of an ultrasonic technique. Circ Res 22:545–548
5. Cieszynski T (1960) Intracardiac method for the investigation of structure of the heart with the aid of ultrasonics. Arch Immun Ter Dosw 8:551–557
6. Daigle RE, Miller CW, Histand MB, McLeod FD, Hokanson DE (1975) Nontraumatic aortic blood flow sensing using an ultrasonic esophageal probe. J Appl Physiol 38:6
7. De Jong N, Lancée CT, Gussenhoven WJ, Bom N, Ligtvoet CM (1985) Transoesofagale echocardiografie. Ultrasonoor Bull 2:231
8. De Jong N, Bom N, Lancée CT (1986) Esophageal echocardiography. IEEE Trans Biomed 8:3–6
9. DiMagno EP, Buxton JL, Regan PT, Hattery RR, Wilson DA, Suarez JR, Green PS (1980) Ultrasonic endoscope. Lancet 1:629
10. Edler I, Hertz CH (1954) The use of ultrasonic reflectroscope for the continuous recording of movements of heart walls. Fysiogr Sallsk Forh 24:1–19
11. Eggleton RC, Townsend C, Herrick J, Templeton G, Mitchell JH (1970) Ultrasonic visualization of left ventricular dynamics. Ultrasonics 17:143–153
12. Frazin L, Talano JV, Stephanides L, Loeb HS, Kopel L, Gunnar RM (1976) Esophageal echocardiography. Circulation 54:102
13. Gussenhoven WJ, Taams MA, Ligtvoet CM, McGhie J, van Herwerden LA, Cahalan MK (1986) Transesophageal twodimensional echocardiography: its role in solving clinical problems. J Am Coll Cardiol 4:975–979
14. Hisanaga K, Hisanaga A, Nagata K, Yoshida S (1977) A new transesophageal real-time two-dimensional echocardiographic system using a flexible tube and its clinical application. Proc Jpn Soc Ultrasonics Med 32:43–44
15. Hisanaga K, Hisanaga A, Ichie Y (1978) A new transesophageal real-time linear scanner and initial clinical results. Proc Jpn Soc Ultrasonics Med 35:115–116
16. Lancée CT (1987) A transesophageal phased array transducer for ultrasonic imaging of the heart. Thesis, University of Rotterdam

17. Lancée CT, Ligtvoet CM, de Jong N (1982) On the design and construction of a transesophageal scanner. In: Hanrath P, Bleifeld W, Souquet J (eds) Cardiovascular diagnosis by ultrasound. Nijhoff, The Hague, pp 260–269
18. Lancée CT, de Jong N, Bom N (1988) Design and construction of an esophageal phased array probe. Med Prog Technol 13:139–148
19. Omoto R, Atsumi K, Suma K, Toyoda T, Sakurai Y, Muroi T, Fujimori Y, et al. (1963) Ultrasonic intravenous sonde – 2nd report. Med Ultrason Jpn 1:11
20. Side CG, Gosling RG (1971) Non-surgical assessment of cardiac function. Nature 232:335
21. Souquet J, Hanrath P, Zitelli L, et al. (1982) Transesophageal phased array for imaging the heart. IEEE Trans Biomed Eng 29:707
22. Stegall HF (1974) Ultrasonic measurement of organ dimension. In: Reneman R (ed) Cardiovascular applications of ultrasound. Excerpta Medica, Amsterdam, pp 150–161

High-Frequency Annular Array Transesophageal Probe for High-Resolution Imaging and Continuous Wave Doppler Measurements

B. A. J. ANGELSEN, J. HOEM, S. DØRUM, J. CHAPMAN, E. GRUBE,
U. GERCKENS, C. A. VISSER, and J. VANDENBOGAERDE

Introduction

In the early 1970s, ultrasonic probes were placed in the esophagus to monitor the blood velocity in the descending aorta, and for measurement of the aortic diameter to estimate the volumetric flow in the descending aorta [1−6]. Later [7−10], a mechanically scanned beam was used for two-dimensional (2-D) ultrasound backscatter imaging of the heart. A 10-MHz linear array mounted on the tip of a gastroscope was reported [11, 12], but the system has had limited application for cardiac imaging, partly because of the field of view and the lack of any ability to use lower frequencies. A phased array transducer mounted on the tip of a gastroscope for transesophageal imaging of the heart was first reported in 1981 [13, 14].

Annular phased array transducers have advantages over linear phased arrays in that:

1. It is easier to produce high-frequency transducers. For a linear phased array, the width of the elements has to be less than $\lambda/2$, where λ is the wavelength of the ultrasound. At 5 MHz, $\lambda/2 = 156$ μm; at 7.5 MHz, $\lambda/2 = 104$ μm; and at 10 MHz, $\lambda/2 = 78$ μm. There is at present a technical problem in cutting the transducer ceramic to such a small size and therefore phased linear array transducers above 5 MHz have not been commercially available until recently. With the annular array, there are fewer elements since it is used for electronic focusing only, and the beam steering is done mechanically. This makes each array element larger than in the linear phased array. Thus it is easier to produce high-frequency transducers, up to 10 MHz.

2. The annular phased array is composed of circular rings, and therefore we obtain a circular, symmetrical, electronically steered focus as illustrated in Fig. 1. With the linear phased array we can only steer the focus in the scan plane, while transverse to the scan plane the focus is fixed. This results in a thinner slice thickness of the scan plane with the annular array, and thus improved resolution.

3. Because the annular array has fewer and larger elements, it is easier to arrange separate transmitting and receiving portions of the transducer with such low capacitive cross-coupling that good continuous wave (CW) Doppler imaging is obtained, even with ultrasound frequencies higher than 5 MHz. This is important diagnostically, since many cardiac lesions produce high-velocity blood jets which require CW Doppler to measure the high velocities.

Transesophageal Echocardiography
Edited by R. Erbel et al.
© Springer-Verlag Berlin Heidelberg 1989

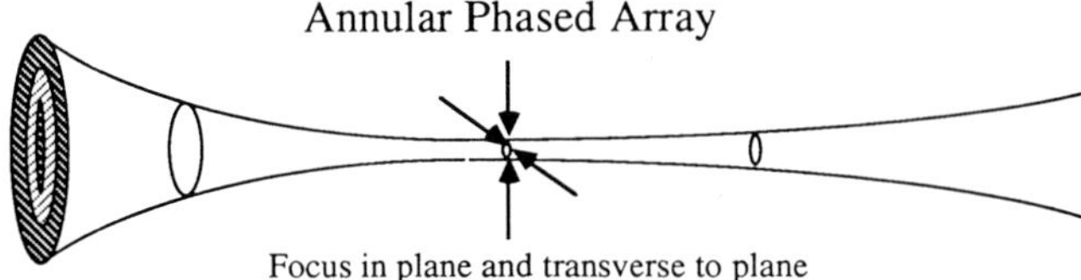

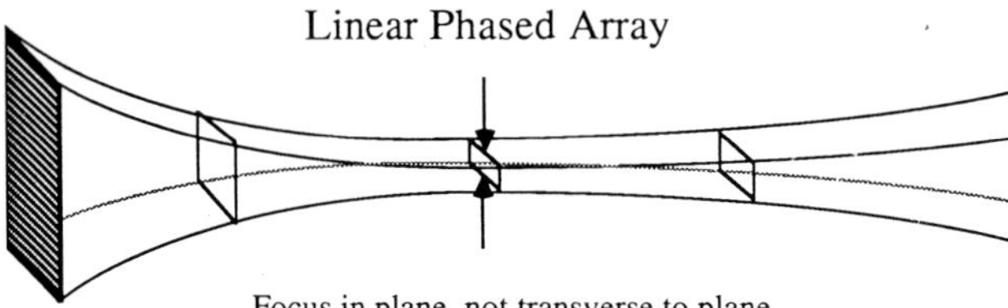

Fig. 1. Illustration of how a symmetrical focus is obtained with an annular array, while the linear phased array only allows electronically steered focus in the scan plane

The first and the third advantages have a practical basis, while the second relies on a fundamental theoretic difference between the methods. The net result for use, however, that the annular array provides higher resolution images and therefore improved diagnosis of small defects such as dissecting aortic aneurysm, thrombus in the left atrium, vegetation on the valves, and coronary artery imaging. CW Doppler measurements allow for quantitation of high velocities.

The problem with annular arrays is that the beam steering is done by mechanically rotating the transducer. The probe tip that can be inserted into the esophagus is limited in size, which presents major challenges in designing such a probe. With the motor drive outside the esophagus, there is the difficult problem of accurate drive transfer of movement from the motor to the probe tip through the flexible gastroscope. The most elegant solution is to use a miniature drive motor and position sensor in the probe tip, but this too presents major challenges in the miniaturization of the motor and position sensor. We chose the last approach, and built a small integral probe assembly that is mounted on the tip of a steerable gastroscope.

Materials and Methods

An overview of the gastroscope and the probe tip with annular array transducer, motor, and position sensor is shown in Fig. 2. The outer diameter of the probe tip is 15 mm and the length is 35 mm. The rotation axis of the transducer is along the gastroscope, so that a beam scan sector that is transverse to the gastroscope axis is obtained, as shown in the figure.

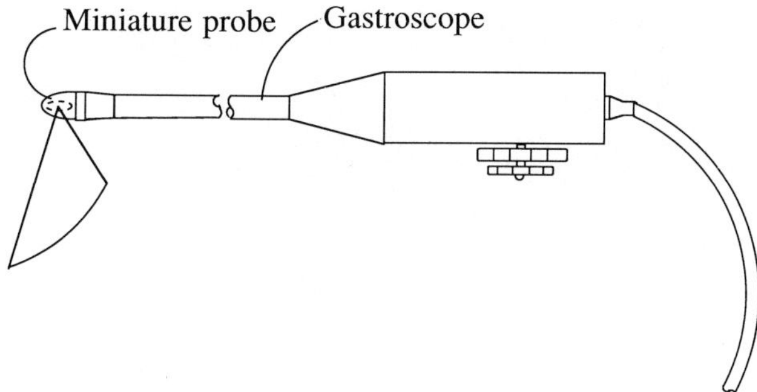

Fig. 2. Schematic overview of gastroscope with probe tip containing annular array transducer, motor, and position sensor. The axis of rotation is along the gastroscope so that an image sector normal to the axis is obtained as illustrated

The outside diameter should be made as large as possible, to get a large transducer aperture for the best possible lateral resolution. The present outer diameter was chosen as a practical compromise between what was felt acceptable for clinical use and the aperture wanted for best resolution. After using the probe in several patients, it was a general experience that the outer diameter could be made larger, because the major cause of discomfort for the patient is that something has been inserted into the esophagus, not the actual dimensions of it.

Figure 3 shows a schematic cross section of the probe tip. The annular array transducer assembly is a circular disk that is mounted directly on the shaft of the motor, which rotates through a limited angle allowing wobbling of the transducer. A miniature position sensor is mounted on the shaft at the other side of the motor, and the angular direction of the motor and the transducer can then be positioned using normal methods of servo feedback control. The probe was connected to a Vingmed Sound CFM 700 annular array color flow mapper with no modifications to the scanner. The instrument and scanner could be operated with 2-D tissue imaging, combined 2-D tissue imaging and color flow imaging, and both pulsed wave (PW) and CW Doppler

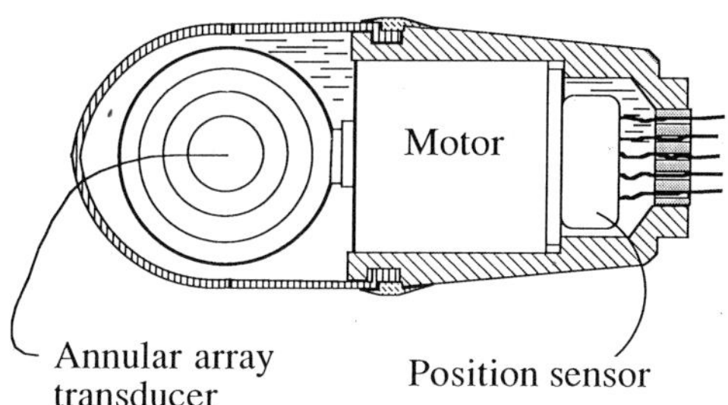

Fig. 3. The probe tip shown in more detail

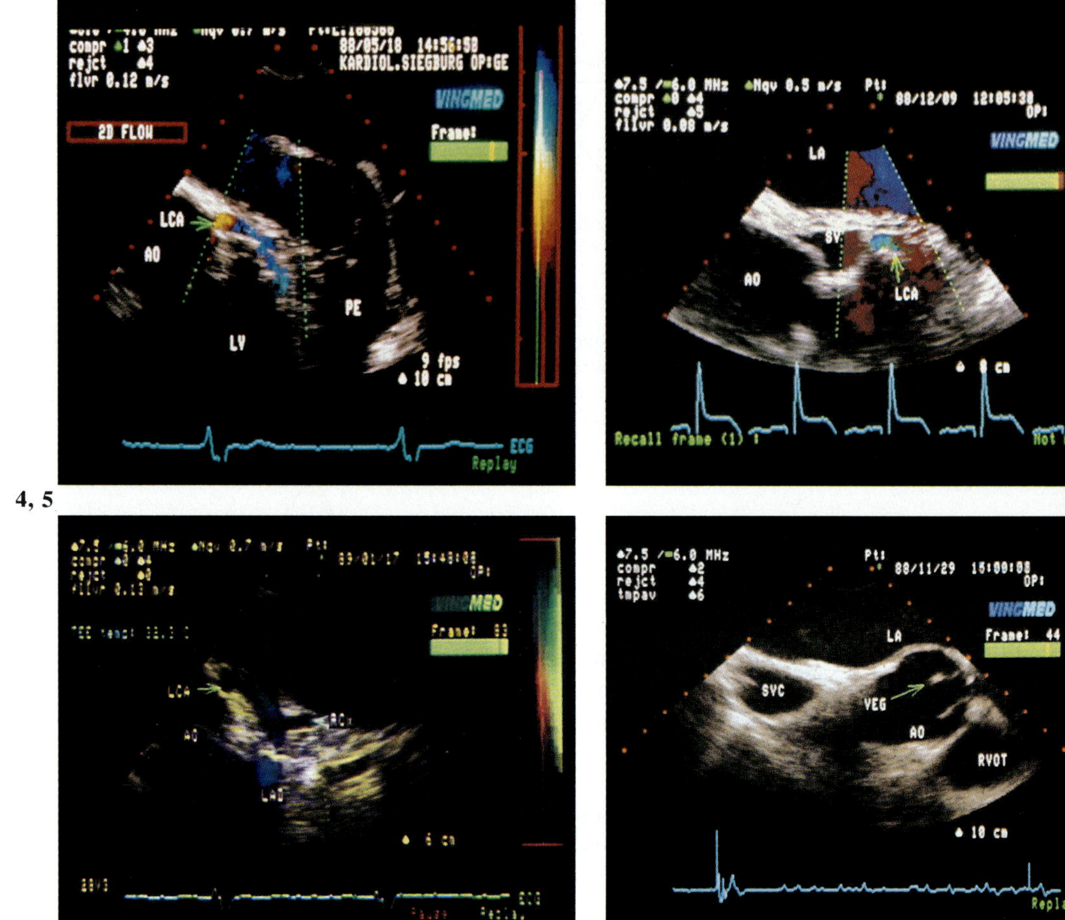

Fig. 4. Proximal portions of the left coronary artery imaged with 7.5-MHZ annular array transesophageal probe. *LCA*, Left coronary artery; *AO*, aorta; *LA*, left atrium; *PE*, pericardial effusion

Fig. 5. Left coronary artery with aneurysm and stenoses shown with green post stenotic region

Fig. 6. Stenoses in the LAD after bypass surgery shown in the tissue image with no green poststenotic region because the graft equalises the pressure across the stenosis

Fig. 7. Thickening of the aortic valve shown with high resolution TEE imaging with a 7.5 MHz transducer

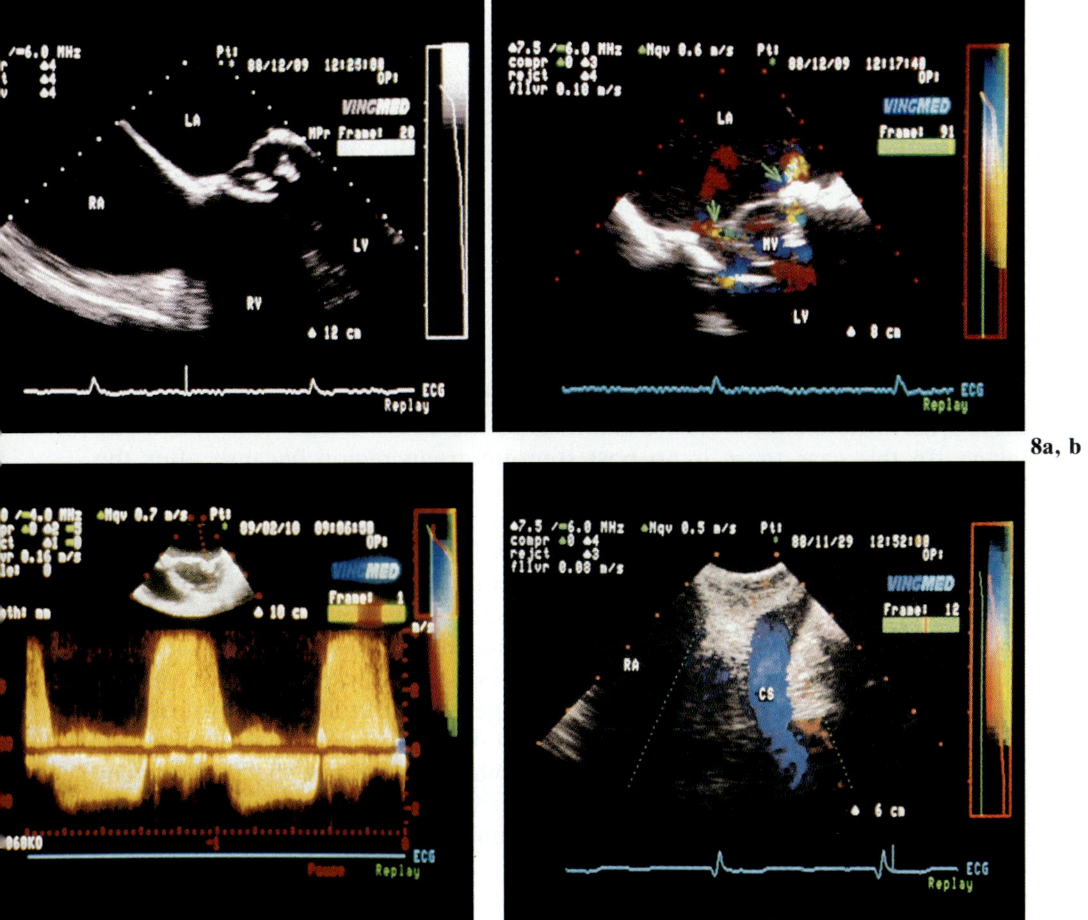

8a, b

9, 10

Fig. 8.a 7.5 MHz tissue image of bioprothesis valve with paravalvular leak, **b** flow image added. The leaking jets are indicated with arrows

Fig. 9. CW Doppler measurement of the jet velocity in combined mitral stenosis and regurgitation

Fig. 10. 7.5 MHz image of flow in the coronary sinus showing crisp edges of the sinus which allows for diameter measurements

measurements of blood velocities. The CW measurements were used to quantify the high velocities found in stenosis and regurgitations [16–18].

The probe was inserted into the esophagus under the guidance of the ultrasound image and was oriented in the esophagus according to standard procedures, as described in [13]. Experimental tests have been conducted with a limited number of patients.

Results

Figure 4 shows the image of the left coronary artery obtained with the 7.5 MHz annular array TEE probe. The red color at the entrance is caused by a flow direction against the transducer, while shortly after the entrance, the flow direction changes so that a blue color for flow away from the probe is obtained. Portions of the bifurcation and a portion of the LAD is also shown until it moves out of the scan plane.

Figure 5 shows a coronary aneurysm together with a stenoses in the left coronary artery obtained with the 7.5 MHz transducer. The post stenotic region is shown with green because turbulence and high velocities with aliasing produces a signal with wide bandwidth.

Figure 6 shows another coronary artery after bypass surgery obtained with the 7.5 MHz transducer were a stenoses in the LAD is shown in the tissue image. In this case there is no post stenotic green region because after the bypass surgery the distal blood pressure is close to the blood pressure proximal to the stenosis. Therefore there is very little acceleration of the blood across the stenosis and no turbulence or aliasing occurs.

Figure 7 is also obtained with 7.5 MHz transducer and shows a thickening of the tips of the aortic cusps which might be vegetation. In this picture the improved resolution with 7.5 MHz ultrasound as well as the thin scanplane with the annular array is necessary to show this small thickening of the valves.

Figure 8a shows a 7.5 MHz tissue image of a mitral valve bioprothesis with paravalvular leak. We see that a penetration of 12 cm is easily obtained. Fig. 8b shows the same case with color image added and the paravalvular leaking jets are clearly indicated.

Figure 9 shows CW Doppler measurements of the blood velocity in combined mitral valve stenosis and regurgitation. A velocity of more than 4 m/sec is obtained which is difficult to measure with pulsed wave Doppler even with high pulse repetition frequency Doppler.

Figure 10 shows a high frequency image of the coronary sinus. We see that the walls of the coronary sinus are well delineated so that the diameter can be measured. This can give a possibility of measuring coronary sinus flow from the esophageal approach.

Discussion

The high frequency capabilities of the annular array gives interesting possibilities for 7.5 and 10 MHz high resolution imaging from the esophagus. The penetration with 7.5 MHz is in the range of 10–14 cm which covers the valve areas, and in many cases also the left ventricle. For diagnosis of defects in the valve area and the atria 7.5 MHz is a good choice, while for the dissecting aortic aneurysm 10 MHz might be a better choice. This is presently under development.

The high frequency imaging gives an interesting possibility for the diagnoses of stenoses in the proximal regions of the coronary arteries. The color image is here very helpful, because the post stenotic turbulence and increase in velocity with frequency aliasing produces a wide band Doppler signal which shows green on the display. This shows up much stronger in the image than tissue details of the stenosis. On the other hand, the patency of a bypass graft can be demonstrated by the lack of a green post stenotic region, showing that the bypass graft keeps up the distal pressure as demonstrated in Fig. 6.

The CW Doppler capabilities of the annular array allows for quantitating very high velocities in jets, which has proven to be of great for estimating pressure drops in valve stenoses and some shunts. With high resolution imaging of regurgitant orifices, the maximum velocity might also be of some use for estimating valve regurgitations.

The high resolution of the coronary sinus with the 7.5 MHz probe gives an interesting possibility of coronary sinus flow measurements. The flow has so low acceleration that a parabolic profile is to be expected, and in this case the mean velocity in the vessel is half the maximum velocity in the vessel. The volumetric flow can then be calculated as the product between this mean velocity and the vessel cross section. The maximum velocity in the vessel can be found as the envelope around the Doppler spectrum, but since the coronary sinus is moving a large distance during the cardiac cycle, it is necessary to use a large range cell so that it covers the central portions of the vessel during the movements.

The experience so far shows an excellent performance of the mechanical scanning of the transducer. The probe tip assembly is small enough so that it can easily be inserted into the esophagus, and the direction of the scanplane manipulated with the gastroscope wires.

References

1. Miller CW, Histand MB, Hokanson DE, McLeod FD, Daigle RE (1973) Atherosclerosis and its effect on thoracic aorta wall motion and peripheral blood velocity patterns. Proc IEEE Ultrason Symp 77−81
2. Olson RM, Skelton DK (1972) A nondestructive technique to measure wall displacement in the thoracic aorta. J Appl Physiol 32:147−151
3. Olson RM, Cooke JP (1974) A nondestructive technique to measure diameter and blood flow in arteries. IEEE Trans Biomed Eng 168−171
4. Duck FA, Hodson CJ, Tomlin PJ (1974) An esophageal Doppler probe for aortic flow velocity monitoring. Ultrasound Med Biol 1:233−241
5. Frazin L, Talano JV, Stephanides L, Loeb HS, Kopel L, Gunnar RM (1976) Esophageal echocardiography. Circulation 54:102−108
6. Wells MK, Histand MB, Reeves JT, Sodal IE, Adamson HP (1979) Ultrasonic transesophageal measurement of hemodynamic parameters in humans. Trans Instrum Soc Am 18 (1):57−61
7. Hisanga K, Hisanga A, Nagata K, Yoshida S (1977) A new transesophageal real-time two-dimensional echocardiographic system using a flexible tube and its clinical application. Proc Jpn Soc Ultrason Med 32:43−44

  8. Hisanga K, Hisanga A, Nagata K, Ichie Y (1980) Transesophageal cross-sectional echocardiography. Am Heart J 100:605−609
  9. Hisanga K, Hisanga A, Hibi N, Nishimura K, Kambe T (1980) High speed rotating scanner for transesophageal cross-sectional echocardiography. Am J Cardiol 46:837−842
 10. Bertini A, Masotti L, Zuppiroli A, Cecchi F (1984) Rotating probe for transesophageal cross-sectional echocardiography. J Nucl Med Allied Sci 28:115−121
 11. Rojogopolan B, DiMagno EP, Greenleaf JF, Regan PT, Buxton J, Green PS, Whitaker JW (1979) Transesophageal ultrasonic imaging of the heart. In: Wang KV Proceedings of the 9th International Conference on Acoustic Imaging 1979. Houston TX, Dec 3−6, 555−567
 12. DiMagno EP, Buxton JL, Regan PT, Hattery RR, Wilson DA, Suarez JR, Green PS (1980) Ultrasonic endoscope. Lancet 1:629−631
 13. Hanrath P, Kremerm P, Langenstein BA, Matsemuoto M, Bleifeld W (1981) Transesophagale Echcardiographie: Ein neues Verfahren zur dynamischen Ventrikkelfunktions-analyse. Dtsch Med Wochenschr 106:523−525
 14. Souquet J, Hanrath P, Zitelli L, Kremer P, Langenstein BA, Schluter M (1982) Transesophageal phased array for imaging of the heart. IEEE Trans Biomed Eng 29:707−712
 15. Seward JB, Khandheira BK, Oh JK, Abel MD, Hughes RW, Edwards WD, Nichols BA, Freeman WK, Tajik J (1988) Transesophageal echocardiography: technique, anatomic correlations, implementation, and clinical applications. Mayo clin Proc 63:649−680
 16. Holen J, Aaslid R, Landmark K, Simonsen S (1976) Determination of pressure gradient in mitral stenosis with non-invasive ultrasound Doppler technique. Acta Med Scand 199:455−460
 17. Hatle L, Angelsen B (1985) Doppler ultrasound in cardiology-Physical principles and clinical applications, 2nd edn. Lea and Febiger, Philadelphia
 18. Angelsen BAJ, Sloerdahl S, Solbakken JE, Samstad S, Linker D, Torp H, Piene H (to be published) Estimation of regurgitant volume and orifice in aortic regurgitation combining CW Doppler and parameter estimation in a Winkessel-like model. IEEE Trans Biomed Eng (to be published)

Recent Technological Progress in Transesophageal Color Doppler Flow Imaging with Special Reference to Newly Developed Biplane and Pediatric Probes

R. OMOTO, S. KYO, M. MATSUMURA, P. SHAH, H. ADACHI, T. MATSUNAKA, and K. TACHIKAWA

Introduction

Color transesophageal Doppler echocardiography (TEE) has made real-time, on-line, beat by beat study of intracardiac events possible without the inconvenience of having a probe in the operative field. The use of transesophageal probes is on the increase and in 1988, at least in our heart center, we hardly used epicardial probes for intraoperative evaluation.

There are many reports of the use of this probe in both the intra- and perioperative periods [1–6]. However, in the present state of the art there are two major limitations. (1) The size of the probe means it is not suitable for use in pediatric patients. (2) Only a transverse view can be obtained at any one given level with the single transducer. In order to further improve the technique, we recently, in close collaboration with Aloka Biomedical engineering department, developed and tested two new probes, a biplane probe and a pediatric probe.

To the best of our knowledge we are the first and the only center where these new probes are being used clinically with good resutls. This is a preliminary communication about these new probes.

Instrumentation

The biplane probe is 13.5 mm in diameter, and transverse and longitudinal transducers are mounted side by side, 1.5 mm apart, on the same transesophageal shaft. There are two types of probe available; one has a longitudinal transducer at the tip, whereas the other probe has a transverse transducer. The tip is 29.5 mm in length, as compared to 13 mm in the conventional probe. The flexible tip can be controlled by the handle on the gastroscope. With this, either transverse or longitudinal scans can be obtained and biplane images can be reproduced simultaneously synchronizing to the R wave of the ECG in cine-memory mode. The pediatric probe is only 6.8 mm in diameter. The difference of size in comparison to conventional adult probes is demonstrated in Figs. 1 and 2. Before we used this probe in patients we checked it intensively in little puppies and tested it in a puppy with a body weight of around 3 kg. After the experiment, the animals were killed and were examined for evidence of any thermal or mechanical injuries. After convinc-

Transesophageal Echocardiography
Edited by R. Erbel et al.
© Springer-Verlag Berlin Heidelberg 1989

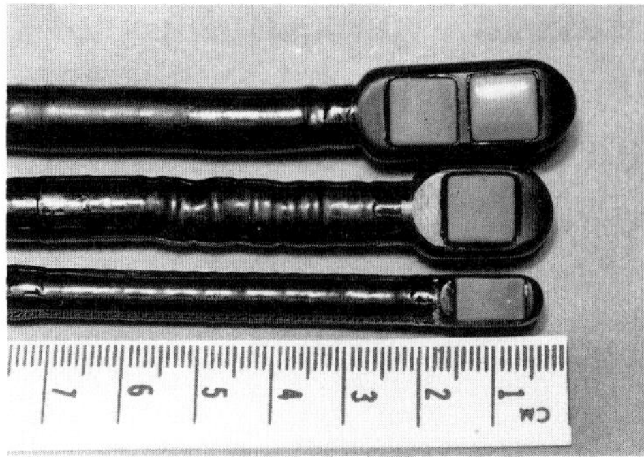

Fig. 1. Various kinds of transesophageal probes. *Upper*, Newly developed biplane probe (5 MHz); *middle*, conventional single-plane probe for transverse imaging; *lower*, newly developed pediatric probe

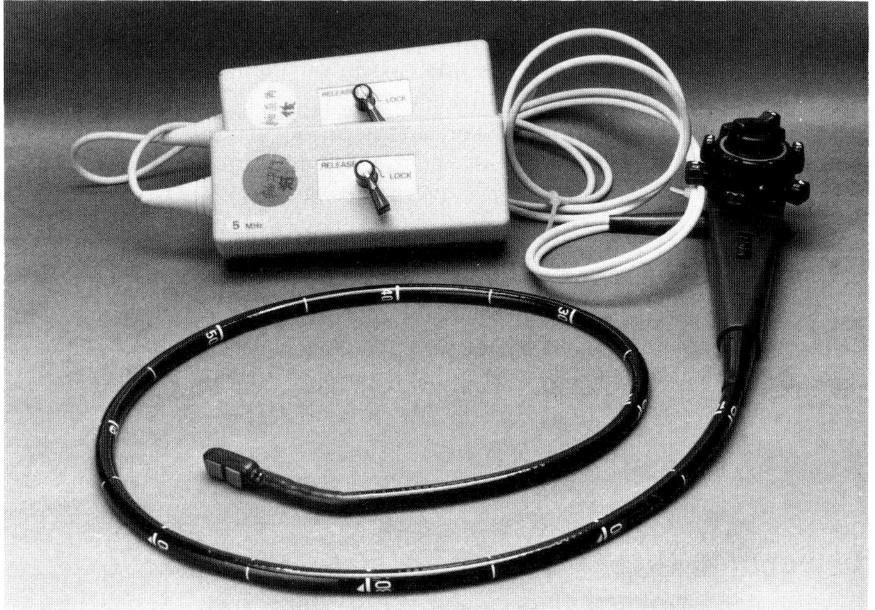

Fig. 2. Biplane probe (5 MHz). Note dual cables and connectors for two transducers

ing ourselves of the safety of the probe, we are now using it intraoperatively in patients. These two kinds of probes can be used with the Aloka SSD-870, which is commercially available.

Initial Clinical Experience

Biplane Probe

Between September and November, 1988, the probe has been successfully used both intra- and postoperatively in 22 adult patients. Three-dimensional

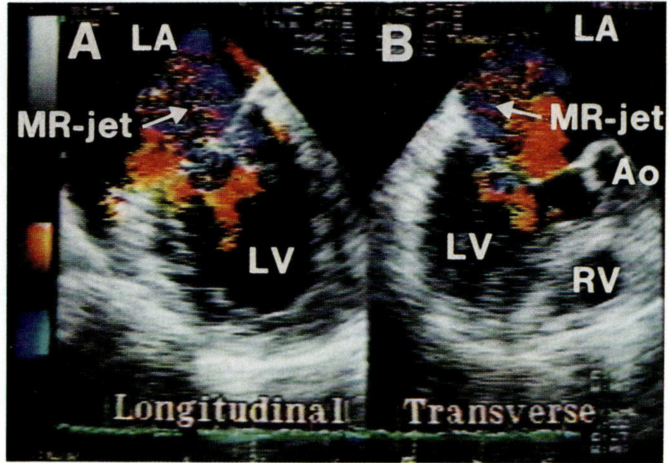

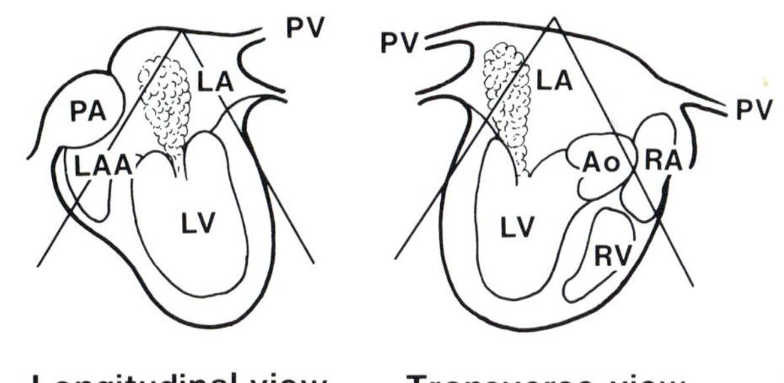

Fig. 3. a Color TEE biplane images in a 57-year-old patient with Sellers' grade 3 mitral regurgitation (*MR-jet*). *A*, Longitudinal view (in systole); *B*, transverse view (in systole). **b** Schematic illustrations of **a.** *LV*, left ventricle; *LA*, left atrium; *RV*, right ventricle; *RA*, right atrium; *Ao*, aorta; *PA*, pulmonary artery; *PV*, pulmonary vein; *LAA*, left atrial auricula

reconstruction of blood flow dynamics was possible in all cases studied with the biplane probe. The further information obtained from the biplane probe, as compared to the standard single-plane probe, is so far as follows: (1) In mitral regurgitation, the information from transverse and longitudinal sections of the heart helps in evaluating the regurgitant jet in a three-dimensional view. An example of a biplane image of mitral regurgitation is given in Fig. 3. With simultaneous biplane images, we can easily and accurately visualize in three-dimensions the mitral regurgitant jet and the site of valvular incompetence [2]. In dissecting aneurysms, one can more accurately visualize the false lumen and the points of entry and exit, all this information being important to a surgeon intraoperatively.

In the thoracic aorta, biplane images offered a CT-equivalent view in transverse sections and angiography-equivalent views in longitudinal sections.

Pediatric Probe

The pediatric probe has been evaluated in eight patients, including an 18-month-old patient with a body weight of 8.9 kg who had a ventricular septal

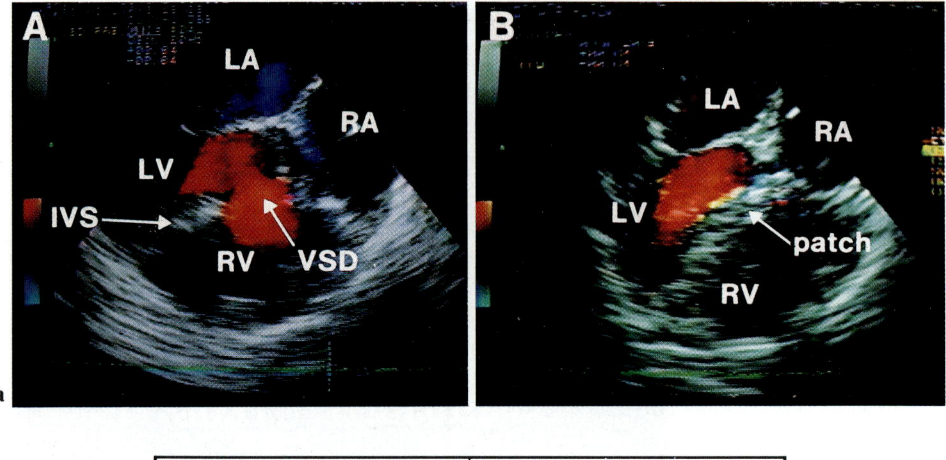

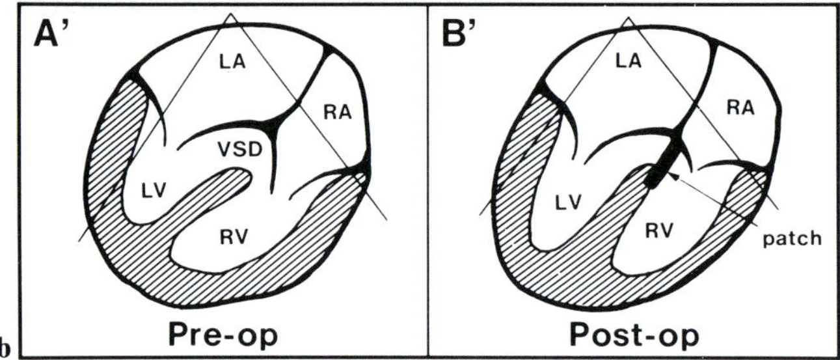

Fig. 4. a Color TEE images in a 19-month-old infant weighing 8.2 kg with ventricular septal defect (VSD), and post-PA banding, using pediatric TEE probe. *A*, Preoperative findings: shunt flow (*arrow*) passing through VSD is imaged in red. *B*, Postoperative findings: the defect was closed successfully by a Teflon patch (*arrow*). **b** Schematic illustrations of **a**. *A'* corresponds to *A* and *B'* to *B*. *LV*, Left ventricle; *LA*, left atrium; *RV*, right ventricle; *RA*, right atrium; *IVS*, interventricular septum

defect. The probe has been found helpful to surgeons in assessing intracardiac repair before closing the chest. The use of the pediatric probe intraoperatively and immediately after the operation provides a lot of useful data: (1) It allows confirmation of preoperative angiographic and two-dimensional transthoracic echocardiographic diagnosis. (2) It provides continuous on-line hemodynamic monitoring. For example, under general anesthesia, shunt reversal may occur in the prebypass period, and immediate treatment may be life saving. (3) In the postbypass period evaluation of repair is very important, and this can be done using the probe. Figure 4 shows an example of color TEE images obtained with the pediatric probe.

Future Aspects

There are several aspects that need to be investigated with the new probe both in normal subjects and in various pathological states. Biplane images are really not familiar to us. Anatomical correlation of the biplane images obtained are being studied in the department using magnetic resonance imaging. In the biplane probe, as the two transducers are separated from each other by 1 cm from center point to center point we had to slightly reposition each transducer to visualize the exact same cardiac segment. If the technology of having two orthogonal planes in realtime with a single transducer [7] can be applied to color transesophageal probes in the future, this limitation will be resolved. In present biplane imaging system, transverse and longitudinal images were stored in cine-loop memory and were visualized half a minute later, off-line, side by side on the TV screen. Thus in a sense it was not true real-time but was reproduced with cine-memory mode. To address this problem we need further technological development, where no cine-memory loop is used, and *real* real-time, on-line images are produced.

Conclusion

In conclusion, the recently developed biplane and pediatric color transesophageal probes have further enhanced our ability to study intracardiac events and help cardiac surgeons to evaluate the procedure performed. The biplane probe provides better information, at least in cases of aortic aneurysms and mitral regurgitation. With the further refinement of true real-time technology, in the near future it will be possible to use a biplane probe in real-time and on-line, both intraoperatively and in the immediate post-operative period. The pediatric probe has expanded the use of TEE into pediatric cardiology field. Further work needs to be done with these new probes.

References

1. Goldman ME, Thys D, Ritter S, Hittel Z, Kaplan J (1986) Trans-esophageal real time doppler flow imaging: a new method for intraoperative cardiac evaluation (abstract). J Am Coll Cardiol 7:1
2. Takamoto S, Kyo S, Matsumura M, Hojo H, Yokote Y, Omoto R (1986) Total visualization of thoracic dissecting aortic aneurysm by transesophageal Doppler color flow mapping (abstract). Circulation 74 (Suppl II):II−132
3. De Bruijn NP, Clements FM, Kisslo JA (1987) Intraoperative transesophageal color flow mapping: inital experience. Anesth Analg 66:386−390
4. Kyo S, Takamoto S, Matsumura M, Asano H, Yokote Y, Motoyama T, Omoto R (1987) Immediate and early postoperative evaluation of results of cardiac surgery by transesophageal two-dimensional Doppler echocardiography. Circulation 76 (Suppl V): V-113-121

5. Omoto R (1987) Intraoperative use of 2-D Doppler. In: Color atlas of real-time two-dimensional Doppler echocardiography, 2nd ed. Shindan-To-Chiryo, Tokyo, p 80, p 112
6. Seward J, Khandheria B, Oh JK, Abel M, Hughes R Jr, Edwards W, Nichols B, Freeman W, Tajik A (1988) Transesophageal echocardiography: technique, anatomic correlations, implementation, and clinical applications. Mayo Clin Proc 63:649−680
7. Snyder JE, Kisslo J, Von Ramm OT (1986) Real-time orthogonal mode scanning of the heart. I. System design. J Am Coll Cardiol 7:1279−1285

Transesophageal Echocardiography: Anatomic Correlations*

A. J. TAJIK, J. B. SEWARD, and B. K. KHANDHERIA

Two-dimensional echocardiography, an accepted noninvasive diagnostic imaging tool, has been increasingly used in various semi-invasive applications such as (1) guiding pericardiocentesis [1], (2) contrast echocardiography [2], (3) intraoperative echocardiography [3], and (4) transesophageal echocardiography [4, 5]. With increasing sophistication and miniaturization of transducers, further refinement and extension of this modality as an invasive tool are being explored [6]. Transesophageal echocardiography has recently received increased interest principally for use in the awake patient because of the availability of high-resolution echocardiographic transducers that incorporate Doppler and color flow imaging capabilities. In this manuscript, we describe from our initial clinical experience with transesophageal echocardiography tomographic anatomic correlations.

Anatomic Correlations

A comprehensive transesophageal examination entails a sequence of transducer positions and tomographic planes of section. Even when a specific clinical problem is being evaluated, a methodologic imaging approach comparable to that recommended for a comprehensive transthoracic two-dimensional echocardiographic examination should be followed [7]. A step-by-step approach is suggested that can be altered on the basis of the clinical situation. During transesophageal echocardiography, two distinct tomographic examinations are performed — namely, of the heart and of the thoracic aorta. For all anatomic correlations to date, horizontal planes of section have been used (Fig. 1). In the future, alternative planes of view, particularly vertical, may ultimately be available.

Cardiac Examination

Step 1 — Basal Short-Axis Scans. The endoscope is initially advanced into the esophagus approximately 25−30 cm from the incisors. This position places the

* Abridged from Seward JB et al. (1988) Transesophageal echocardiography: technique, anatomic correlations, implementation, and clinical applications. Mayo Clin Proc 63:649−680

Transesophageal Echocardiography
Edited by R. Erbel et al.
© Springer-Verlag Berlin Heidelberg 1989

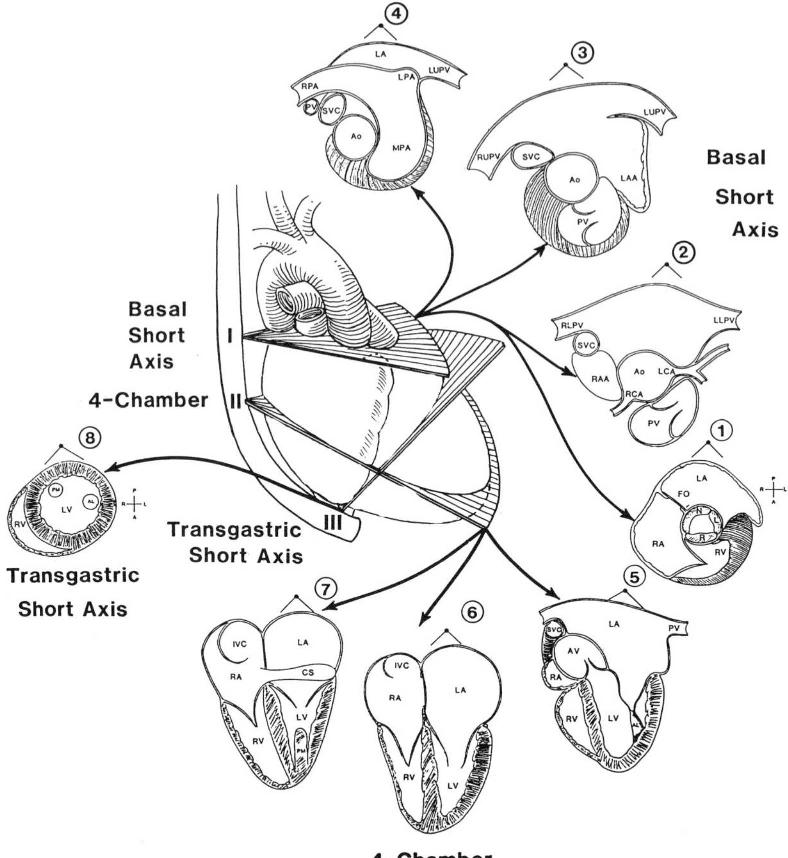

Fig. 1. Planes of section for transesophageal echocardiography. Three primary tomographic planes are obtained. Basal short-axis planes (*I*) are initially obtained, usually at 25- to 30-cm distance of transducer tip from incisors. Four-chamber (frontal) planes (*II*) are obtained by retroflexion or slight advancement of tip of endoscope (or both) from position I (approximately 30 cm from incisors). Transgastric short-axis planes (*III*) are obtained from within fundus of stomach, 35−45 cm from incisors. (From [12])

transducer posterior to the left atrium. Gains are set high, and landmarks such as the thoracic aorta and left atrium are sought for orientation. The initial image obtained is usually a short-axis scan at the base of the heart (Fig. 2). By tilting the tip superiorly or by slightly withdrawing the transducer, sequential basal short-axis scans are obtained. Basal short-axis scans sequentially depict the aortic valve, proximal ascending aorta, proximal coronary arteries, atrial appendages, superior vena cava, atrial septum, pulmonary veins, and proximal pulmonary arteries.

The image orientation for the basal short-axis scan, which we have used, corresponds to a frontal dissection of the heart. On the video screen, anterior structures are at the bottom, and posterior structures are at the top; left-sided structures are to the viewer's right. This orientation is comparable to viewing

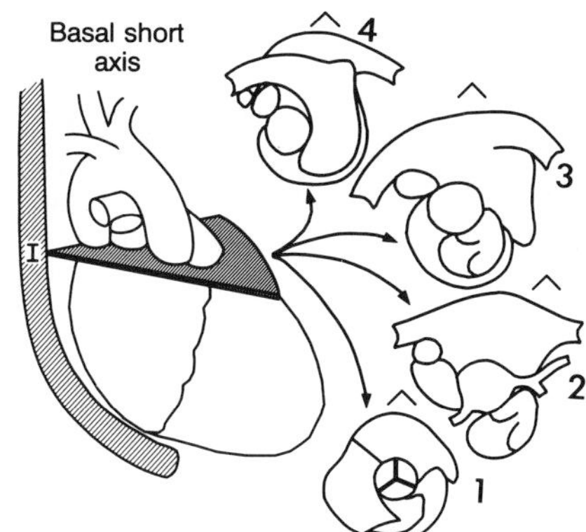

Fig. 2. Diagram of common scan planes. I: *1*, basal short-axis aortic root; *2*, coronary arteries; *3*, left atrial appendage; *4*, pulmonary artery bifurcation

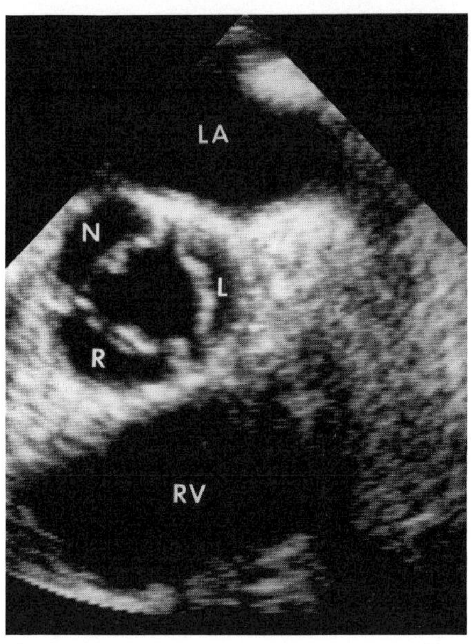

Fig. 3. Transesophageal echocardiographic basal short-axis scan of *aortic root*. Centrally, aortic cusps are evident (*L* left, *N* non-, *R* right coronary cusps). Atrial septum, commonly at level of foramen ovale, can usually be seen. Anteriorly, right ventricle (*RV*), right ventricular outflow tract, pulmonary valve, and proximal pulmonary artery may be seen, depending on orientation of heart and endoscope. Left atrium (*LA*) is adjacent to the transducer. (From [12])

the frontal aspect of the heart. (Older instruments provided views that can be conceptualized only as looking from the posterior or inferior surface of the heart [8]).

The *aortic root* and the *aortic valve cusps* are usually scanned in a short-axis plane (Fig. 3). On the video screen, the left cusp is rightward, the right cusp is depicted inferiorly, and the noncoronary cusp is to the left of the image. The atrial septum, with its central thin fossa ovalis membrane, separates the left and right atria. Anteriorly (inferiorly on the screen), portions of the right ventricle are evident.

The *coronary arteries* (Fig. 4) are above the aortic cusps, and high-resolution images of the proximal coronary arteries can be obtained in most patients

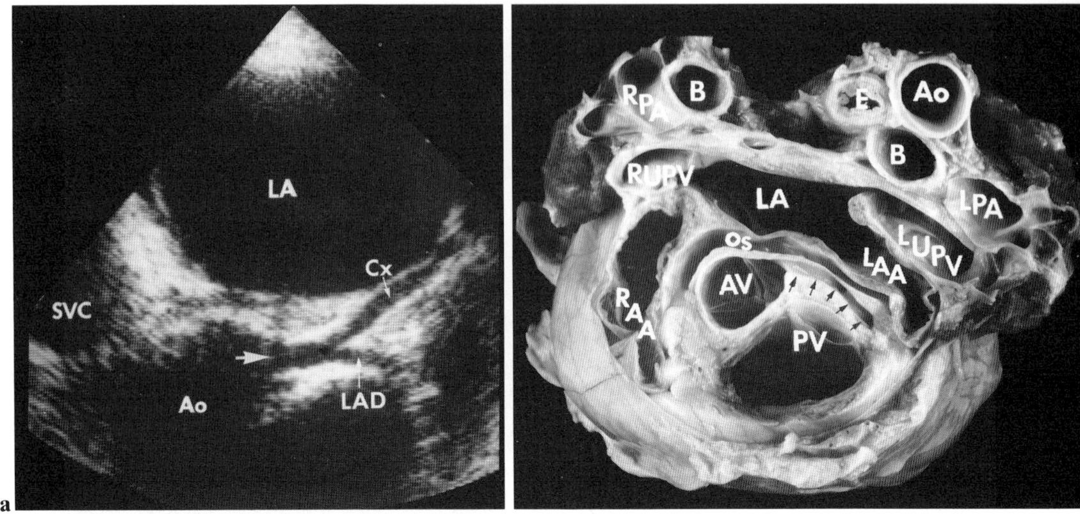

Fig. 4. a Transesophageal echocardiographic basal short-axis scan of left coronary artery. Left main coronary artery (*large arrow*) is imaged just above left aortic cusp. Bifurcation into circumflex artery (*Cx*) (circling posteriorly) and left anterior descending coronary artery (*LAD*) (anteriorly) is shown. Right coronary artery is usually depicted in a different tomographic plane. *SVC*, Superior vena cava. **b** Anatomic specimen sectioned in same basal short-axis plane is shown in **a,** demonstrating relationship of left coronary artery (*arrows*), aortic valve (*AV*), pulmonary valve (*PV*), and left atrial appendage (*LAA*). At level of LAA and right atrial appendage (*RAA*), right and left upper pulmonary veins (*RUPV* and *LUPV*) are visible. Note relationship of descending thoracic aorta (*Ao*) and left atrium (*LA*) to esophagus (*E*). *B*, Bronchus; *LPA*, left pulmonary artery; *os*, oblique sinus; *RPA*, right pulmonary artery. (From [12])

with upward tilt of the tip of the endoscope. The origin of the left coronary artery from the left aortic sinus and its course beneath the left arterial appendage to its bifurcation into the circumflex and left anterior descending coronary arteries can frequently be seen. These images are consistently superior to those obtained by standard surface echocardiography. The right coronary artery arises, usually at a tomographic level different from that of the left coronary artery. Superior and inferior tilting of the transducer is necessary in order to best visualize the coronary arteries.

Further superior tilting of the tip of the endoscope will allow consistent imaging of the *atrial appendages* (Fig. 5). The left atrial appendage appears as a triangular extension of the left atrium. Muscular ridges (pectinate muscles) within the appendage are easily visible and should not be confused with thrombi. The left atrial appendage overlies the left coronary artery. The orifice of this appendage is anterior to the left upper pulmonary vein, and the two are separated by a distinct ridgelike infolding of the wall (Fig. 4 b). The right atrial appendage (Figs. 4 b, 5 b) is anterior to the superior vena cava.

The *superior vena cava*, visible at several levels, enters the dome of the right atrium (Fig. 6).

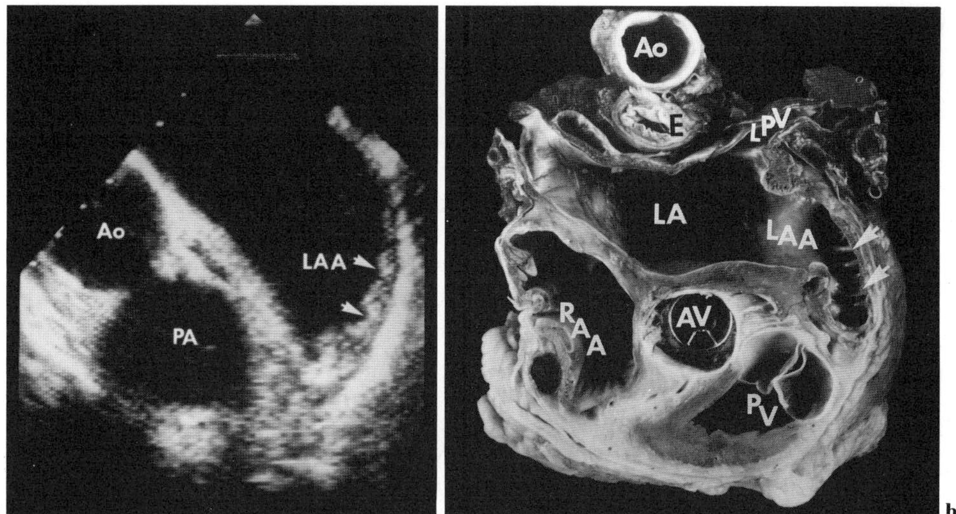

Fig. 5. a Transesophageal echocardiographic basal short-axis scan of left atrial appendage (*LAA*). LAA is consistently imaged superior to left coronary artery, anterior to left pulmonary vein, and left of aortic root (*Ao*) and proximal pulmonary artery (*PA*) and valve. At apex of LAA, pectinate muscles are frequently visible (*arrows*). **b** Anatomic specimen sectioned in same basal short-axis plane as shown in **a**. Pectinate muscles (*arrows*) of LAA can be seen; when prominent, these can be a source of dense echoes in LAA. Right atrial appendage (*RAA*) can usually be imaged at same level. Note close relationship of esophagus (*E*) to left atrium (*LA*) and descending thoracic aorta (*Ao*). (This specimen has an aortic disk prosthesis, *AV*.) *LPV*, left pulmonary vein; *PV*, pulmonary valve. (From [12])

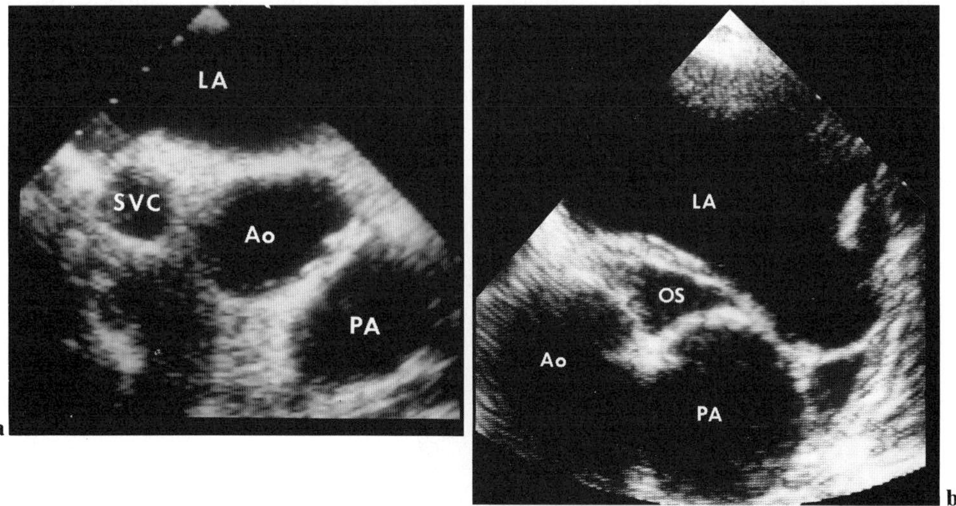

Fig. 6a, b. Transesophageal echocardiographic basal short-axis scans of superior vena cava (*SVC*). **a** Three circular structures [SVC, aortic root (*Ao*), and proximal pulmonary artery (*PA*)] are imaged at base of heart. *LA*, Left atrium. **b** Note oblique sinus (*OS*), an echo-free space interposed between aorta anteriorly and LA posteriorly. This space is the posterior extension of the pericardial sac (also see Fig. 4) and should not be misinterpreted as a vessel or abnormal cavity. (From [12])

The superior vena cava appears as an ovoid structure adjacent to the ascending aorta. The right upper pulmonary vein courses posteriorly and is orthogonal to the superior vena cava. Occasionally, the azygos vein can be seen where it enters the posteromedial aspect of the superior vena cava. More superiorly, the right pulmonary artery courses posteriorly. The *inferior vena cava*, which can be seen by retroflexion of the transducer toward the floor of the right atrium, is most commonly imaged in the four-chamber planes of section (see Fig. 15 b).

The *atrial septum* (Fig. 7) is evident in multiple short-axis and four-chamber transesophageal tomographic projections. The thin membrane of the fossa ovalis may also be imaged on the left atrial surface of the atrial septal limbus. In most patients, a complete scan of the atrial septum can be obtained by tilting and alternately withdrawing and advancing the tip of the endoscope.

The upper *pulmonary veins* course anteroposteriorly into the left atrium at the same level as the left and right atrial appendages (Fig. 8). The inferior pulmonary veins are scanned by rotating the endoscope posteriorly and advancing it 1 or 2 cm into the esophagus. The lower pulmonary veins enter the posterolateral area of the left atrial cavity.

The right ventricular outflow tract lies anterior to the aortic root. The *pulmonary valve* is anterior, leftward, and orthogonal to the aortic valve and is normally scanned in an oblique projection (Fig. 9). By tilting and withdrawing the transducer superiorly, the main and proximal right and left *pulmonary arteries* can be imaged. The left pulmonary artery lies anterior to the descending thoracic aorta and courses posterolaterally. Usually, only the proximal portion of the left pulmonary artery is visible. The right pulmonary artery passes beneath the aortic arch, posterior to the ascending aorta, and is posterosuperior to the left atrial cavity. This vessel also lies behind the superior vena cava and superior to the right upper pulmonary vein. The right pulmonary artery can be imaged for several centimeters towards the right hilum.

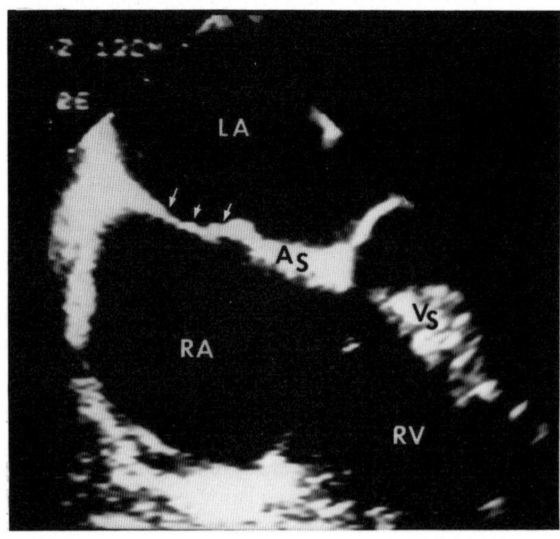

Fig. 7. Transesophageal echocardiogram of atrial septum (*AS*), structure that is evident in both four-chamber plane and basal short-axis scans. Thin valve of fossa ovalis (*arrows*) can be consistently imaged. Limbus of AS is highly refractile and noticeably thicker. Complete imaging of AS necessitates use of multiple planes of section. *LA*, Left atrium; *RA*, right atrium; *RV*, right ventricle; *VS*, ventricular septum. (From [12])

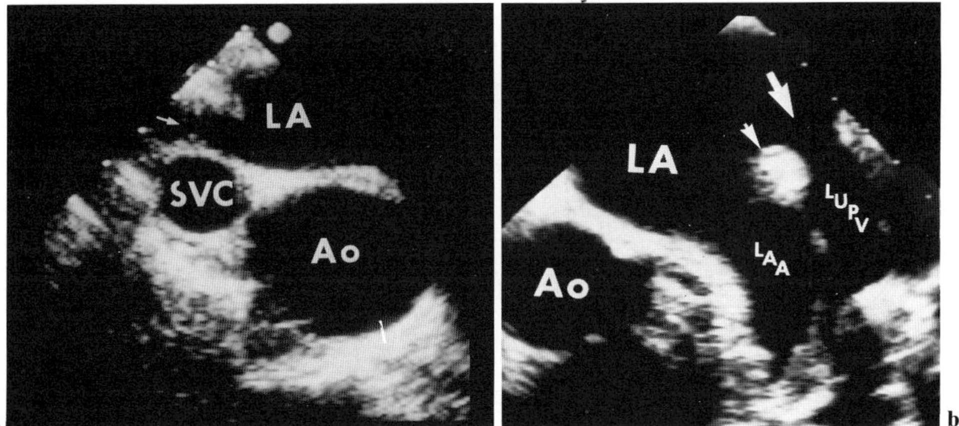

Fig. 8 a, b. Transesophageal echocardiographic basal short-axis scans of pulmonary veins. **a** Right upper pulmonary vein (*arrow*). *Ao*, Aorta; *SVC*, superior vena cava. **b** Most easily imaged pulmonary vein is left upper pulmonary vein (*LUPV*), whose orifice (*large arrow*) lies posterolateral to orifice of left atrial appendage (*LAA*). Distinct wall (*small arrow*) separates pulmonary vein orifice from atrial appendage. Upper pulmonary veins enter left atrium (*LA*) in anteroposterior direction. (From [12])

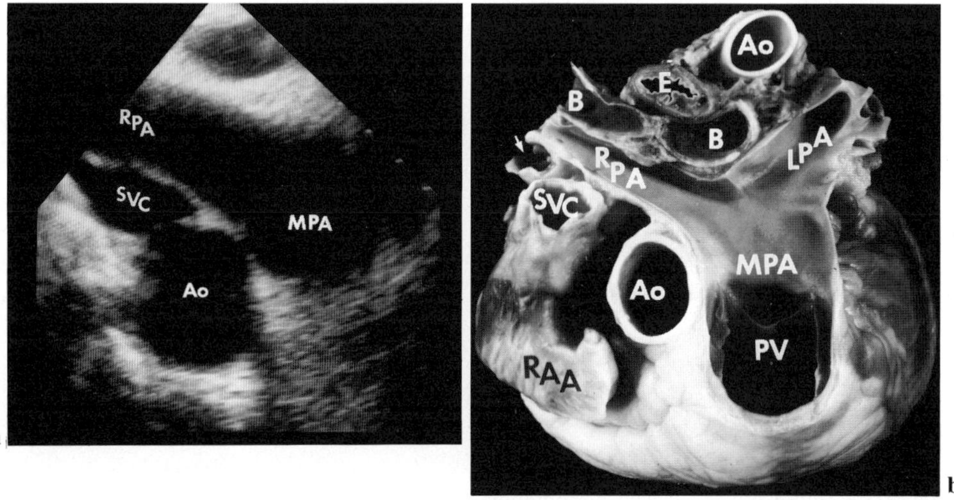

Fig. 9. a Transesophageal echocardiographic basal short-axis scan of main pulmonary artery and bifurcation. Right pulmonary artery (*RPA*) courses superior to left atrium, and posterior to superior vena cava (*SVC*). Only proximal portion of left pulmonary artery is evident. Main pulmonary artery (*MPA*) courses in anteroposterior direction and lateral to aortic root (*Ao*). At this level, trachea lies very close to tip of endoscope and may limit optimal imaging of pulmonary artery bifurcation. **b** Anatomic specimen cut in same basal short-axis plane as shown in **a.** Pulmonary valve (*PV*), *MPA*, and proximal *RPA* and left pulmonary artery (*LPA*) are displayed in this tomographic section. RPA courses posterior to SVC and right upper pulmonary vein (*arrow*) and anterior to right bronchus (*B*). Note close proximity of esophagus (*E*) and tracheal bifurcation at this level. *RAA*, Right atrial appendage. (From [12])

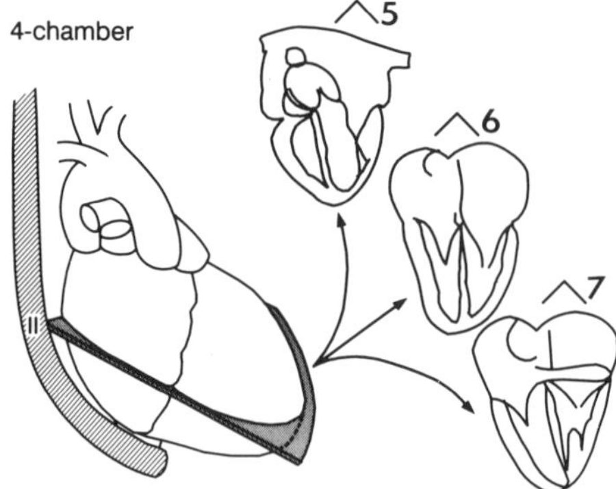

Fig. 10. Diagram of scan planes. II: Four-chamber (frontal long axis) 5, Left ventricular outflow; 6, four-chamber; 7, coronary sinus view

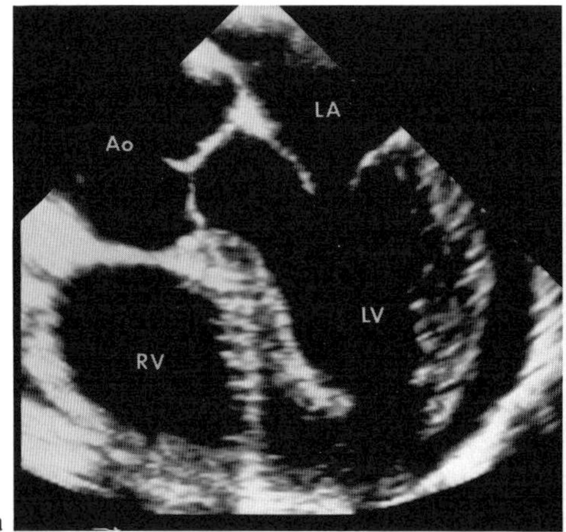

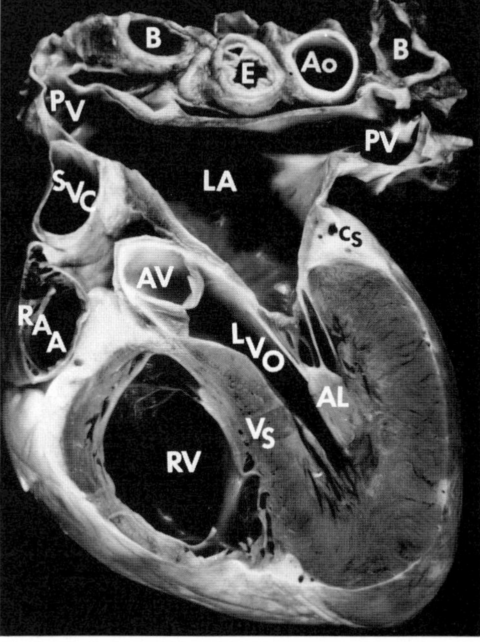

Fig. 11. a Transesophageal echocardiographic frontal long-axis view of left ventricular outflow tract. This scan is an anterior tangential section of left ventricle (*LV*), showing aortic valve, left ventricular outflow tract, anterior portions of mitral valve apparatus, and anterolateral papillary muscle. Portions of right ventricular (*RV*) inflow can also be seen. *Ao*, Aorta; *LA*, left atrium. **b** Anatomic specimen cut in same plane as shown in **a**. LV can usually be depicted from apex to base, including anterolateral papillary muscle (*AL*). Both mitral leaflets along with chordal apparatus and two aortic cusps are clearly evident. Note proximity of esophagus (*E*) to LA and descending thoracic aorta (*Ao*). *AV*, Aortic valve; *B*, bronchi; *CS*, coronary sinus surrounded by fat pad in left atrioventricular groove; *LVO*, left ventricular outflow tract; *PV*, pulmonary veins; *RAA*, right atrial appendage; *SVC*, superior vena cava; *VS*, ventricular septum. (From [12])

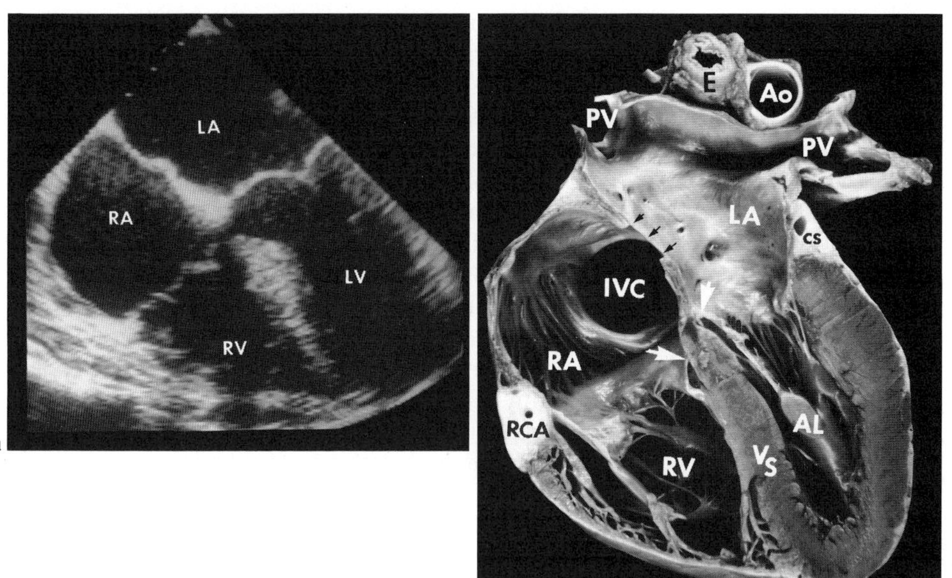

Fig. 12. a Transesophageal echocardiographic frontal long-axis four-chamber view of heart. This view is obtained by advancement and retroflexion of tip of endoscope. All four cardiac chambers are imaged simultaneously along with respective septa and atrioventricular valve, analogous to apical four-chamber view. *LA*, Left atrium; *LV*, left ventricle; *RA*, right atrium; *RV*, right ventricle. **b** Anatomic specimen cut along same plane as shown in **a**. Internal cardiac crux − atrial septum, ventricular septum (*VS*), septal leaflet of tricuspid valve, and septal attachment of anterior mitral leaflet − is best depicted in this projection. Note that mitral valve inserts higher than tricuspid valve (*large white arrows*). Valve of fossa ovalis (*small black arrows*) is thin central membrane of atrial septum. Anterolateral papillary muscle (*AL*) is visible within left ventricle. Note prominent amount of fat in both atrioventricular grooves, surrounding coronary sinus (*cs*) on left and right coronary artery (*RCA*) on right. *Ao*, Descending thoracic aorta; *E*, esophagus; *IVC*, inferior vena cava; *PV*, lower right and left pulmonary veins. (From [12])

Step 2 − Four-Chamber Scans. With further advancement of the endoscope into the esophagus (approximately 30 cm from the incisors) or retroflexion of the endoscope (or both), four-chamber (frontal) scans of the heart are obtained (Fig. 10). These tomographic scans image the atrioventricular valves and support apparatus, ventricles, left ventricular outflow tract, and coronary sinus. Color flow assessment for regurgitation of atrioventricular and aortic valves is best performed from this transducer position.

The image orientation which we have used is apex down with the left ventricle to the right on the video screen [8]. This orientation conforms to option 1 from the American Society of Echocardiography, with the apex oriented downward [8, 9].

The left ventricle is projected to the right on the screen, and the right ventricle is to the left on the screen, as though viewing a frontal projection of the heart [8].

By retroflexion of the tip of the endoscope, sequential long-axis views of the left ventricle can be obtained. From the basal short-axis view at the aortic valve (Fig. 3), retroflexion of the transducer will initially display the left ventricular outflow tract and a long-axis view of the aortic cusps (Fig. 11). This view is comparable to a transthoracic apical four-chamber view with anterior tilt of the transducer toward the aorta [9, 10].

With yet further retroflexion and/or advancement of the scope, a conventional four-chamber view is obtained (Fig. 12). The morphologic characteristics of the internal cardiac crux [10] can be appreciated in this projection. The atrial septum (limbus and fossa ovalis) can also be imaged in the four-chamber plane of section. Using both the basal short-axis views (see "Step 1 − basal short axis scans") and the four-chamber views provides a comprehensive assessment of the atrial septum.

Anatomic and functional abnormalities of the mitral annulus, leaflets, and subvalvular apparatus can be readily imaged in this four-chamber plane of sec-

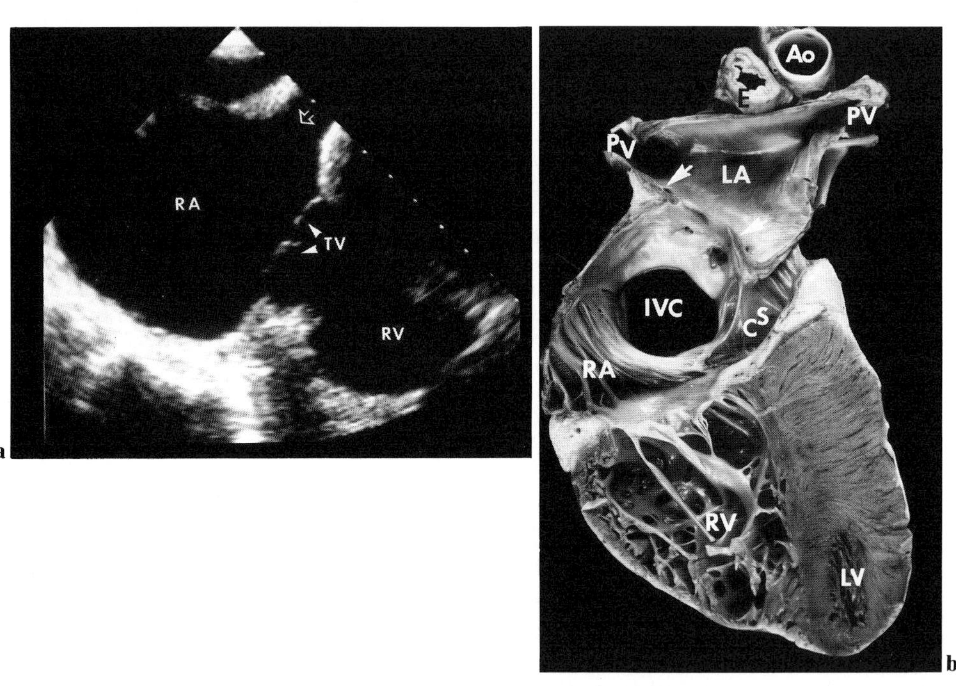

Fig. 13. a Transesophageal echocardiographic frontal long-axis view of coronary sinus. Usually, right atrium (*RA*) and oblique view of right ventricle (*RV*) and tricuspid valve (*TV*) are visible when scan is optimized for coronary sinus (*open arrow*). This view is obtained with extreme retroflexion of tip of endoscope at gastroesophageal junction. Orifice of inferior vena cava can also be seen. **b** Anatomic specimen cut to demonstrate coronary sinus (*CS*). This tomographic section is far posterior in cardiac specimen and excludes most of the left ventricle (*LV*). CS courses in atrioventricular groove and enters RA at lower margin of atrial septum (*arrow*). *Ao,* Descending thoracic aorta; *E,* esophagus; *IVC,* inferior vena cava; *LA,* left atrium; *PV,* pulmonary vein

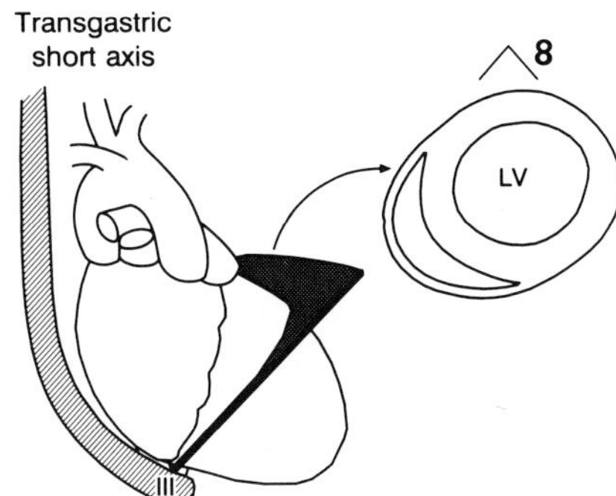

Fig. 14. Diagram of common scan planes. III: *8*, transgastric short-axis

tion. Although the anterolateral papillary muscle is most easily imaged in the anterior four-chamber plane, the posteromedial papillary muscle can be visualized only with extreme retroflexion of the endoscope. Because the mitral valve orifice is parallel to the ultrasound beam in this view, excellent pulsed Doppler and color flow imaging examinations can be performed.

Tricuspid valve leaflets are also imaged in the long-axis projection; however, the orifice is oblique to the plane of section. Because the orifice is off axis, an accurate Doppler examination cannot be performed without angle correction. Color flow imaging, however, can be used to evaluate tricuspid valve regurgitation semiquantitatively.

Extreme retroflexion and further advancement of the endoscope in the four-chamber plane will view the coronary sinus in its long axis (Fig. 13). This structure can be seen in the left atrioventricular groove with the orifice into the right atrial cavity.

Step 3 – Transgastric Short-Axis Scans. With the endoscope controls in a neutral position, the instrument is advanced further (35–40 cm from the incisors) into the stomach and anteflexed to image the short axis of the heart from the fundus of the stomach (that is, transgastric view) and the left lobe of the liver (Fig. 14). This position is most frequently used intraoperatively to monitor global and regional myocardial function.

We display the left ventricle to the right and the right ventricle to the left (Figs. 15, 16), an orientation similar to that recommended by the American Society of Echocardiography for display of ventricular short-axis views. This orientation projects the heart as if viewed from the apex toward the base [9].

Examination of Thoracic Aorta (Step 4)

The endoscope, usually in a neutral position, is withdrawn back into the esophagus. Through the vertical extent of the esophagus, most of the thoracic aorta can be systematically imaged (Fig. 17). The aortic root, 2–3 cm of the

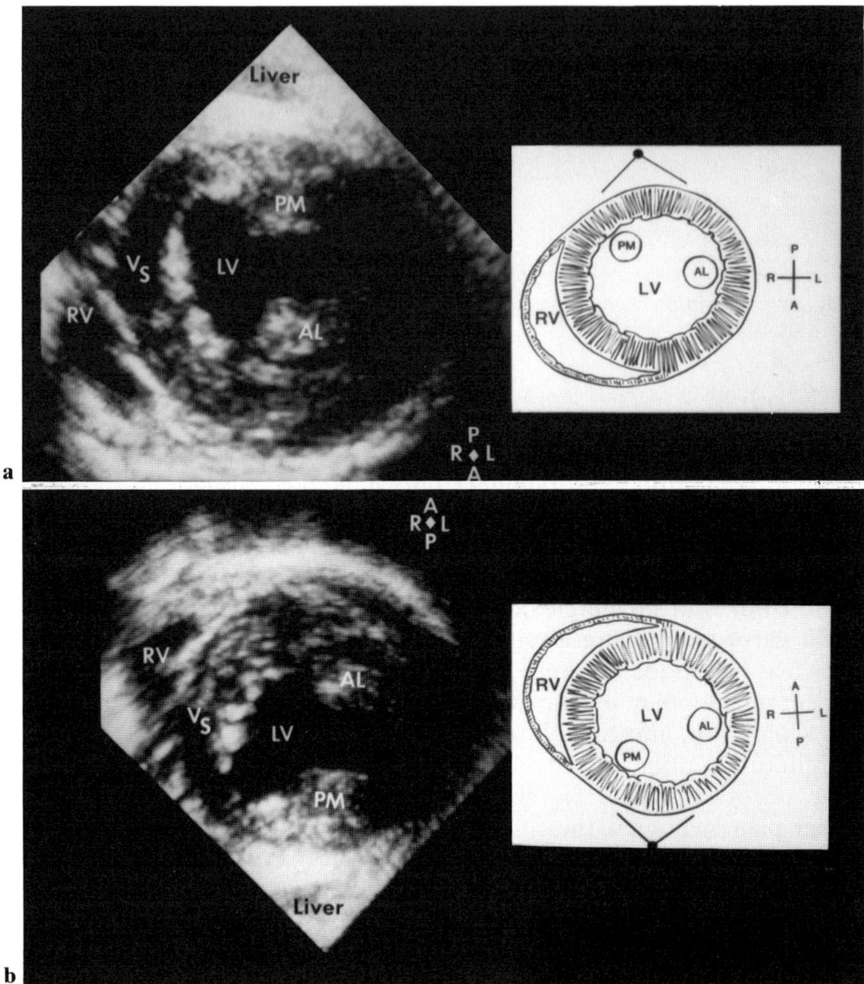

Fig. 15. a Transgastric short-axis echocardiographic scan of heart; posterior structures are at the *top* of image. This view projects heart as though looking from base toward apex. **b** Posterior structures are oriented downward on video screen, and heart is projected as though looking from apex toward base. This view corresponds to American Society of Echocardiography short-axis projection of left ventricle and is obtained by electronic inversion of two-dimensional echocardiographic image [45]. *VS*, Ventricular septum; *LV*, left ventricle; *AL*, antrolateral papillary muscle; *PM*, posteromedial papillary muscle; *RV*, right ventricle; *A* anterior; *P*, posterior; *L*, left; *R*, right. (From [12])

supravalvular ascending aorta, transverse aortic arch, left carotid and left subclavian arteries, entire descending thoracic aorta, and upper abdominal aorta can be systematically imaged (Figs. 18, 19). A *blind zone* for transesophageal echocardiography is the upper portion of the ascending aorta. In this region, the air-filled trachea is directly interposed between the esophagus and the ascending aorta and therefore obscures the anterior structures. Thus, a complete

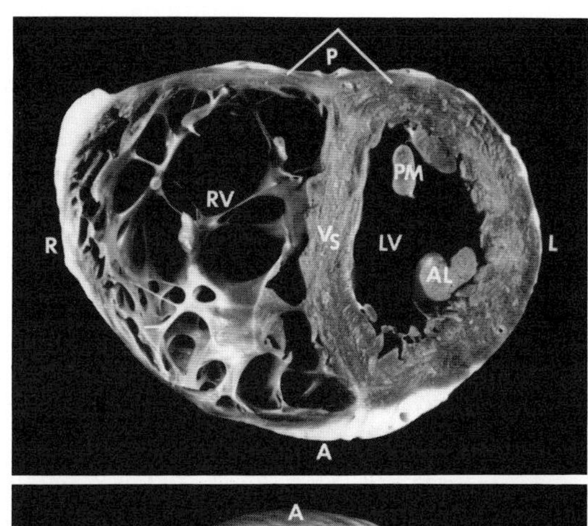

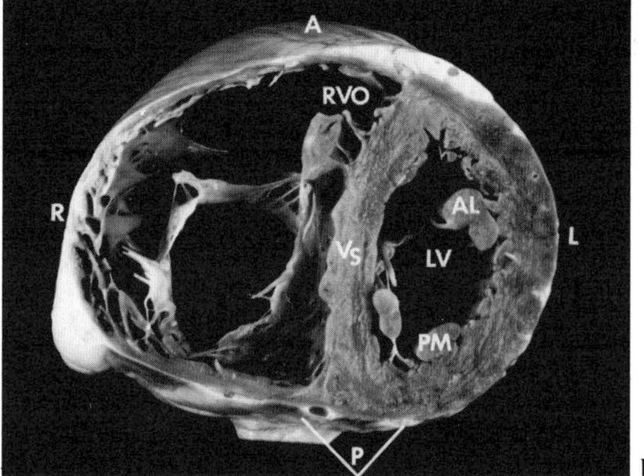

Fig. 16 a, b. Anatomic sections of left ventricle at level of papillary muscle, corresponding to transgastric plane of view. **a** Specimen has been photographed to correspond to preset orientation of two-dimensional echocardiographic image. In this projection, posterior surface is displayed at top of screen, and structures are displayed as though viewing from cardiac base toward apex. **b** Other half of same specimen, now viewed from midventricle (*MV*) toward base. Posterior structures are displayed *downward*. *RVO*, Right ventricular outflow tract; *VS*, ventricular septum. For explanation of other abbreviations, see legend for Fig. 15. (From [12])

examination of the entire aorta is accomplished only with combined precordial and transesophageal echocardiographic approaches [11].

Because the relationship between the esophagus and the aorta changes at various levels in the thorax (Fig. 17), the image orientation relative to other imaging modalities has not been standardized. Lack of distinct anatomic landmarks behooves the examiner to record the depth of insertion of the endoscope and to use standard, unchanging image orientation. From the midthorax, the endoscope is rotated to the patient's left (counterclockwise), and a tomographic short-axis image of the mid-descending aorta is obtained (Fig. 17). The tip of the transducer is then advanced while the descending thoracic aorta is imaged. As the endoscope enters the stomach, the tip will be oriented posteriorly (counterclockwise rotation) because the esophagus lies anterior to the aorta at this level. From this distal position, the endoscope is then slowly withdrawn while the aorta is kept in view. As the endoscope passes from the stomach to the thorax, the tip is rotated clockwise. Slight anteflexion of the tip helps maintain good contact with the esophageal-aortic interface. Depth, in centimeters from the incisors, is substantiated throughout the withdrawal and used to determine the site of observed pathologic changes.

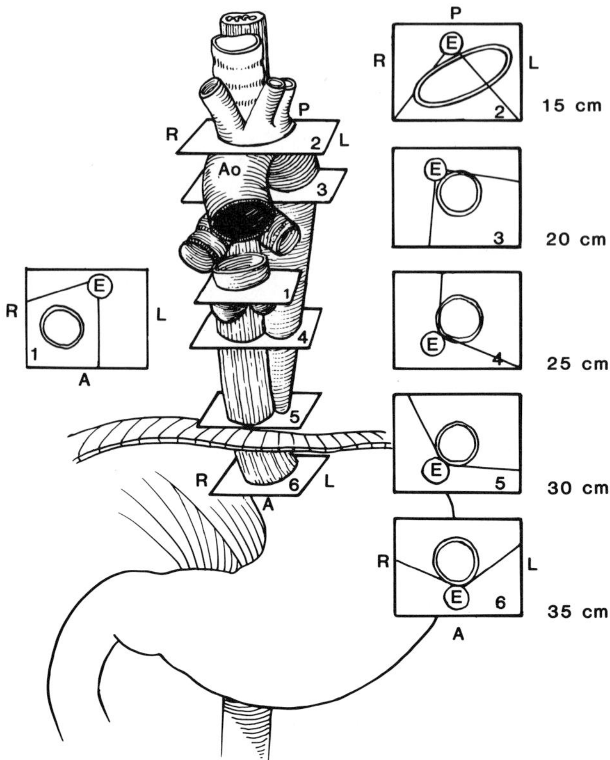

Fig. 17. Anatomic relationships of aorta (*Ao*), trachea, and esophagus (*E*). Also shown are various levels of horizontal scan planes of thoracic aorta: *1*, aortic root; *2*, transverse aortic arch; *3*, upper descending aorta; *4, 5*, mid-thoracic aorta; and *6*, upper abdominal aorta. Note that esophagus lies anterior to aorta and diaphragm and posterior at level of transverse arch. Portion of ascending aorta directly anterior to trachea is a blind area for transesophageal echocardiography. Few internal landmarks accurately allow examiner to designate anterior-posterior and right-left orientation of mid-thoracic aorta. Examiner must record, in centimeters, depth of tip of transducer and must relate orientation to an anatomic depiction, such as that shown in this diagram. Approximate incisor-to-tip distance for adults is shown. *A*, Anterior; *L*, left; *P*, posterior; *R*, right. (From [12])

Descending Thoracic Aorta

Between the upper abdomen and the aortic arch, the esophagus and aorta change their anterior-to-posterior relationships (Figs. 17, 18) − at the diaphragm, the esophagus lies anterior to the aorta; at mid-thorax, it is medially located; and at aortic arch, it is posterior. This gently intertwining relationship will alter the orientation of the displayed aortic walls, depending on the level of the tip of the endoscope in the esophagus (Fig. 17).

Aortic Arch

The esophagus lies posterior to the aortic arch (Fig. 19). In horizontal planes of section, the transverse aortic arch is displayed with the ascending arch to the left of the screen. With the patient in a left decubitus position, most of the transverse aortic arch can usually be seen. With the endoscope at the level of the transverse aortic arch, the patient will usually experience an increased gag and cough reflex, which prevents prolonged imaging in this position. If the aortic and cardiac scan planes are considered suitable, the endoscope is

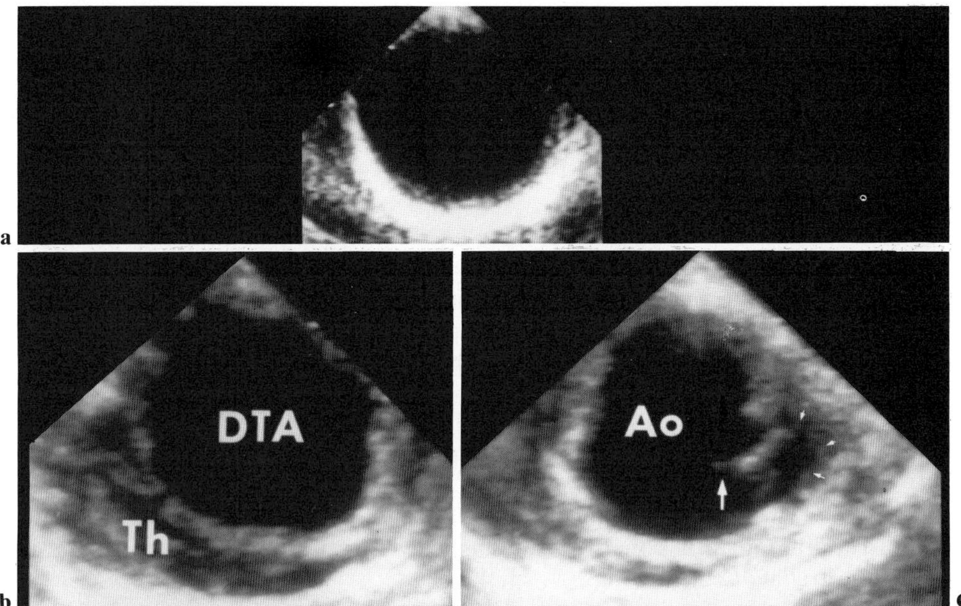

Fig. 18a–c. Transesophageal echocardiography, descending thoracic aorta can be clearly imaged from transverse aortic arch to upper abdomen. It is important to record depth of insertion of transducer and relate orientation to relative position within thorax (see Fig. 19). **a** Two-dimensional image of normal descending thoracic aorta. **b** Atherosclerotic changes and intimal thickening or thrombus (*Th*) evident in descending thoracic aorta (*DTA*). Intimal pathologic changes can be detected and accurately mapped by transesophageal echocardiography. **c** Small intimal flap (*large arrow*). Penetrating atheromatous ulcer (*small arrows*) and small intimal hematoma were evident in aorta (*Ao*). (From [12])

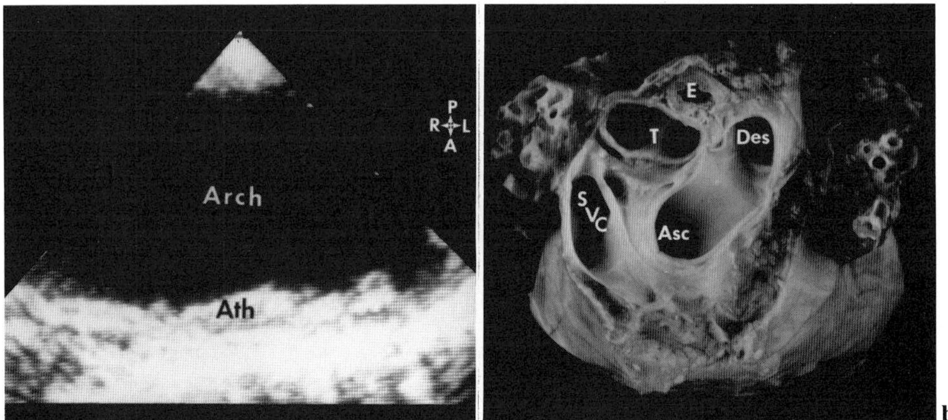

Fig. 19. **a** Transesophageal echocardiographic scan of aortic arch. *Ath*, Atheromatous change in vessel wall. *A*, Anterior; *L*, left; *P*, posterior; *R*, right. Tomographic sections of transverse aortic arch are obtained by gradually advancing and withdrawing endoscope at level of tracheal carina. **b** Anatomic specimen cut in same plane as shown in a. Note that trachea (*T*) lies anterior to esophagus (*E*) and can interfere with assessment of upper part of ascending aorta (*Asc*). *Des*, Descending thoracic aorta; *SVC*, superior vena cava. (From [12])

then withdrawn to the base of the transverse aortic arch, and the proximal left subclavian artery and left carotid artery are imaged on withdrawal. As the tip of the endoscope approaches the posterior pharynx, the gag and cough reflex will appreciably increase.

Upper Ascending Aorta

Because the trachea lies between the esophagus and the ascending aorta, esophageal imaging of the upper ascending aorta is usually not possible [11]. Standard precordial (high left or right parasternal window) examination is used to complete the scanning of this portion of the aorta.

Aortic Root and Proximal Ascending Aorta

The segment of the thoracic aorta that consists of the aortic root and the proximal ascending aorta is consistently imaged when the tip of the endoscope is below the tracheal carina (Figs. 3, 11, 17).

Upper Abdominal Aorta

The stomach and lower part of the esophagus lie anterior to the aorta at the level of the diaphragm. Occasionally, the superior mesenteric and celiac arteries can be scanned with the tip of the transducer in the stomach.

Brachiocephalic Vessels

The left common carotid artery and the proximal left subclavian artery can usually be imaged as the endoscope is withdrawn superior to the aortic arch. The innominate artery is usually not visible because of the interposed trachea. When the endoscope is withdrawn superiorly, it should be rotated counterclockwise (leftward) to scan the left subclavian artery, which courses away from the transducer (leftward and inferiorly on the video screen). The left carotid artery is more medial and is imaged in the short-axis views. The left jugular vein lies anterior (at the bottom of the video screen) to the left common carotid artery.

Conclusion

Ultrasound as an imaging medium has been further advanced by the introduction of new high-resolution transesophageal transducers. This application should promote the development of an entire new line of future devices. Centainly, transesophageal echocardiography is a feasible technology to introduce into a cardiologist-supervised echocardiographic laboratory. Rapid generation of high-resolution images with minimal preparation of the patient makes this an appealing technique. To learn the procedure, the cardiovascular specialist must become familiar with new tomographic anatomic sections and image orientation.

References

1. Callahan JA, Seward JB, Nishimura RA, Miller FA Jr, Reeder GS, Shub C, Callahan MJ, Schattenberg TT, Tajik AJ (1985) Two-dimensional echocardiographically guided pericardiocentesis: experience in 117 consecutive patients. Am J Cardiol 55:476−479
2. Meltzer RS, Roelandt J (eds) (1982) Contrast Echocardiography. The Hague, Martinus Nijhoff, 2 The Hague
3. Currie PJ, Seward JB, Hagler DJ, Tajik AJ (1986) Two-dimensional/Doppler echocardiography and its relationship to cardiac catheterization for diagnosis and management of congenital heart disease. Cardiovasc Clin 17:301−322
4. Hisanaga K, Hisanaga A, Hibi N, Nishimura K, Kambe T (1980) High speed rotating scanner for transesophageal cross-sectional echocardiography. Am J Cardiol 46:837−842
5. Hanrath P, Kremer P, Langenstein BA, Matsumoto M, Bleifeld W (1981) Transösophageale Echokardiographie: Ein neues Verfahren zur dynamischen Ventrikelfunktionsanalyse. Dtsch Med Wochenschr 106:523−525
6. Yock PG, Linker DT, Thapliyal HV, Arenson JW, Samstad S, Saether O, Angelsen BAJ (1988) Real-time two-dimensional catheter ultrasound: a new technique for high-resolution intravascular imaging (abstract). J Am Coll Cardiol 11(Suppl A):130A
7. Tajik AJ, Seward JB, Hagler DJ, Mair DD, Lie JT (1978) Two-dimensional real-time ultrasonic imaging of the heart and great vessels: technique, image orientation, structure identification, and validation. Mayo Clin Proc 53:271−303
8. Seward JB, Tajik AJ, Edwards WD, Hagler DJ (eds) (1987) Two-dimensional echocardiographic atlas, Vol 1, Congenital heart disease. Springer, Berlin Heidelberg New York
9. Henry WL, DeMaria A, Gramiak R, King DL, Kisslo JA, Popp RL, Sahn DJ, Schiller NB, Tajik A, Teichholz LE, Weyman AE (1980) Report of the American Society of Echocardiography Committee on Nomenclature and Standards in Two-Dimensional Echocardiography. Circulation 62:212−217
10. Seward JB, Tajik AJ, Hagler DJ, Edwards WD (1984) Internal cardiac crux: two-dimensional echocardiography of normal and congenitally abnormal hearts. Ultrasound Med Biol 10:735−745
11. Erbel R, Börner N, Steller D, Brunier J, Thelen M, Pfeiffer C, Mohr-Kahaly S, Iversen S, Oelert H, Meyer J (1987) Detection of aortic dissection by transesophageal echocardiography. Br Heart J 58:45−51
12. Seward JB, Khandheria BK, Oh JK, et al. (1988) Transesophageal echocardiography: technique, anatomic correlations, implementation, and clinical applications. Mayo Clin Proc 63:649−680

Congenital Heart, Valvular Heart,
Ischemic Heart Disease

The Role of Transesophageal Echocardiography in Adolescents and Adults with Congenital Heart Disease

G. R. SUTHERLAND

Introduction

Transoesophageal echocardiography (TEE) is rapidly gaining acceptance as a semi-invasive diagnostic approach in adults in whom an adequate precordial ultrasound examination is impossible due to lung disease, chest deformity or mechanical ventilation [1, 2]. Transoesophageal imaging is increasingly used as the approach of choice in the adult cardiac outpatient clinic for the investigation of atrial mass lesions [3], in the evaluation of mitral prosthetic valve function [4], in the assessment of endocarditis and its complications [5, 6] and in the evaluation of thoracic aortic pathology [7, 8]. However, little has yet been reported on its potential role in the evaluation of the complexities of congenital heart disease.

At present both transducer size and the semi-invasive nature of the procedure appear to preclude its use in non-sedated or non-anaesthetised conscious children. Even when general anaesthesia is used to allow probe insertion and placement, probe size will normally not allow children of less than 5 years to be investigated with safety. Fortunately, using a combination of precordial and subcostal high resolution cross-sectional imaging (i.e. 5.0 or 7.5 MHz) allied to spectral Doppler (pulsed and continuous wave) plus colour flow mapping studies diagnostic information can be derived in virtually all unoperated infants and young children (i.e. those less than 5 years), and thus recourse to the alternative transoesophageal approach is rarely required in this age group. However, as more children are operated on at a young age for complex heart disease a non-invasive technique is required for the sequential evaluation of the results of cardiac surgery and the identification of residual or newly acquired lesions. The precordial ultrasound window is frequently restricted in such operated patients with midline thoracotomies as a direct consequence of acquired fibrous adhesions following cardiac surgery. In addition, ultrasound imaging in all children becomes more difficult with age due to increasing chest and cardiac size and the natural reduction in the ultrasound window. Ultrasound studies of complex congenital heart disease in the adolescent and adult population present many difficulties. In addition, complex heart disease is frequently associated with either cardiac malpositions, where the heart is completely or partially obscured by the sternum and rib cage, or significant spinal or thoracic cage abnormalities which make ultrasound examination difficult.

Transesophageal Echocardiography
Edited by R. Erbel et al.
© Springer-Verlag Berlin Heidelberg 1989

Certain structures themselves are poorly visualised from the precordial approach. Atrial appendage anatomy is inadequately visualised. Individual pulmonary veins are not well seen. Sinus venosus atrial septal defects may prove difficult to visualise. The visualisation of right atrial to pulmonary artery, or right atrial-right ventricular connections inherent in a Fontan or modified Fontan procedure are further good examples of morphology which is difficult to evaluate from the precordial approach. Other examples include right ventricular-pulmonary artery valved conduits, atrial baffle function following a Mustard or Senning procedure, and the precise arrangement of atrioventricular valve chordae with respect to the ventricular septal defect in the so called "criss-cross heart". Many more examples could be cited. In the majority of these cases better evaluation might be achieved from the transesophageal approach using a combination of high resolution imaging to evaluate structure and colour flow mapping to define any associated flow abnormalities.

We therefore used TEE to attempt to define its potential role (both advantages and limitations) in adolescents and adults with congenital heart disease. We report our initial experience of its use over a wide spectrum of simple and complex congenital heart defects.

Patients and Methods

Between 1984 and 1988, a total of 681 transoesophageal cross-sectional imaging studies were carried out in the Thoraxcentre. Until 1987, 5.6 MHz transoesophageal cross-sectional imaging alone was available. Since 1987, cross-sectional imaging plus colour flow mapping at either 3.75 MHz or 5.6 MHz has been available. During this time period 77 outpatients (11% of the total patient population undergoing transoesophageal studies) were referred for the evaluation of varying aspects of congenital heart disease. Their ages ranged from 12 to 78 years (mean age 32 years). The range of morphologic diagnoses (which varied from possible subaortic membrane to extremely complex cyanotic congenital heart disease) is given in Table 1. Fifty-three patients were initially studied prior to cardiac surgery and a further 24 were studied some months or years after the surgical procedure was carried out to evaluate the late results of surgery. In every case information on the clinical history, electrocardiogram and chest X-ray was available prior to the TEE study. All subsequently underwent correlative angiography.

An initial precordial ultrasound study was routinely carried out using either 2.5-, 3.75- or 5-MHz cross-sectional imaging (Toshiba SSH 65A; Hewlett Packard or Toshiba SSH 160 or Vingmed 770 scanning equipment). A comprehensive assessment of the atrial situs, intracardiac connections and the great vessel morphology was undertaken in every case. Each study included the routine use of multiple transducer positions (i.e. subcostal or suprasternal) to derive the maximal information on cardiac morphology. Continuous wave and pulsed Doppler information on the intracardiac flow patterns and velocity waveforms was routinely recorded, as was the information derived

Table 1. Primary morphologic diagnosis in each patient studied (other associated abnormalities were present in some patients)

Fibromuscular subaoartic obstruction	8
Fontan circulation	5[a]
TGA, post Mustard procedure	6
Secundum atrial septal defect	6[b]
Sinus venosus atrial septal defect	2
Atrioventricular defect	3
Atrioventricular discordance	5
LSVC −coronary sinus	3
LSVC +coronary sinus ASD	1
Fallot (preop)	3
Marfan aorta	7
Aortic coarctation	5
Cor triatriatum	1
Double inlet ventricle	2
"Criss-cross" heart	2
Ebstein	4
Double outlet right ventricle	2
PDA + endocarditis	1
VSD	7
Supraaortic stenosis	2
Subaortic tunnel	2
Total	77

[a] Three patients with coexisting Glenn anastomosis.
[b] Two patients with associated atrial myxomas.
TGA, transposed great arteries; LSVC, left-sided vena cava; ASD, atrial septal defect; PDA, patent ductus arteriosus; VSD, ventricular septal defect.

from colour flow mapping at 2.5- MHz or 3.75-MHz. On the basis of the above information, in each case the echocardiographer and the referring physician (following joint discussion) decided that certain important clinical questions remained unanswered or were only partially answered. A joint decision was made that more information was both essential to the management of the patient and that the required information might be obtained from a transoesophageal study. The patient was then given an appointment to return for such a study.

All 77 transoesophageal studies were carried out in the outpatient clinic, after the patient had fasted for 4 prior to the procedure. No prior antibiotic prophylaxis was given, as is our standard practice. Local anaesthetic in the form of lidocaine spray was administered to the hypopharynx to abolish the gag reflex, but no sedation was used. Patients were studied lying in the left lateral decubitus position. The probe was introduced and manipulated within the oesophagus in the manner described previously in our work. In every case the heart and thoracic aorta was viusalised and scanned, with special attention being paid to the specific area(s) of interest. The cross-sectional imaging study was supplemented in the last 34 patients by a complete colour flow mapping study. Where appropriate selective pulsed Doppler recordings were made of pulmonary vein flow, mitral flow and pulmonary artery flow. No other pulsed Doppler recordings were normally attempted because of poor alignment to flow across the majority of other intracardiac structures.

In every case an attempt was made to define atrial appendage anatomy, the pattern of systemic and pulmonary venous drainage, the integrity of the atrial septum, the mode of atrioventricular connection, atrioventricular valve structure and function, the integrity of the ventricular septum, the morphology of the ventricular outflows and semilunar valves and the morphology of the thoracic aorta and proximal pulmonary arteries. Apart from mild retching, normally only following probe introduction, no complication was noted during the study. All patients had continuous electrocardiographic monitoring but no other form of continuous monitoring was carried out.

Results

Cardiac Position and Atrial Situs

Of the 77 patients studied, five had hearts in the right chest, four had midline hearts and 66 had hearts in the left chest. Atrial situs solitus was present in 74 cases and atrial situs inversus was present in three cases. An abnormal cardiac position did not create major problems in completing the study although a different transducer manipulation technique had to be evolved to cope with hearts in the midline or right chest. These changes in transducer manipulation were relatively easy to learn and a full imaging study was carried out in every case.

Identification of Atrial Appendage Anatomy

In all patients studied both atrial appendages could be visualised with care despite the cardiac position or degree of cardiac rotation. Three cases of abnormal atrial situs (all three inversus) were found in this series. All subsequently had high kV filter films to determine the bronchus morphology and thus confirm atrial situs. There were no cases of atrial isomerism nor was there a case of juxtaposed appendages. Atrial appendage anatomy was reliably identified since the long, crescentic, crenellated left atrial appendage, consistently was easily differentiated from the short blunt right atrial appendage. Although only three cases of abnormal atrial situs were studied it is our impression that such is the clarity with which the appendage morphology is visualised that the transoesophageal technique may prove to be the most reliable in vivo technique for the definition of atrial situs.

Identification of Normal and Abnormal Systemic Venous Drainage

In all 77 cases a superior vena cava was identified entering the right atrium superiorly in the normal position. This could be scanned within the thorax in a series of short axis cuts by positioning the probe at differing levels within the oesophagus. In three of the cases of absent right atrioventricular connection a functioning Glenn anastomosis was present. The transoesophageal colour flow mapping images clearly demonstrated the direct communication between the upper dilated portion of the superior vena cava and the distal portion of the transected right pulmonary artery. In both cases pulsed Doppler was used to confirm the nature of the flow across the anastomosis. The site of the superior vena caval interruption was easily identified as was the lower patent position of the superior vena cava attached to the right atrium. None of the above information in these three cases was available from the prior precordial imaging study.

Although the orifice of the inferior vena cava entering the floor of the right atrium could be visualised in all 77 cases, thus confirming its presence, no further part of the inferior vena cava could be studied in these patients without causing them discomfort. No case of azygos continuation of the inferior vena cava, draining the superior caval veins, was enountered in this series.

Identification of a second superior vena cava entering the heart either directly to the superior aspect of the left atrium (one case) or by an anastomosis with the coronary sinus and draining by this structure to the right atrium (four cases) was present in five patients. In the latter four cases the prior precordial studies had suggested the diagnosis but the diagnosis had been missed in the case where the left superior vena cava drained directly to the left atrial roof. Colour flow mapping was of value in all four cases as an adjunct to the imaging diagnosis, confirming the abnormal site of venous flow drainage and excluding any related transatrial flow in three cases where drainage was via the coronary sinus to the right atrium. In the remaining case the presence of a coronary sinus atrial septal defect was confirmed when a defect was clearly visualised between the two atria around the normal site of the coronary sinus.

Identification of Normal and Abnormal Pulmonary Venous Drainage

A sinus venosus atrial septal defect was present in the other two cases in whom prior precordial studies had failed to demonstrate the site of the transatrial flow despite a clinical examination which strongly suggested the presence of an atrial septal defect. In both cases the transoesophageal study imaged a defect in the superior portion of the atrial septum roofed by the free atrial wall. In both cases an abnormal site of drainage of the right upper pulmonary vein was identified. In one case, drainage was to the roof of the right atrium close to its junction with the superior vena cava and in the second it was directly to the superior vena cava. The morphologic diagnosis of both the transatrial flow and the site of drainage of the anomalous pulmonary vein was enhanced by confirming the associated flow abnormality on colour flow mapping.

In the remaining 75 patients with presumed normal pulmonary venous drainage an analysis of the ability of the transoesophageal approach to visualise individual pulmonary veins was undertaken. Upon analysing the tapes it became clear that the ability of the investigator to visualise these structures improved with experience at transducer manipulation and was additionally improved when colour flow mapping identification of individual pulmonary vein inflow into the left atrium could be used as a marker to guide transducer manipulation. Bearing these caveats in mind, in the last 40 cases studied in whom an attempt was made to visualise every pulmonary vein the individual pulmonary veins were visualised, using appropriate (and different) transducer orientations with the following frequency: left upper 100%; right upper 90%; left lower 62%; right lower 23%. In every case the left upper pulmonary vein and left atrial appendage were clearly imaged and distinguished from each other. This was frequently impossible using the precordial imaging approach.

Identification of Abnormalities of the Atrial Septum

Twelve patients in this series had a defect in the atrial septum as their primary morphologic abnormality (six secundum defects, three partial atrioventricular defects, two sinus venosus defect and one coronary sinus defect). In two of the secundum defects and atrial myxoma was present attached to the defect edge. In both cases the myxoma was predominantly sited in the right atrium but in one this prolapsed back and forward through the defect during the cardiac cycle. In every case the patient had been referred for the transoesophageal study because of poor quality or ambiguity in the precordial images. In all these 12 cases the site of the defect in the atrial septum was clearly imaged, as was the abnormal transatrial flow in the four cases in which colour flow mapping was available. Associated abnormalities such as partial anomalous pulmonary venous drainage (see previous section), atrial septum accessory tissue tags or atrial septum aneurysm formation, associated left superior vena cava, adherent myxomas and the classic abnormal atrioventricular valve abnormalities associated with an atrioventricular defect were all visualised with a clarity not normally associated with precordial ultrasound studies in these older patients with congenital heart disease.

A further 17 patients with more complex morphologic lesions (e.g. Ebstein's anomaly, Fallot, etc.) were also noted to have bidirectional or right to left shunting across a patent foramen ovale. In five, there was a persistent defect at the lower end of the thin membrane which covers the foramen ovale; bidirectional (four cases) or right to left (one case) transseptal flow was confirmed by pulsed Doppler interrogation or colour flow mapping. In the other 12 patients the thin membrane across the foramen ovale appeared intact but mobile, but colour flow mapping demonstrated a definite bidirectional shunt across the atrial septum in this position. This varied in some cases with the phase of respiration. In none of the last 17 cases was an atrial shunt suspected on the precordial examination.

Atrioventricular Junction Abnormalities

Twenty-one patients with major abnormalities of the atrioventricular were studied, five with absent right atrioventricular connections, five with atrioventricular discordance, three with atrioventricular defects, two with double inlet left ventricle, two with "criss-cross" heart (both in the setting of atrioventricular discordance) and four with Ebstein's anomaly to the tricuspid valve. In 19 cases the primary morphologic diagnosis had been correctly made at the prior precordial study. In the remaining two cases (both with dextrocardia and "criss-cross" hearts) the precordial examination had produced ambiguous results. Apart from imparting a remarkable degree of detail to the images, the transoesophageal approach contributed no significant new diagnostic information on either absent right connection or double inlet ventricle, but it did provide unique information in the evaluation of the morphology of any associated Fontan circulation (five cases) and in the assessment of the degree of related atrioventricular valve incompetence in both the double inlet and absent connection groups.

A detailed description of the information obtained in the patients with a Fontan-type circulation is outwith the scope of this article, but suffice it to say that the transoesophageal approach allowed direct visualisation of the Glenn anastomosis, right atrial morphology and flow characteristics, the direct atriopulmonary communication (where this was present) and the central pulmonary arteries. In every case very high quality pulsed Doppler tracings of the velocity profiles from each of these structures could be recorded for subsequent detailed analysis. This information had not been obtained from the precordial study. The only problem in this group of patients occurred in those with a conduit-type connection between right atrium and an anterior right ventricular chamber. In the two patients with this morphology, transoesophageal echo failed to visualise the conduit and the valve it contained. This, however, might have been predicted prior to the commencement of the study as we have long recognised the inability of the transoesophageal approach to visualise the anterior portion of the trabecular septum as well as the apex of the heart.

Transoesophageal imaging in these Fontan patients allowed accurate use of pulsed Doppler to record the velocity waveforms in the Glenn anastomoses, the vena cava, right atrium, the morphologic right ventricle (when this was incorporated into the right-sided circulation), the direct right atrial-pulmonary artery anastomosis and the central pulmonary arteries. In these patients, a further series of pulsed Doppler recordings were routinely made from the following left heart sites: left and right upper pulmonary veins, mid-lift atrial flow, and transmitral flow. These unique velocity waveforms consistently provided remarkable new insights into the haemodynamics of the Fontan circulation in individual patients. Again, this pulsed Doppler information had been only partially derived from the preceeding precordial studies and the precordial waveforms did not have the high quality of those obtained from the transoesophageal approach.

The Ventricular Septum

Precordial echocardiography is remarkably accurate in identifying the presence of single ventricular septal defects using a combination of cross-sectional imaging, continuous wave Doppler and colour flow mapping. The only problem area inherent in the precordial assessment is in distinguishing between single and multiple defects. Thus it might be predicted that the transoesophageal approach would have little additional to offer in their identification. In fcat there are major problems inherent in using the transoesophageal approach. Precordial cross-sectional imaging is a good technique to visualise moderate or large-sized defects as multiple transducer positions and transducer orientations can be combined to interrogate the septum in a large number of planes. In an echogenic patient every part of the septum can be scanned from the precordium. Compare this with the transoesophageal window − the transducer is very limited in its scan planes and in addition large areas of the trabecular septum (the apex, anterior trabecular and outlet septum) are blind areas to the oesophageal probe. In fact, only the perimembranous area can be consistently imaged. This is of some value as the majority of moderate or large ventricular septal defects wholly or partially involve this region and thus can be imaged from the oesophagus. However, problems exist with false-positive areas of echo "drop-out" occurring in normal patients. Problems are also created by the image moving in and out of the scan plane. In our experience transoesophageal imaging is a poor substitute for good quality precordial ultrasound studies in the evaluation of congenital ventricular septal defects. The problem is even worse when the transoesophageal technique is used to attempt to visualise central trabecular or apical postinfarction ventricular septal defects. Because these are blind areas even very large defects may be missed by esophageal imaging (inferolateral left ventricular pseudoaneurysms pose identical problems for transoesophageal imaging for the same reasons).

Ventriculoarterial Connections

Transoesophageal imaging provided no additional diagnostic information on the morphology of the ventriculoarterial connection in the patients studied when compared to the prior precordial studies. However, in patients with transposed or malpositioned great vessels some new insights into the relationships of the great vessels to the ventricles and any underlying ventricular septal defect were of value.

Ventricular Outflow Tracts

Transoesophageal imaging provides excellent imaging of the left ventricular outflow tract but virtually no information on the right ventricular outflow tract. On the left side transoesophageal imaging allied to colour flow mapping is superb at demonstrating the range of subvalve obstruction encountered in congenital heart disease. In this series it provided more information of the morphology of discrete fibromuscular subaortic obstruction ("subaortic membrane") and its associated abnormalities than the precordial approach. Some 17 such patients have now been investigated in our combined study and the findings confirm that not only is this the diagnostic method of choice in adult patients with this lesion but also that the spectrum of abnormalities encountered is far greater than those in the paediatric population. This would suggest that this may be a progressive lesion. Substantially more information may also be gained by transoesophageal imaging in the spectrum of abnormalities which include tunnel subaortic stenosis and hypertrophic obstructive myopathies.

The Morphology of the Great Vessels

Transoesophageal imaging provides excellent visualisation of the aortic valve (albeit viewed in an oblique sectioning plane), proximal left and right coronary arteries and the proximal two-thirds of the ascending aorta. Due to interposition of the bronchus between the oesophagus and the aorta the distal third of the ascending aorta and the proximal position of the aortic arch may not be well visualised. However, the distal aortic arch and descending thoracic aortic can be easily imaged in every patient. Clear advantages gained by transoesophageal versus precordial images in visualising the ascending aorta in this patient group were: (1) definition of proximal coronary anatomy (the origin of the left anterior descending coronary artery from the left main could be confirmed in every patient in whom this was attempted − this is of relevance in patients with tetralogy of Fallot who have variable coronary anatomy); (2) identification of supravalvar aortic stenosis (this is frequently impossible to visualise from the precordial approach); (3) exclusion of acute ascending aortic dilatation or localised areas of dissection in Marfan's syndrome; and (4) the visualisation of descending aortic pathology (i.e. coarctation, patent ductus arteriosus or multiple aortopulmonary vessels). No difficulties arose in the definition of the ascending aortic pathology in the seven patients with Marfan's syndrome but major problems were encountered in the definition of descending aortic lesions. In three patients a small patent ductus arteriosus was present. In none of the three did imaging alone identify its presence although a diagnostic flow disturbance was recorded in the central pulmonary arteries on colour flow mapping. In the five patients with descending aortic coarctation an area of abnormal aortic lumen narrowing was identified in every case but in three cases the precise morphology of the narrowed segment was not demonstrated due to the complex tortuous nature of the lesion. In the remaining two cases, both with discrete short segment "ring-type" coarctations the morphology was accurately demonstrated. In all five cases transoesophageal imaging gained no information which was not present from the prior suprasternal scan and in three cases supplied considerably less information. Angiography or magnetic resonance imaging would appear to be superior diagnostic techniques in the definition of complex coarctations.

In two patients, two or more descending aortic collateral vessels were present which supplied lung tissue. In both cases these multiple vessels were seen to arise from the anterior or lateral aspect of the descending aorta. However, in neither case did transoesophageal imaging correctly predict either the number of morphology of the aorta-pulmonary collaterals.

Conclusion

In conclusion, this initial experience has convinced us that transoesophageal imaging is a major advance in the evaluation of certain aspects of congenital heart disease in the adolescent and adult patient. It is not a procedure to be undertaken lightly as the studies are complex and can last much longer than a routine study. Such studies should only be undertaken when precordial imaging has failed to provide the information required and the lesion to be studied can be scanned from the oesophageal approach. An experienced echocardiographer should perform the study. He should be fully conversant with the morphology and haemodynamics of complex congenital cardiac malformations. Sedation should be given to these patients for two reasons: (1) the time taken to perform such studies and (2) young patients tolerate the procedure less well than older patients. The studies require very detailed analysis as they can contain so much information.

However, it is clear that a suprising amount of new information can be gained by use of the transoesophageal approach (compared to precordial imaging) in the following lesions: (1) abnormalities of systemic and pulmonary venous drainage, (2) atrial lesions, (3) atrial baffle function, (4) the Fontan circulation, (5) atrioventricular valve morphology and function, (6) "criss-cross heart", (7) chordal straddling, (8) subaortic obstruction (especially discrete fibromuscular obstruction), (9) supraaortic stenosis, (10) the ascending aorta in Marfan's syndrome, and (11) types of descending aortic pathology.

References

1. Schluter, M. Langenstein BA, Polster J et al. (1982) Transesophageal cross-sectional echocardiography with a phased array transducer system: technique and initial clinical results. Br Heart J 48:62–72
2. Gussenhoven EJ, Taams MA, Roelandt JRTC et al. (1986) Transesophageal two-dimensional echocardiography: its role in solving clinical problems. J Am Coll Cardiol 8: 975–79

3. Aschenberg W, Schluter M, Kremer P et al. (1986) Transesophageal two-dimensional echocardiography for the detection of left atrial appendage thrombus. J Am Coll Cardiol 7 (1):163–66
4. Taams M, Gussenhoven E, Cahalan M et al. (1989) Transesophageal Doppler color flow imaging in the detection of native and Bjork-Shiley mitral valve regurgitation. J Am Coll Cardiol 13 (1):95–99
5. Drexler M, Erbel R, Rohmann S et al. (1987) Diagnostic value of two-dimensional transesophageal versus transthoracic echocardiography in patients with infective endocarditis. Eur Heart J 8 [Suppl 1]:303–06
6. Erbel R, Rohman S, Drexler M et al. (1988) Improved diagnostic value of echocardiography in patients with infective endocarditis by transoesophageal approach. A prospective study. Eur Heart J 9 (1):43–53
7. Borner N, Erbel R, Braun B et al. (1984) Diagnosis of aortic dissection by transesophageal echocardiography. Am J Cardiol 54:1157–58
8. Erbel R, Mohr-Kahaly S, Rennoliet H et al. (1987) Diagnosis of aortic dissection: the value of transesophageal echocardiography. Thorac Cardiovasc Surg 35 (2):126–33

Is the Quantification of Mitral Stenosis and Aortic Stenosis by Transesophageal Echocardiography Feasible?

E. Grube, U. Gerckens, and N. Cattelaens

The quantification of gradients in patients with mitral and aortic stenosis by conventional transthoracic Doppler echocardiography is well accepted in clinical diagnostic routine. Studies comparing it with angiography showed it produced excellent results in the determination of mean and maximum transmitral gradients. In patients with aortic stenosis, measurements of transaortic mean and maximum instantaneous gradients were highly reproducible and when mean aortic gradients were compared with those obtained by other methods, results were also quite satisfactory.

Occasionally, however, the transthoracic approach for the determination of mitral and aortic gradients is impossible because of poor signal quality for anatomic reasons.

In order to evaluate whether the determination of gradients by transesophageal echocardiography is feasible, we examined patients with mitral and aortic valve lesions by transesophageal echocardiography with integrated pulsed and continuous Doppler facilities. These studies in particular should answer the question whether quantification of mitral and aortic stenosis by transesophageal echocardiography is possible or even necessary, and whether this approach offers any advantages for clinical decision making. Furthermore, the study should elucidate in which patients this technique should be considered as an alternative and complementary diagnostic procedure.

We examined 42 patients with mitral valve disease with a mean age of 48 years (range 23–72 years). Twenty-five patients had pure mitral stenosis, 17 had mixed mitral lesions, and 12 had combined mitral and aortic lesions.

Transthoracic echocardiography was performed in all patients using commercially available color flow ultrasonic equipment (Aloka 860/880, Vingmed CFM 700) with integrated pulse wave (PW) and continuose wave (CW) Doppler facilities. In all patients, transesophageal echocardiography with integrated PW and CW Doppler facilities was also performed.

In order to compare these results with invasive data, cardiac catheterization as well as biplane angiography and aortography were performed in all patients. The following hemodynamic and anatomic variables were determined by transthoracic and transesophageal echocardiography:

- Mean transmitral gradient (mmHg)
- Maximum transmitral gradient (mmHg)
- Degree of mitral insufficiency (1–4)
- Valve morphology (mobility and calcification)
- The presence of left atrial thrombi

Transesophageal Echocardiography
Edited by R. Erbel et al.
© Springer-Verlag Berlin Heidelberg 1989

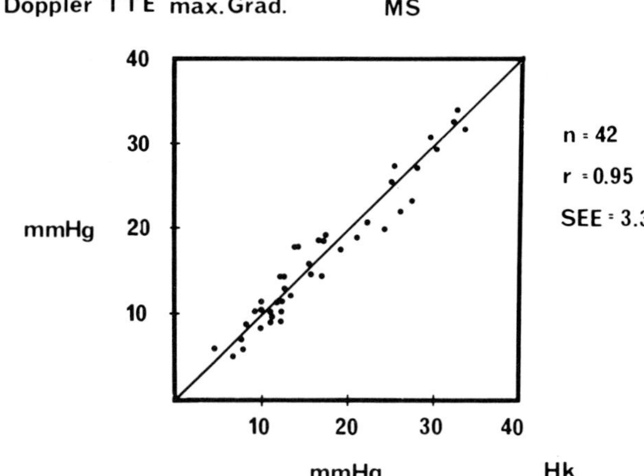

Fig. 1. Correlation of maximum transmitral gradients in patients with mitral stenosis (*MS*), comparing transthoracic echocardiographic (*TTE*) and invasive *Hk*) data

During cardiac catheterization, the degree of mitral insufficiency (Sellers 1—4) and pressure data (mean and maximum mitral gradient) were also determined.

When maximum transmitral gradients are compared, the results from transthoracic, transesophageal, and angiographic examination correlate well. The *r* value between maximum transthoracic gradients measured by echocardiography and invasively was 0.95 and the standard error of the estimate (SEE) was 3.3 mmHg (Fig. 1). For transesophageal and angiographic maximum mitral gradients the *r* value was 0.96 and the SEE slightly lower, at 2.8 mmHg (Fig. 2). The presence of mitral insufficiency was diagnosed by transthoracic echocardiography in 13, by transesophageal echocardiography in 19, and by angiography in 17. Left atrial thrombi were detected by trans-

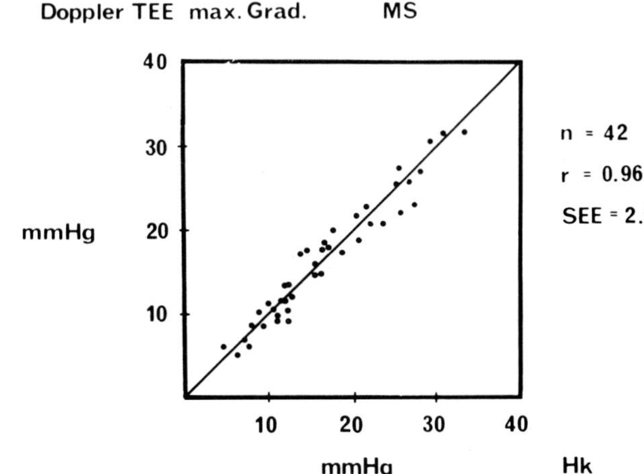

Fig. 2. Correlation of maximum transmitral gradients in patients with mitral stenosis (*MS*) comparing transesophageal echocardiography (*TEE*) and cardiac catheterization (*Hk*) data

                                                          E. Grube et al.

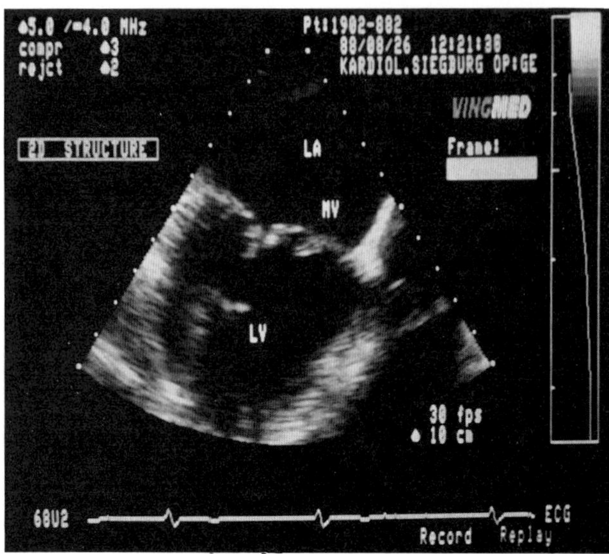

Fig. 3. Transesophageal echocardiogram in a patient with mitral stenosis. Note the thickened mitral valve leaflets in the near field of the echocardiographic probe. *LA*, left atrium; *MV*, mitral valve; *LV*, left ventricle

esophageal echocardiography in 12 patients and by transthoracic echocardiography in only four patients; with angiography, as would be expected, no atrial thrombus could be documented.

We concluded that, in comparison with transthoracic echocardiography, transesophageal echocardiography gives more detailed information about valve morphology, particularly mobility and calcification (Fig. 3), the pre-

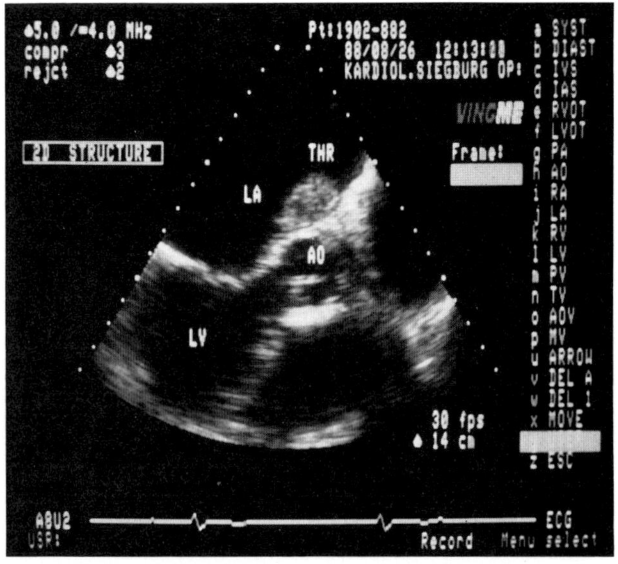

Fig. 4. Transesophageal echocardiogram in a patient with mitral stenosis and a wall-adherent left atrial thrombus (*THR*). *LA*, left atrium; *LV*, left ventricle; *AO*, aorta

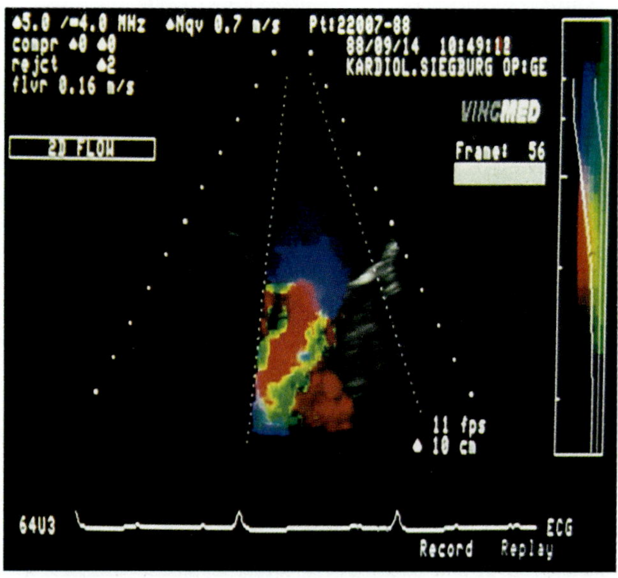

Fig. 5. Transesophageal color flow map of a patient with mitral stenosis. Note the high turbulent left ventricular inflow with central aliasing. This image is typical for a color transesophageal echocardiogram in patients with mitral stenosis

sence of left atrial thrombi (Fig. 4), left ventricular inflow pattern (Fig. 5), and accompanying mitral insufficiency (Fig. 6). Moreover, in patients with mitral stenosis, transesophageal echocardiography can be used to reliably calculate mean and maximum transmitral gradients as in compared to transthoracic and angiographic techniques (Fig. 7). As regards mean mitral gradients, transesophageal echocardiography and transthoracic echocardiography compare favorably with invasive techniques, with correlation coefficients of $r = 0.96$ and an SEE of 1.34 mmHg, and $r = 0.95$ and an SEE of 1.79 mmHg, respectively. Mitral gradients are shown in Table 1 (Fig. 1, Fig. 2). In order to compare the transthoracic and transesophageal approaches in patients with aortic stenosis, we examined 39 patients with a mean age of 52 years (range 32−82 years). Twenty-nine patients had pure aortic stenosis, ten

Table 1. Mitral Stenosis ($n = 42$)

	TTE	TEE	Angiography
Mean gradient (r)	0.95	0.96	
Max. gradient (r)	0.92	0.91	
Mitral insufficiency			
Presence (n)	13	19	17
Left atrial thrombi (n)	4	12	−

TTE transthoracic echocardiography; TEE transesophageal echocardiography

                                                                E. Grube et al.

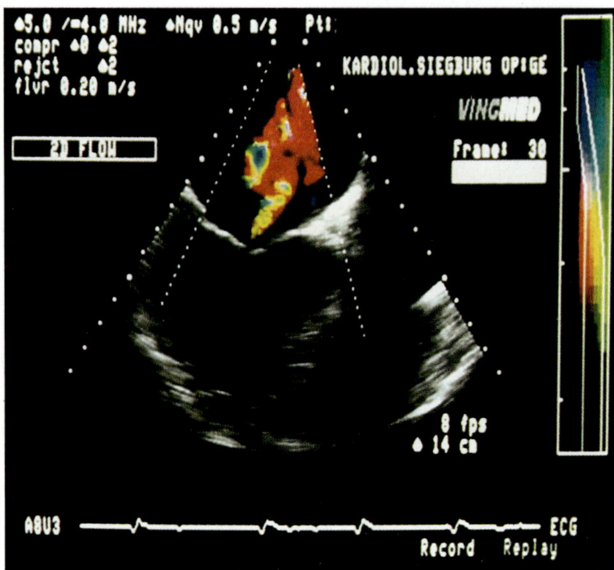

Fig. 6. The same patient as in Fig. 5: note the regurgitant jet (*yellow*) as a part of the combined mitral lesion

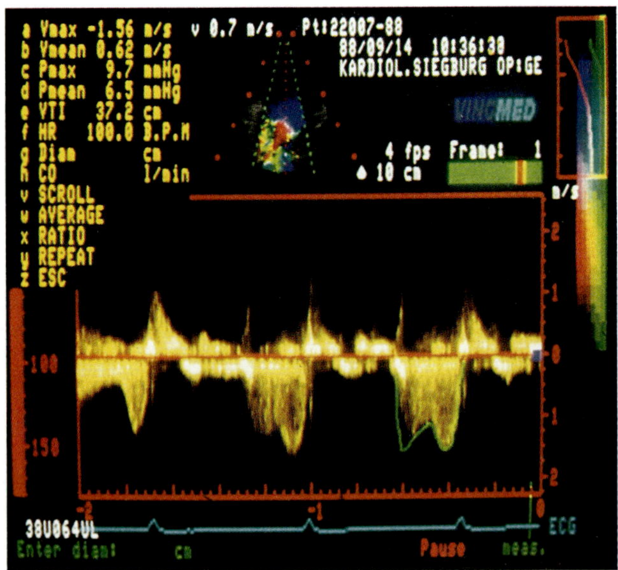

Fig. 7. CW transesophageal Doppler echocardiography in a patient with mitral stenosis. Note the exact delineation of highly turbulent areas with the calculation of mean and maximum transmitral gradients. In the *upper part* of the picture, the highly turbulent left ventricular inflow in the color flow map can be seen

had mixed aortic lesions, and twelve had combined aortic-mitral lesions. All 39 patients were examined by transthoracic echocardiography using PW and CW Doppler (Aloka 860/880, Vingmed CFM 700) and by transesophageal echocardiography with integrated PW and CW Doppler facilities (Vingmed CFM 700). In all 39 patients, cardiac catheterization and subsequently calculation of gradients, aortography, and ventriculography were performed.

The following hemodynamic and anatomic variables were compared: mean transaortic gradient (mmHg), maximum transaortic gradient (mmHg) and peak-to-peak gradient (mmHg), measured by cardiac catheterization; mean transaortic gradient and maximum instantaneous transaortic gradient measured by Doppler echocardiography. The degree of aortic insufficiency $(1-4)$ as well as valve morphology (mobility and calcification) were also determined by angiography and Doppler echocardiography. Transthoracic measurement of Doppler gradients using the modified Bernoulli equation $[\Delta p = 4 \times (v_2^2 - v_1^2)]$ (Δp, gradient; v_1, prestenotic velocity; v_2, poststenotic, velocity) was performed using the apical four-chamber view, from the right sternal or the suprasternal approach with a pencil probe. In transesophageal echocardiography the plane of the aortic valve was displayed, and the best possible interrogation by the CW beam of the ejection jet was searched for. The following correlations were found. For maximum instantaneous gradients, transthoracic echocardiography and invasive techniques revealed a good correlation, with $r = 0.88$ and a SEE of 13.7 mmHg (Fig. 8). If we compare transesophageal echocardiography with cardiac catheterization, the correlation is considerably worse, with an r value of 0,64, although four patients showed excellent correlations with data on the line of identity (Fig. 9).

If we compare transesophageal and transthoracic maximal gradients, the correlations shows a wide scatter with an r value of 0.68, transesophageal echocardiographic consistently underestimating gradients as compared to transthoracic echocardiography. Correlation coefficients are shown in Table 2. Aortic insufficiency was detected in ten patients by angiography and transthoracic echocardiography as opposed to 13 patients with transesophageal echocardiography.

We concluded that in most patients with aortic stenosis, the routine transthoracic approach yields adequate results for estimating aortic valve gradients and for clinical decision making. In about $10\% - 15\%$ of patients, transthoracic echocardiography is not able to quantify gradients reliably, mostly for anatomic reasons. In these patients, however, transesophageal echocardiography with integrated CW Doppler facilities might be a useful alternative to determine quality and direction of ejection jets and to calculate gradients. Invasive data correlate with these measurements with a r value of $0.64-0.68$. As with mitral stenosis, transesophageal echocardiography gives more detailed and extensive information about accompanying aortic valve insufficiency as well as about aortic valve morphology (mobility and calcification). Moreover, aortic valve and aortic root pathology (such as dissection, aneurysms, and thrombi) can be better diagnosed by transesophageal echocardiography.

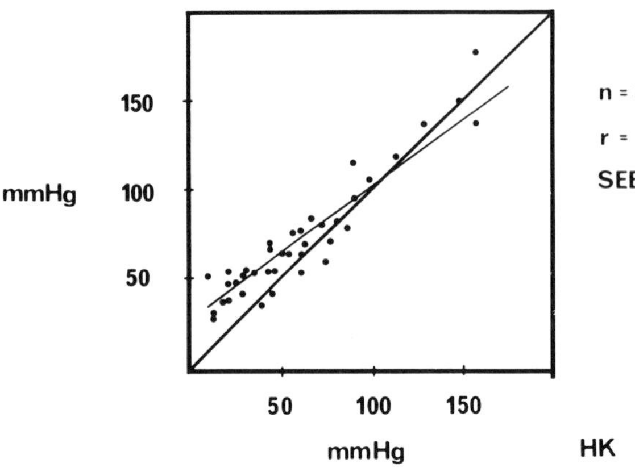

Fig. 8. Correlation of maximum instantaneous gradients in patients with aortic stenosis (*AS*), comparing transthoracic echocardiographic (*TTE*) and invasive data (*HK*)

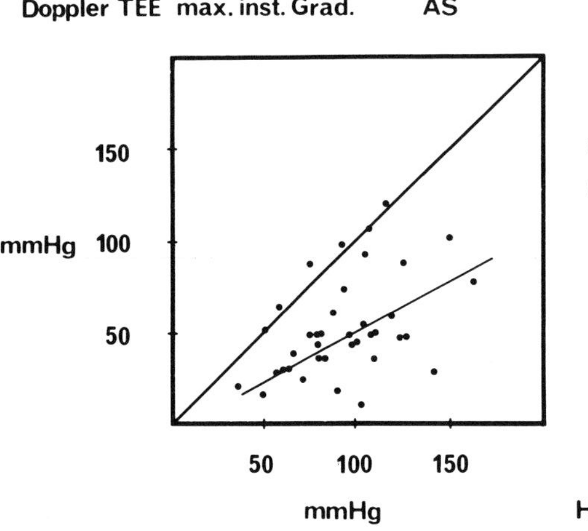

Fig. 9. Correlation of maximum instantaneous gradients in patients with aortic stenosis (*AS*), comparing transesophageal echocardiography (*TEE*) and cardiac catheterization (*HK*)

Table 2. Aortic Stenosis (*n* = 39)

	TTE	TEE	Angiography
Mean gradient (*r*)	0.25	0.61	
Max. gradient (*r*)	0.80	0.59	
Max. instantaneous gradient (*r*)	0.88	0.64	
Aortic insufficiency			
Presence (*n*)	10	13	10

We conclude that in patients with mitral stenosis, transesophageal echocardiography should be considered if detailed information about valve morphology, left atrial thrombi, accompanying mitral insufficiency, and gradients is of any clinical importance.

Transesophageal echocardiography is the most comprehensive and most reliable noninvasive approach in this patient population. In most patients with aortic stenosis, transesophageal echocardiography is not able to predict aortic valve gradients reliably as compared to invasive measurements; correlations showing a wide scatter.

In individual patients, however, transesophageal echocardiography is superior for the diagnosis and quantification of aortic valve disease, because the direction of the ejection jets allows better alignment to the transesophageal CW probe. Transesophageal echocardiography should always be considered if transthoracic echocardiography gives technically inadequate results, or if there is a discrepancy with clinical findings.

Transsesophageal Echocardiography in the Assessment of the Severity of Aortic Stenosis

C. STÖLLBERGER, E. SEHNAL, R. KARNIK, and J. SLANY

Introduction

Transthoracic and Doppler echocardiography provide useful information about the severity of aortic stenosis. According to recently published reports, the problems in assessing the degree of stenosis seem to be solved by the application of several formulas (continuity equation and modified Bernoulli equation) (Harrison et al. 1988; Oh et al. 1988). But in reality, there are always patients in whom echo and Doppler studies are impossible to perform or inconclusive due to emphysema, thoracic deformities, inability to obtain a good visualization of the valves, or an adaequate Doppler signal (Krafchek et al. 1985; Dennig et al. 1986). In addition, a complete Doppler study may require half an hour, which cannot be tolerated by patients in advanced stages of heart failure.

These problems are frequently found in a geriatric population. However advances in surgery and development of percutaneous valvuloplasty do offer therapeutic possibilities for elderly patients with aortic stenosis (Bessone et al. 1985; Cribier et al. 1986).

Hofmann et al. published in 1987 their results on the determination of aortic valve orifice area in aortic valve stenosis by two-dimensional transesophageal echocardiography. They found a good correlation between the aortic valve area as determined by transesophageal echocardiography (TEE) and the valve area calculated with Gorlin's formula using a catheter. Hofmann et al.'s report inspired us to perform TEE in all patients with clinically suspected aortic stenosis. We wanted to know if TEE can help in estimating the degree of aortic stenosis in these patients.

Patients and Methods

Within 18 months, TEE was performed in 60 patients with clinically suspected aortic stenosis. There were 38 women and 22 men, aged from 27 to 88 years with a mean of 72 years. Half of the study population was older than 74 years. All patients had clinical symptoms and each had one or more of the classical symptoms of angina, syncope, or heart failure. Twenty patients were in NYHA stage I or II and 40 were in NYHA stage III and IV at the time of echocardiography.

Transesophageal Echocardiography
Edited by R. Erbel et al.
© Springer-Verlag Berlin Heidelberg 1989

TEE was performed using a Varian 3400 R with a commercially available 3.5-MHz transducer. After obtaining a transesophageal four-chamber view of the heart, the transducer was pulled back $3-5$ cm and tilted $70°-90°$ to the front and $70°-90°$ to the right side to get a cross-sectional view of the aortic valve area. The valve area was defined as the smallest orifice area found at any cross-sectional view in early systole. A valve area smaller than 0.75 cm^2 was classified as severe stenosis, between 0.75 and 1.0 cm^2 as moderate stenosis, and larger than 1.0 cm^2 as mild stenosis. The time required for the transesophageal study was $5-8$ min.

Results

Figure 1 shows an example of a patient with a mild stenosis. The valves are calcified and thickened, and the valve area is 1.3 cm^2. Figure 2 shows a patient with a moderate aortic stenosis with an orifice area of 0.9 cm^2 by TEE and 0.95 cm^2 by catheter. In Figures 3 and 4, a case of severe aortic stenosis, it is impossible to define the orifice area. Only the heavily calcified valves can be seen; they do not move and have nearly the same shape during systole and diastole.

In 34 patients, left heart catheterization was performed after echocardiography. In order to minimize the invasive procedure in these elderly patients, right heart catheterization and estimation of cardiac output were not performed in each patient. Thus, in the majority of patients, orifice area could not be calculated. The severity of aortic stenosis was therefore quantified according to the systolic peak to peak gradient (Table 1). A patient having a gradient of less than 30 mmHg was classed as having a mild stenosis, one with a gradient between 30 and 59 mmHg as having moderate stenosis, and one with 60 mmHg or more as having severe stenosis. Ten patients died before catheterization could be performed, and the severity of aortic stenosis was

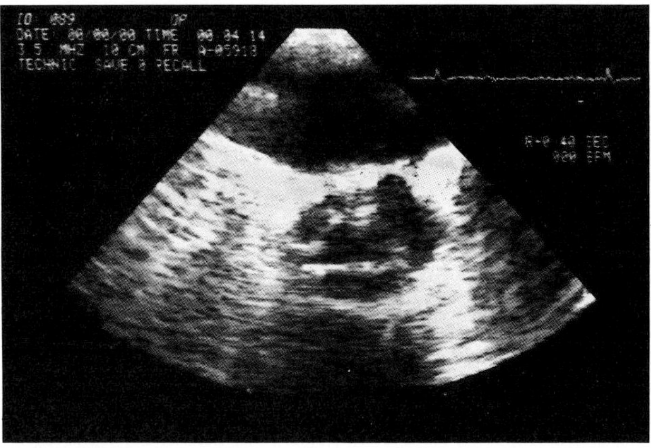

Fig. 1. TEE image from a patient with mild aortic stenosis

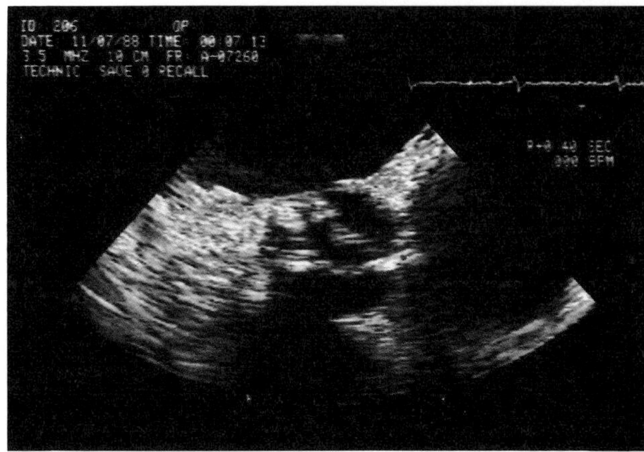

Fig. 2. TEE image from a patient with moderate aortic stenosis

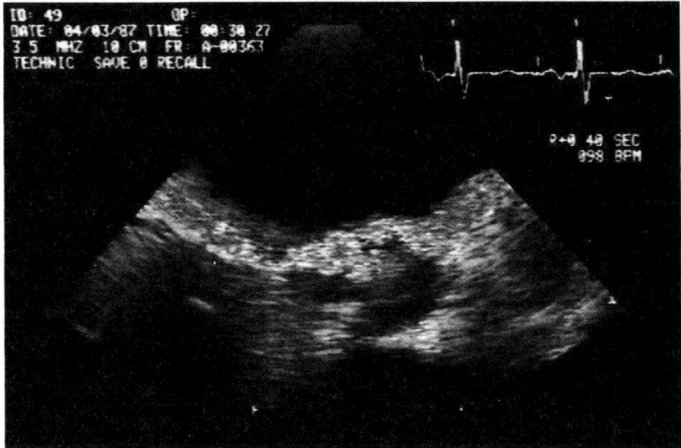

Fig. 3. TEE image from a patient with severe aortic stenosis

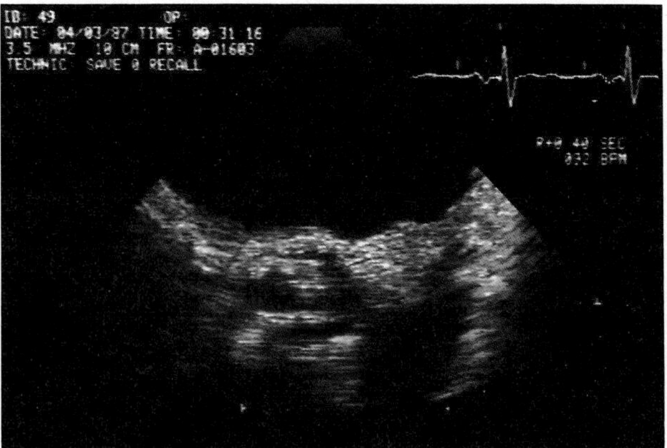

Fig. 4. TEE image from the patient in Fig. 3

assessed by the pathologist. In 16 patients, no cardiac catheterization was performed. Clinically and by TEE, eight cases were classed as mild and eight cases as moderate stenosis. All these patients are still alive and clinically stable. The measurement of the valvular orifice area was possible in only 36 cases. Eleven were classed as mild, 15 as moderate, and ten as severe. In the remaining 24 cases, no reliable measurement could be performed due to poor picture quality, no visualization of the cross-section area, artifacts due to heavily calcified valves, or no visible orifice area. In these cases, an estimation of the severity was made from the videotape by two independent observers unaware of the findings in the patients.

TEE allowed correct assessment of the severity of aortic stenosis in all but five of the catheter and autopsy proven cases (Table 2). In one case − a young woman with a congential aortic stenosis − TEE underestimated the degree of stenosis severely because of lack of calcification of the valves. There was one case of overestimation: a patient with very poor left ventricular function and calcified valves. Transthoracic and Doppler studies were impossible or inconclusive in 14 of these 44 cases (Table 3). In nine patients transthoracic echocardiography underestimated the severity, and in seven cases overestimated the severity. Only in 14 cases was it possible to classify the degree of stenosis correctly by transthoracic echocardiography.

Table 1. Severity of aortic stenosis and confirmation by catheter or autopsy

	No.
Catheter ($n = 34$)	
Mild (syst. gradient < 30 mm Hg)	7
Moderate (syst. gradient 30−59 mm Hg)	7
Severe (syst. gradient ≥ 60 mm Hg	20
Autopsy ($n = 10$)	
Mild	2
Moderate	2
Severe	6
No confirmation ($n = 16$)	
8 mild, 8 moderate cases, all alive at follow-up	

Table 2. Estimation of severity of aortic stenosis by TEE and by catheter or at autopsy ($n = 44$)

		TEE			
		+	+ +	+ + +	Total
Catheter	(Autopsy)				
	+	6(2)	1		7(2)
	+ +		7(2)		7(2)
	+ + +	1	3	16(6)	20(6)
	Total	7(2)	11(2)	16(6)	34(10)

+, Mild; + +, moderate; + + +, severe

Table 3. Estimation of severity of aortic stenosis by transthoracic echocardiography (TTE) plus Doppler and by catheter or at autopsy ($n = 44$)

		TTE + Doppler				
		?	+	+ +	+ + +	Total
Catheter	(Autopsy)					
	+	1(2)	1	2	3	7(2)
	+ +	4(1)		2	1(1)	7(2)
	+ + +	4(2)	2	4(3)	10(1)	20(6)
	Total	9(5)	3	8(3)	14(2)	34(10)

?, Impossible or inconclusive; +, mild; + + moderate; + + +, severe

Discussion

Unlike Hofmann et al. in their study, we were not able to correlate orifice areas found with TEE with orifice areas derived by catheterization. Estimation of the severity of aortic stenosis by using only the systolic peak to peak gradient is controversial. In our series which included mainly elderly patients with impaired left ventricular function and lack of significant aortic regurgitation, the systolic peak to peak gradient may sometimes have underestimated the severity. Additionally, in 16 patients no catheterization was performed. The clinical follow-up of these cases with mild or moderate stenosis showed that these patients were in a stable condition and suggests that we did not overlook a severe stenosis in these patients.

As Hofmann et al. pointed out in their paper, it is not possible to determine the orifice area in all patients. In their series it was impossible in 17%. Especially in patients with heavily calcified valves, no orifice area can be found. However, even in those cases where the orifice cannot be measured, the transesophageal approach allows evaluation of the morphology of the valves and their mobility during the cardiac cycle, and differentiation between sclerosis and stenosis.

Conclusion

TEE allows aortic stenosis to be quantified in most patients in whom transthoracic studies are technically inadequate. The valve orifice cannot be measured in all cases, especially when valves are severely calcified. A source of pitfalls may be patients with congenital stenosis and valves which are not calcified. Because of the better picture quality and the limited time required for the examination, TEE can also be performed in patients with advanced heart failure.

References

Bessone LN, Puppello FD, Blantz HR, Lopez-Cuenca E, Hiro PS, Ebra G (1985) Valve replacement in the elderly: a long term appraisal. J Cardiovasc Surg 26:417–425

Cribier A, Saoudi N, Savin T, Rocha P, Letac B (1986) Percutaneous transluminal valvuloplasty of acquired aortic stenosis in elderly patients: an alternative to valve replacement? Lancet 1:63–67

Dennig K, Krans F, Rudolph W (1986) Doppler-echokardiographische Bestimmung der Öffnungsfläche bei Aortenklappenstenose unter Anwendung der Kontinitätsgleichung. Herz 11:309–317

Harrison MR, Gurley JC, Smith MD, Grayburn PA De Maria (1988) A practical application of Doppler echocardiography for the assessment of severity of aortic stenosis. Am Heart J 115:622–628

Hofmann T, Kasper W, Meinertz T, Spillner G, Schlosser V, Just H (1987) Determination of aortic valve orifice area in aortic valve stenosis by two-dimensional transesophageal echocardiography. Am J Cardiol 59:330–335

Krafchek J, Robertson JH, Radford M, Adams D, Kisslo J (1985) A reconsideration of Doppler assessed gradients in suspected aortic stenosis. Am Heart J 110:765–773

Oh JK, Taliercio CP, Halmes DR, Reeder GS, Bailey KR, Seward JB, Tajik AJ (1988) Prediction of the severity of aortic stenosis by Doppler aortic valve area determination: prospective Doppler-catheterization correlation in 100 patients. J Am Coll Cardiol 11:1227–1234

Assessment of Etiology and Severity of Mitral Regurgitation by Transesophageal Echocardiography

J. Kisslo

Assessment of the etiology and severity of mitral regurgitation is particularly suited for evaluation by transesophageal echocardiography. with the transducer located just behind the left atrium and without intervening chest wall to attenuate or distort the ultrasound signals, images are invariably of excellent quality.

Indications for Transesophageal Echocardiography in Mitral Disease

Transesophageal echocardiography is indicated in patients with suspected mitral valve disease whenever images from the chest wall are inadequate for proper interpretation. This commonly occurs in the elderly, patients with chronic obstructive lung disease, patients in intensive care units, and patients with prosthetic mitral valves or any condition where image quality is impaired.

Prosthetic mitral valves impair the transmission of ultrasound because of marked reflection or sound attenuation. As a consequence, it is frequently impossible to obtain adequate flow images from any position on the chest wall. In fact, when any prosthetic valve is interposed between the transducer and the left atrium, no conclusion as to the presence or severity of mitral regurgitation should be made in routine clinical situations. In this setting, transesophageal echocardiography is most revealing.

Figure 1 shows a transesophageal color flow image from a patient with a prosthetic valve. No adequate images could be made from the chest wall and the transesophageal color flow image shows significant mitral regurgitation from a periprosthetic leak as the jet moves to the left along the interatrial septum posteriorly toward the transducer.

In cases where adequate diagnostic data are, however, available from the chest wall, transesophageal echocardiography is not necessary. Temperate use of this diagnostic modality should be exercised in this setting so as not to result in undue patient risk or discomfort. For example, if a patient severely short of breath is evaluated from the chest wall and a clearly rocking prosthesis is present the clinical situation obviously points to mitral valve dehiscence. Logical clinical judgement indicates that transesophageal echocardiography will reveal severe mitral regurgitation and it is questionable whether

Transesophageal Echocardiography
Edited by R. Erbel et al.
© Springer-Verlag Berlin Heidelberg 1989

such a study will provide any further information necessary to decide in favor of mitral valve replacement.

Such obvious cases do exist and the performance of studies from the transesophageal approach simply to provide better pictures is not always clinically necessary. Thus, a decision in favor of transesophageal echocardiography should be made in the context of whether it will obtain data directly useful for the patients benefit.

Assessment of Etiology

Lessons from transthoracic echocardiography can be directly applied to transesophageal echocardiography. Any diagnosis made from the chest wall can also be made with the transducer positioned in the esophagus, including rheumatic mitral prolapse, vegetative endocarditis, mitral tumor and others. Figure 2 shows a myxoma attached to the mid-portion of the interatrial septum in a difficult-to-image patient with clinical mitral regurgitation. The findings of atrial tumor were available only from the transesophageal echocardiogram.

Transesophageal echocardiography is occasionally helpful in evaluating patients as candidates for mitral valve repair since the quality of images is so much better than those obtained from the chest wall. In such a setting, however, such detailed analysis can usually be performed in the operative setting and patients rarely need to be exposed to their initial examination while ambulatory.

In the setting of infective endocarditis and when a valve ring abscess is suspected, transesophageal echocardiography is most helpful. This diagnosis is rarely established even with high-quality chest wall studies. Such information can be very helpful in the clinical decision-making process for or against surgical intervention in such patients.

Assessment of Severity

Rules concerning the assessment of severity of regurgitation are roughly comparable to those used from the chest wall. Figure 3 shows readily identifiable moderate aortic regurgitation (left panel) and mild mitral regurgitation (right panel) from the chest wall. In this patient, no transesophageal echocardiogram was required.

Figure 4 shows mild mitral regurgitation from a transesophageal echocardiogram in a patient with ischemic heart disease. Such small degrees of mitral regurgitation are frequently encountered and should be considered normal for most patients.

It should be recognized that the area of flow disturbance, and thus the degree of mitral regurgitation, will always appear somewhat larger from the transesophageal approach when compared to the images obtained from the

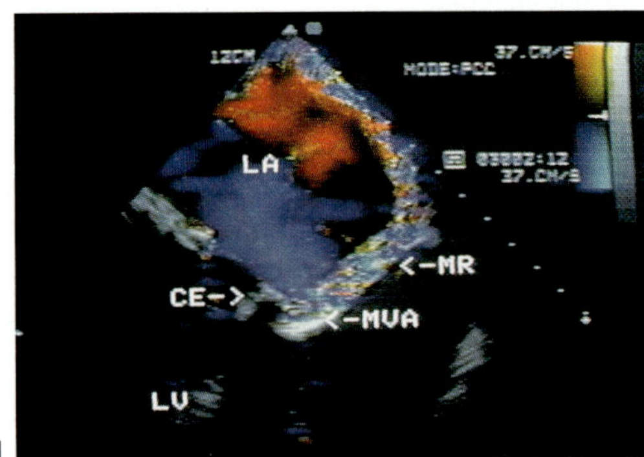

Fig. 1

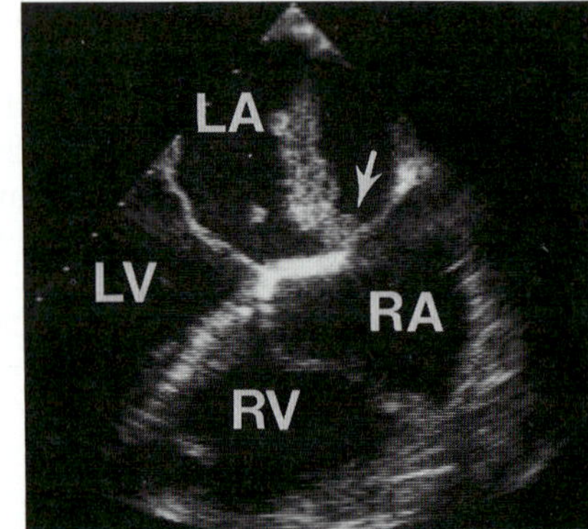

Fig. 2

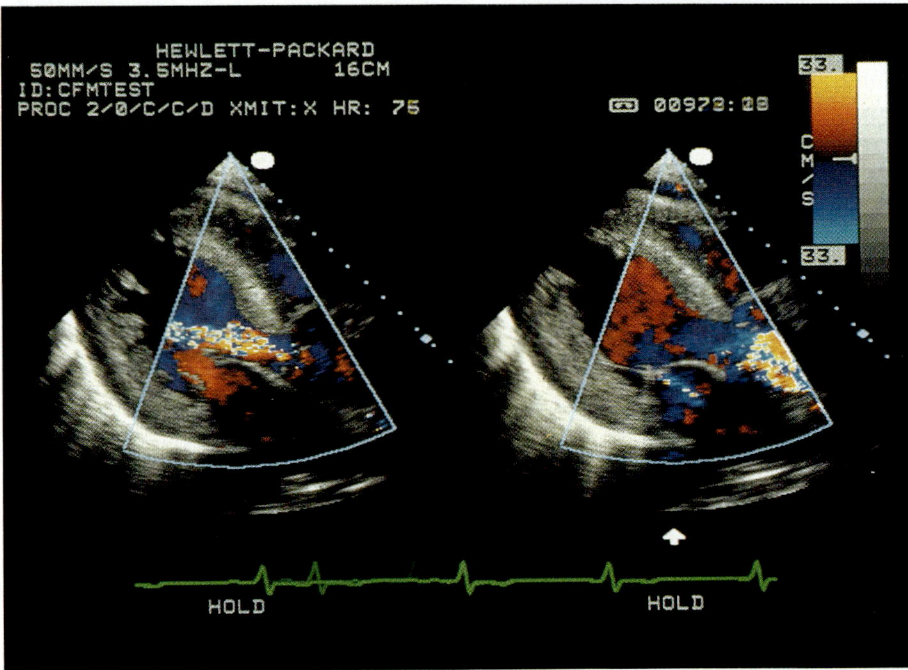

Fig. 3

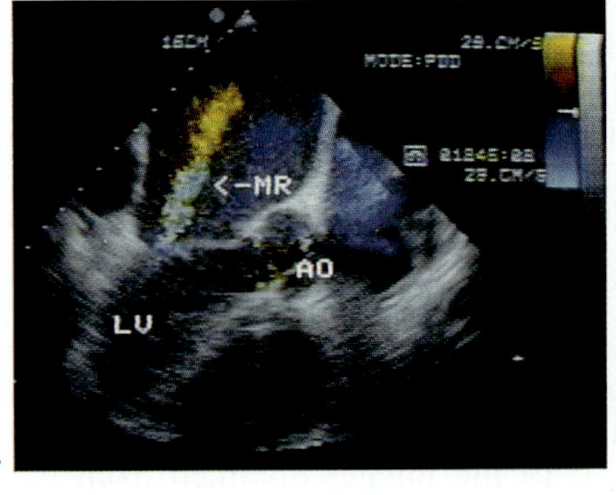

Fig. 4

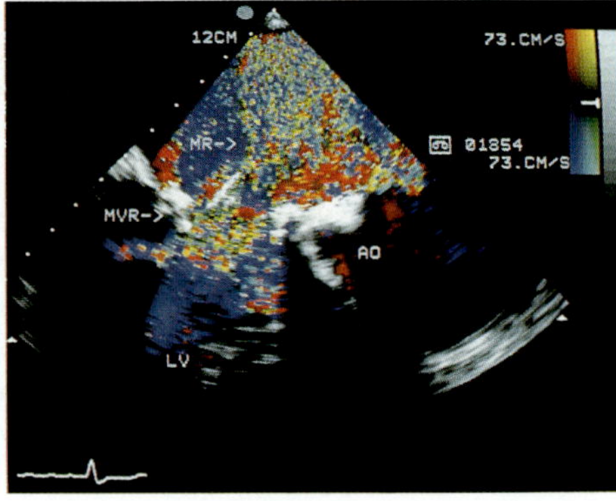

Fig. 5

chest wall. Such observations are logical given the ability of the chest wall to attenuate sound waves. No firm rules currently exist for such comparisons given the marked patient variability in chest wall attenuation characteristics.

Small degrees of mitral regurgitation are usually seen in an area just adjacent to the coaptation point of the valve. Moderate mitral regurgitation generally fills nearly half the left atrial cavity. Severe mitral regurgitation fills more than half of the atrium.

These general comments are made with the obvious provision that the area of the flow disturbance noted by color flow imaging alone does not proved adequate information for estimation of the severity of valvular regurgitation. Observation of the duration of the jet is also required. For example, notation of a jet disturbance of one half the area of the atrium on only one video frame does not constitute adequate diagnostic data to establish a diagnosis moderate mitral regurgitation. Jets of moderate severity usually last the entirety of cardiac systole.

Almost all prosthetic valves will have at least some small degree of mitral regurgitation. Porcine valves always have a central core of mild regurgitation. Tilting disc prostheses may have two tiny jets at either extreme of the circumference of the valve. St. Jude prostheses always have three noticeable tiny flame-like jets. Likewise, Starr-Edwards valves have a noticeable early systolic small degree of regurgitation that rarely lasts after the ball seats properly.

Once adequate experience is achieved with these methods, estimations of the severity of mitral regurgitation can be reliably made by most observers. Figure 5 shows severe mitral regurgitation resulting from disruption of a Carpentier-Edwards prosthetic valve in a patient impossible to image from the chest wall. Such findings obviated the need for cardiac catheterization and resulted in immediate mitral valve replacement.

Fig. 1. Transesophageal color flow image showing mitral regurgitation (*MR*) between the sewing ring of a Carpentier-Edwards (*CE*) prosthesis and the native mitral valve annulus (*MA*). The regurgitant jet is seen to move posteriorly into the left atrium (*LA*). No flow images could be obtained from the chest wall in this patient due to "masking" from the prosthesis. *LV*, left ventricle

Fig. 2. Transesophageal echocardiogram from a patient with an atrial myxoma attached at the mid-portion of the atrial septum (*arrow*). *LA*, left atrium; *LV*, left ventricle; *RA*, right atrium; *RV*, right ventricle

Fig. 3. Parasternal long axis views of moderate aortic regurtitation (*left*) and mild mitral regurgitation (*right*) from an easy to image patient

Fig. 4. Transesophageal color flow image from a patient with mild ischemic mitral regurgitation (*MR*). *AO*, aortic root; *LV*, left ventricle

Fig. 5. Transesophageal color flow image from a patient with severe prosthetic mitral regurgitation (*MR*). *AO*, aortic root; *LV*, left ventricle; *MVR*, mitral valve ring

Implications for Patient Care

Given prudent use of the transesophageal probe, useful data can now be obtained in many clinical settings where quality echocardiographic data could not previously be obtained. When mitral valve disease and regurgitation are clinically suspected and chest wall echo cardiography is either wholly unrewarding or indicates further study, a transesophageal echocardiogram is indicated.

Is Tricuspid Regurgitation Underestimated as a Clinical Problem in Valvular Heart Disease?

E. C. CHERIEX, H. LAMBREGTS, F. PIETERS, and P. BRUGADA

Introduction

In the first years of heart surgery, it was generally believed that tricuspid regurgitation was only a consequence of left valvular heart disease and reversible after correction of the left heart problem. This assumption was overruled by clinical observations in patients who developed untreatable right heart congestion after mitral valve surgery.

Symptoms of tricuspid regurgitation are usually present when malfunction of the right ventricle occurs. Cardiac output declines and right heart congestion develops. Symptoms include tiredness, ascites, peripheral edema, painful congestive hepatomegaly and occasionally throbbing pulsations in the neck [1]. Depending on the underlying cause and the severity of right ventricular dysfunction, correction of tricuspid regurgitation can have a beneficial effect on the clinical course. Proper identification of right heart disease is essential for the future of the patient with valvular heart disease.

Diagnosis of tricuspid regurgitation has traditionally been made by physical examination and hemodynamic and angiographic findings, or through phonocardiographic examination of the jugular venous pulse in combination with a positive liver pulse. Contrast echocardiography was a major "noninvasive" breakthrough showing V-synchronous contrast in the presence of tricuspid regurgitation [3]. Doppler echocardiography and particularly color Doppler echocardiography have made detection of tricuspid regurgitation easier. These Doppler recordings also allow us to estimate the pressure gradient between the right ventricle and right atrium [10] and the volume and direction of the regurgitant flow. Miyatake et al. [4] showed that pulsed Doppler flow mapping can successfully be used to grade the severity of tricuspid regurgitation.

Color-coded Doppler, a multiple pulsed Doppler technique, can directly display the spatial relation and direction of regurgitant flow. The grading systems using these techniques measure the extent of the regurgitant flow into the right atrium. In this system, grade I regurgitation is defined as backflow into the right atrium for less than 1/4 of the atrial length. Grade II regurgitation is defined as back flow up to 1/2, grade III up to 3/4, and grade IV up to the total right atrial length. Continuous Doppler allows calculation of the maximal blood velocity between ventricle and atrium, but can also give an impression of the number of blood particles passing the valvular plane [2]. A specific grading system based on continuous wave Doppler has not been introduced yet.

Transesophageal Echocardiography
Edited by R. Erbel et al.
© Springer-Verlag Berlin Heidelberg 1989

As already mentioned, systolic venous pulsations are generally accepted as a sign of significant tricuspid regurgitation. Jugular venous pulse tracings have today been replaced by Doppler recordings of venous regurgitant flow. Sakai et al. [8] described three main flow patterns in the vena hepatica, dividing the third pattern into six subpatterns. Others have tried to simplify the grading system by using 4 grades of severity [7, 11].

The clinical importance of tricuspid incompetence depends on many factors, including whether the patient has sinus rhythm or suffers atrial arhythmias like atrial fibrillation. Also, mean right atrial pressure plays an important role as a marker for diastolic pressures in the right ventricle and filling pressures. As shown by others [6, 9], most patients with tricuspid regurgitation are in atrial fibrillation. In a study using contrast echocardiography, the diameter of the inferior vena cava was larger in patients with tricuspid regurgitaion than in patients without regurgitation [3]. This study probably underestimated non-clinical tricuspid regurgitation, because of the insensitivity of the method in detecting small regurgitations, particularly in patients with sinus rhythm. Transesophageal echocardiography is another method to estimate the severity of tricuspid regurgitation. This method, however, can only detect intraatrially located regurgitant flow and gives no real impression of the involvement of the venous system in the regurgitation. The use of transesophageal echocardiography for perioperative evaluation of the effect of a certain surgical procedure in correcting tricuspid regurgitation is probably a major advantage of this technique.

Study Objectives

Before the use of transesophageal echocardiography in tricuspid valvular disease is considered, it is essential to know what factors make tricuspid regurgitation hemodynamically significant. In order to avoid postoperative right heart problems, decisions must be taken preoperatively about wether to correct tricuspid regurgitation during surgery for mitral valve disease. When surgical correction is indicated, different kinds of procedures can be used which may yield different results. The potential role of transesophageal echocardiography in the evaluation of successful correction is controversial. Our purpose was to try to answer the following questions:

1. Which are the main factors making tricuspid regurgitation clinically significant?
2. How many patients who underwent surgery for left valvular heart disease have tricuspid regurgitation after the operation, indicating underestimation of their tricuspid disease?
3. What are the effects of correction of left valvular heart disease on tricuspid insufficiency?

Methods

In order to evaluate the severity of tricuspid regurgitation, the following studies were undertaken

1. Left ventricular function, type and severity of left valvular disease, heart rate, and rhythm were assessed.
2. Tricuspid regurgitation was graded using the following methods:
a) Color Doppler grading in four grades of severity (listed above).
b) Continuous wave Doppler using the opacification of the regurgitant jet in a semiquantitive way (Fig. 1). Using a small continuous wave probe of 2.5 MHz, an acoustic window giving optimal recordings of tricuspid flow patterns was searched for. The gain setting of the continuous wave recording was chosen to be optimal for antegrade flow across the tricuspid orifice. Grade I regurgitation was defined as a regurgitant jet staining enough for its presence to be detected, but not enough to get a clear delineation. Grade II regurgitation was thought to be present when a complete jet could just be seen, grade III when a clear darkening of the jet was visible but still a difference in density in comparison to antegrade flow. Grade IV was preserved for the dark-stained jets.
3. The maximal velocity of the tricuspid incompetence was calculated using continuous Doppler, if possible with angle correction using color Doppler.
4. The tricuspid annulus diameter and right atrial length and area were measured. An area length method was used to estimate right atrial volume. All measurements were made using the apical four-chamber view, placing the transducer as apical as possible at the right ventricular apex. A systolic still frame was used to measure the right atrial length and area, and a diastolic frame for calculation of the tricuspid anulus diameter.
5. Measurement of the diameter and collapse index of the inferior vena cava during maximal inspiration. The collapse index was calculated as: [(maximal diameter minus diameter during inspiration)/maximal diameter] ×

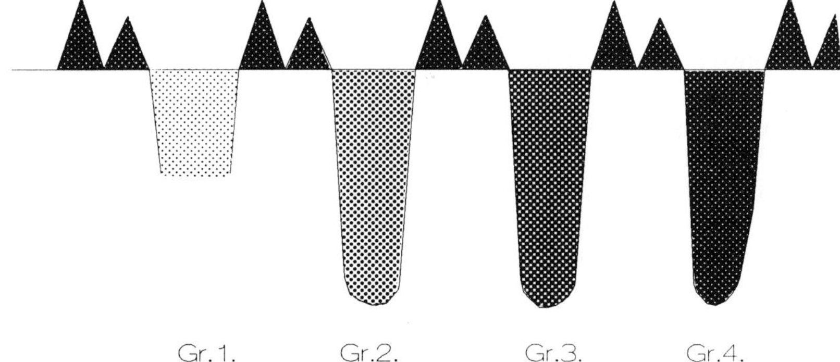

Fig. 1. Continuous semiquantitative Doppler grading system. Flow above the zeroline is antegrade flow from atrium to ventricle. The regurgitant volume is graded according to the density of the regurgitant jet

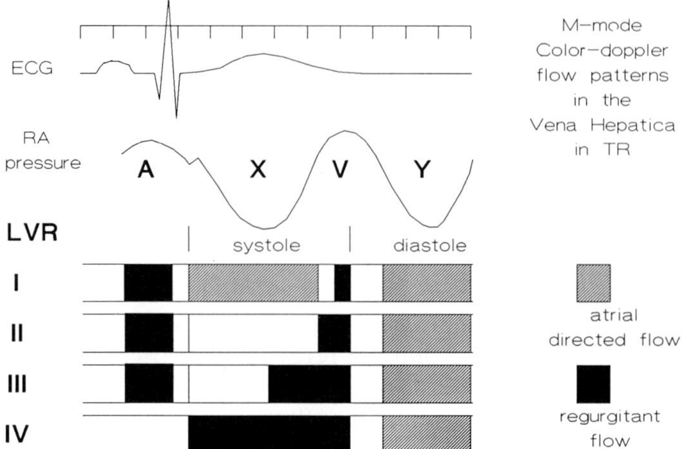

Fig. 2. Grading system used for estimation of the severity of regurgitation into the hepatic vein. Hepatic vein regurgitation (*HVR*) grade 1 is considered normal. Most patients with grade IV regurgitation are in atrial fibrillation (absence of A-wave flow). *TR*, tricuspid regurgitation

100). All the diameters were measured at the beginning of the P wave (or beginning of the QRS complex in patients with atrial fibrillation). An inspiratory collapse of less than 40% was held to be indicative of mean right atrial pressures of more than 7 mmHg [5].

6. In order to simplify the method of grading the hepatic vein regurgitant flow, color-coded Doppler was used, giving a color M-mode scan of the hepatic veins. To visualize the hepatic vein, the transducer was placed in the subxiphoideal region, searching for veins nearly parallel to blood flow. The grading system used is shown in Fig. 2. Flow coming to the transducer was coded in red and could be A-wave synchronous or holo-, mid- or end-systolic flow away from the right atrium. X- or Y-wave synchronous flow going away from the transducer was coded in blue.

Group I consisted of 80 patients with tricuspid regurgitation. All the above-named variables were measured in these patients. Group II consisted of 90 patients who underwent surgery and received a mitral disc prosthesis and 30 patients who received a bioprosthesis. These operations were performed in seven different centers for thoracic surgery. No significant dysfunction of the prosthetic valve was present in this group of patients. Group III consisted of 21 patients who underwent surgery and had an optimal recording of their preoperative "stable" tricuspid regurgitation. The effect of surgery on the regurgitant flow was evaluated using transthoracic echocardiography within two weeks after surgery. Transesophageal echocardiographic evaluation was performed perioperatively in a subgroup of these patients.

Results

Continuous wave Doppler was the more sensitive method for the detection of tricuspid regurgitation in all the patient groups. The main reason was the inability to obtain optimal two-dimensional images in all patients. The better the quality of the two-dimensional echocardiographic images, the better the correlation was between the continuous wave and color-Doppler grading. This correlation was excellent in 50% of all patients and reasonably good (not more than one grade difference) in an additional 20%. In 20% of all patients with continuous wave-proven tricuspid regurgitation, we were not able to find tricuspid incompetence using color Doppler. Continuous wave Doppler was used as the best method to define the presence of tricuspid regurgitation in this study.

In the patients of group I, most remarkable observations were made. The results are shown in Figs. 3, 4 and Tables 1, 2. Figure 3 shows the distribution of sinusrhythm and atrial fibrillation (four patients with a pacemaker with a right ventricular lead) in the 80 patients. It can be seen that hepatic vein regurgitation of grades III or IV was observed in 65% of patients with tricuspid regurgitation of grade II or more and atrial fibrillation, as compared to 20% of patients with the same degree of tricuspid insufficiency and sinusrhythm. Of patients with tricuspid regurgitation and hepatic vein regurgitation grades III or IV, 75%–85% had inspiratory collapse of the inferior vena cava of less than 40%. Using an inferior vena cava collapse index of less than 40% as the second most important parameter (Fig. 4) after heart rhythm, hepatic vein regurgitation of grades III or IV was present in 81% of all patients with atrial fibrillation and tricuspid regurgitation greater than grade II, as compared to 32% of patients with sinus rhythm and tricuspid regurgitation greater than grade II. As shown in Table 1, no significant differences were present between the velocities of the tricuspid regurgitant jet in patients with tricuspid regurgitation grade I, grade II, or more than grade II.

In the group of patients with hemodynamically significant tricuspid regurgitation, the right ventricular pressure was higher because of the higher mean right atrial pressures as indicated by the decreased vena cava collapse indices in these subgroups. A significant difference was present between estimated right atrial volume in patients with tricuspid regurgitation grade I, grade II, or more than grade II. Particularly in patients with atrial fibrillation, right atrial volume was markedly larger than in patients with sinus rhythm (Table 2).

The mean follow-up period of patients of group II after surgery was 57 ± 60 months for the 90 patients who had a mitral disc prosthesis and 59 ± 41 weeks in the 30 patients who had a bioprosthesis. 78% of patients with a disc prosthesis and 83% of patients with a bioprosthesis still had tricuspid regurgitation after surgery. The tricuspid regurgitation was graded higher than grade II in 67% of the mitral disc group and 53% in the bioprosthesis group, indicating that a considerable underestimation of tricuspid incompetence must have taken place before and during surgery. In 70% of patients with tricuspid regur-

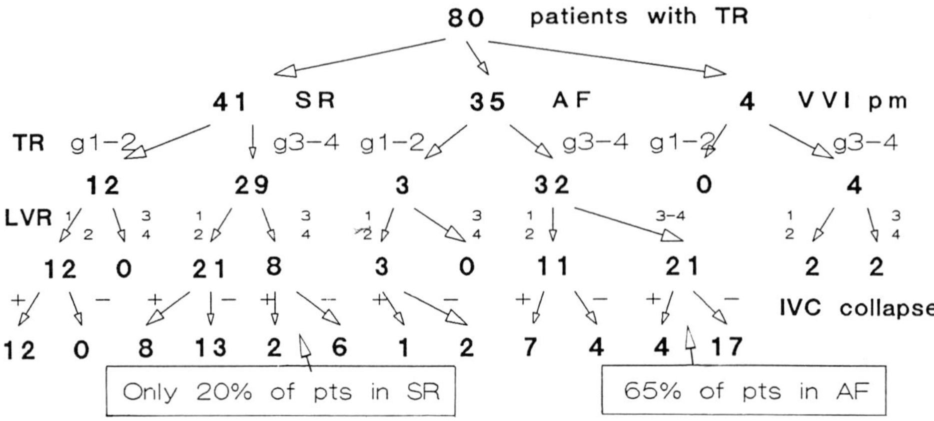

Fig. 3. Chart showing the relation between rhythm (*AF*, atrial fibrillation; *SR*, sinus rhythm, tricuspid regurgitation (*TR*), liver vein regurgitation (*LVR*), and inferior vena cava (*IVC*) index. Only 20% of patients with sinus rhythm and tricuspid regurgitation grade II or more had hepatic vein regurgitation grades III or IV. In patients with atrial fibrillation, the corresponding figure was 65%. Of patients with hepatic vein regurgitation grades III or IV, 75%−80% showed decreased collapse of the inferior vena cava

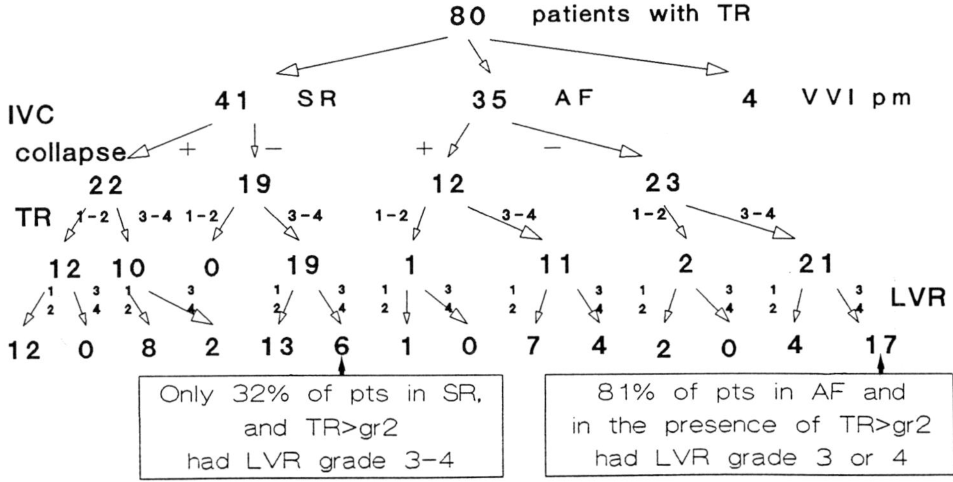

Fig. 4 . Chart showing the relation between atrail rhythm, inferior vena cava collapse, and tricuspid and hepatic vein regurgitaion (abbreviations as in Fig. 3). Only 32% of patients with sinus rhythm, decreased collapse of the inferior vena cava, and tricuspid regurgitation grade II or more had hepatic vein regurgitation grades III or IV. The corresponding percentage for patients in atrial fibrillation was 81%

gitation greater than grade II, collapse of the inferior vena cava of less than 40% was present, indicating elevated mean right atrial pressures.

In patient group III, tricuspid incompetence did not change significantly after surgery (mean grade before surgery 2.6 ± 0.9 vs 2.6 ± 0.7 after surgery). The cardiac surgeon only corrected the valvular incompetence if

Table 1. Relation between the severity of tricuspid incompetence (TR), the velocity of the regurgitant jet (V, m/s) and the liver vein regurgitation (LVR) grade (no significant differences between V data, $p \leq 0.05$ between all LVR data)

	V	LVR	No. of patients
TR grade I	2.9 ± 0.3	1.0 ± 0.0	11
grade II	3.0 ± 0.6	1.9 ± 1.1	24
grade III, IV	3.0 ± 0.5	2.7 ± 1.3	45

Table 2. Comparison between data of patients in sinus rhythm (SR) and atrial fibrillation (AF)

	SR	AF	
Number	34	25	
Age (years)	56 ± 15	66 ± 7	$p \leq 0.005$
MR (I−IV)	1.5 ± 1	1.5 ± 1	ns
IVC diameter (mm)	19 ± 6	23 ± 4	$p = 0.005$
IVC collapse index (%)	53 ± 23	32 ± 19	$p \leq 0.000$
TR (I−IV)	2.1 ± 1.3	3.0 ± 0.5	$p \leq 0.005$
V (m/s)	2.9 ± 0.5	3.0 ± 0.5	ns
LVR (I−IV)	1.4 ± 0.9	3.1 ± 1.1	$p \leq 0.000$
RAL (cm)	5.7 ± 1.3	7.6 ± 1.2	$p \leq 0.000$
RAA (cm^2)	25 ± 9	39 ± 11	$p \leq 0.000$
RAV (ml)	91 ± 51	169 ± 71	$p \leq 0.000$
TAD (cm)	2.9 ± 0.5	3.2 ± 0.4	ns

Abbreviations: MR, mitral regurgitation; IVC, inferior vena cava; TR, tricuspid regurgitation; V, velocity of TR; LVR, liver vein regurgitation; RAL, right atrial length; RAA, right atrial area, RAV, right atrial volume, TAD, tricuspid anulus diameter

tricuspid regurgitation was palpable with his fingertip. This was possible in only 24% of the patients, leading to a decrease of regurgitation equal to or more than one grade in 60%. Only 31% (5/16) of patients who had not received correction of their tricuspid apparatus showed a decrease of the regurgitant jet, leaving 69% of the uncorrected patients with a regurgitation at least as large as before surgery, even though tricuspid velocities decreased from 3.2 ± 0.5 m/s to 2.8 ± 0.5 m/s. It is not surprising that 71% of these patients had atrial fibrillation. Perioperative transesophageal echocardiography in the patients undergoing corrective procedures showed a clear decrease of tricuspid regurgitant volume, parallel with the surgeon's being unable to detect regurgitation with his fingertip. 71% of the patients used diuretics during the postoperative evaluation.

Discussion

As has been shown by the results of our study, tricuspid regurgitation is present in nearly 80% of all patients who underwent surgical correction of left mitral valvular disease in the past. Correction of tricuspid incompetence, even when its presence was known, was not performed in 76% of the patients in our study group III, leaving the regurgitation unaltered in 69% of the group without correction. These data shows that tricuspid regurgitation is a valvular disease which was poorly recognized in the past and is still underestimated at present.

Continuous wave grading of tricuspid regurgitation in the hands of our team seems to detect more regurgitant jets than color Doppler when optimal image resolution is not present. Semiquantitive grading using the staining of the regurgitant jet had the best sensitivity as compared to color Doppler. The possible advantage of this grading system is that tricuspid insufficiency is graded independently from atrial size. Larger tricuspid regurgitations will cause an increase of antegrade flow over the tricuspid orifice, necessitating gain reduction and making it nearly impossible to get a density of the regurgitant jet equal to the antegrade flow. Further studies are required to determine the real value of this grading system.

When tricuspid regurgitation grade III or IV was present causing clear systolic backflow in the liver veins, the right atrium was significantly larger than in patients with grade I regurgitant flow, particularly when atrial fibrillation and high right atrial pressures were present. This was an expected finding. When right atrial size increases, the atrial wall loses its compliance and is more prone to fibrillation. The stiffer, noncompliant atrium is not able to accept any regurgitant flow within its borders, irrespective of its volume, and passes the incoming volume directly into the vessels supplying it. The persistence of tricuspid insufficiency could theoretically lead to earlier dilatation of the right atrium, earlier atrial fibrillation, and thus to more right sided congestive problems. As was shown by van Lakwijk [11], tricuspid valvular corrections (especially Kay's anuloplasty) had fairly good results in correcting tricuspid incompetence without too much conduction disturbance (11%) and without much overcorrection leading to some functional tricuspid stenosis. Transesophageal echocardiography in our small subgroup did not allow optimal prediction of the real postoperative results. Manipulating the tricuspid anulus during surgery, changing pre- and afterload, a not fully stretched atrium, and differences in cardiac rhythm can markedly influence the perioperative impression of the result of correction of the tricuspid apparatus. A good preoperative evaluation of tricuspid regurgitation with all its variables is in our opinion the best indicator of the necessity of surgical correction of tricuspid insufficiency.

Conclusions

Tricuspid regurgitation is an underestimated valvular disease. As a direct consequence, correction is not performed routinely in subgroups of patients. Subgroup analysis shows that patients with atrial fibrillation, decreased respiratory collapse of the inferior vena cava, and tricuspid regurgitation higher than grade II would benefit the most. This subgroup also showed marked enlargement of the right atrium. Transesophageal echocardiography is of potential use in these corrective procedures if thoracic surgeons are willing to accept the results of Doppler examinations.

References

1. Braunwald E (1984) Valvular heart disease. In: Braunwald E (ed) Heart disease: a textbook of cardiovascular medicine, 2nd edn. Saunders, Philadelphia, pp 1149−1153
2. Hatle L (1982) Doppler ultrasound in cardiology. Lea and Febinger, Philadelphia, pp 113−121
3. Meltzer RS, van Hoogenhuyze D, Serruys PW, Haalebos HMP, Hugenholtz PG, Roelandt J (1981) Diagnosis of tricuspid regurgitation by contrast echocardiography. Circulation 63:1093−1099
4. Miyatake K, Omoto M, Kinoshiba N (1982) Evaluation of tricuspid regurgitation by pulsed Doppler and two-dimensional echocardiography. Circulation 66:777−784
5. Moreno F, Hagan A, Holmen J, Pryor T, Strickland R, Castle C (1984) Evaluation of size and dynamics of the inferior vena cava as an index of right sided cardiac function. Am J Cardiol 53:579−585
6. Müller O, Shillingford J (1954) Tricuspid incompetence. Br Heart J 16:195
7. Pennestri F, Loperfido F, Pellegrino-Salvatori M, Mongiardo R, Ferrazza A, Guccione P, Manzoli V (1984) Assessment of tricuspid regurgitation by pulsed Doppler ultrasonography of the hepatic veins. Am J Cardiol 54:363−368
8. Sakai K, Nakamura K, Satomi G, Kondo M, Hinosana K (1984) Evaluation of tricuspid regurgitation by blood flow pattern in the hepatic vein using pulsed Doppler technique. Am Heart J 108:516−522
9. Sepuveda G, Lukas D (1955) The diagnosis of tricuspid insufficiency: clinical features in 60 cases with associated mitral valve disease. Cirulation 11:552
10. Skaerpe T, Hatle L (1981) Diagnosis and assessment of tricuspid regurgitation with Doppler ultrasound. In: Rijsterborgh H (ed) Echocardiology. Martinus Nijhoff, The Hague, pp 299−304
11. van Lakwijk-Chondrovicová E (1987) Tricuspid regurgitation. Thesis, Katholic University of Nymegen. The Netherlands

Visualization of the Coronary Artery
Using Transesophageal Echocardiography

S. ILICETO, C. MEMMOLA, G. DE MARTINO, G. PICCINNI, and P. RIZZON

The left main coronary artery, its bifurcation, and the proximal part of both the left anterior descending and the circumflex coronary arteries can be visualized by two-dimensional echocardiography (Chen et al. 1980; Douglas et al. 1988; Presti et al. 1987; Rink et al. 1982; Rogers et al. 1980a, b; Ryan et al. 1986). Several studies have demonstrated that this technique enables one to investigate the proximal left coronary tree and to diagnose significant coronary artery disease with variable sensitivity and specificity by recognising high-intensity infraluminal echoes which are very probably due to the calcification of the arterial walls (Presti et al. 1987; Rink et al. 1982; Rogers et al. 1980; Ryan et al. 1986).

Although attractive, this diagnostic approach is not yet commonly used in clinical settings. Ultrasound exploration of coronary arteries is, in fact, considerably hampered by two major technical and practical limitations. First, the quality of the echocardiographic image obtained during routine ultrasound exploration of coronary arteries is very often limited and, therefore, unsatisfactory for the evaluation of anatomic structures as small as coronary arteries. Second, review and interpretation of examinations has always been troublesome, because, due to heart movements during the cardiac cycle, the coronary arteries are only imaged for a few consecutive frames and then disappear, to reappear again in the following cycle. This latter problem has been completely solved by the advent of digital technology, which allows a certain number of selected consecutive frames to be reviewed in a cine loop format, thus making it easier to recognise the anatomy and alterations of the proximal left coronary vessel (Douglas et al. 1988; Presti et al. 1987; Ryan et al. 1986).

The first of the two above-mentioned problems has, by contrast, only been partially solved. New probe innovations (focused annular array transducers; Douglas et al. 1988) give echocardiographic images a decidedly better resolution, making a more accurate analysis in a larger proportion of patients possible. Unfortunately, this is not always possible in all patients, the transthoracic examination still very often being inadequate for analysis because of frequent concomitant lung diseases or particular chest configurations.

Transesophageal echocardiography is an emerging application of cardiac ultrasound that has increasingly and successfully been used in the last few years to evaluate many kinds of cardiovascular disease (Borner et al. 1984; Daniel et al. 1988; Gussenhoven et al. 1987; Shively and Schiller 1987; Topol et al. 1984). Its great potential lies mainly in the decidedly high quality and resolution of the echocardiographic images obtained. The superior quality of the images is due: (a) to ultrasound transmission through cardiac structures

Transesophageal Echocardiography
Edited by R. Erbel et al.
© Springer-Verlag Berlin Heidelberg 1989

being greatly facilitated because of the absence of lung interposition between the source of the ultrasound beams and the heart; and (b) to the possibility of using high emission frequency transducers because of the short distance between the esophagus and the posterior cardiac structures.

The above characteristics mean that transesophageal echocardiography might well be an ideal technique for noninvasively evaluating coronary arteries. We undertook this study to assess its potential. A consecutive series of patients undergoing coronary angiography for diagnostic purposes was also prospectively evaluated by means of transesophageal echocardiography.

Material and Methods

Fifty-six patients undergoing diagnostic coronary angiography in our institute were all scheduled for transthoracic and transesophageal echocardiogaphy. Transesophageal echocardiographic studies were performed 2−3 days before coronary angiography using a Hewlett-Packard transesophageal probe (21362A) connected to a Hewlett-Packard 77020 two-dimensional echocardiographic color Doppler instrument. Transthoracic echocardiographic examinations were performed with the same ultrasound equipment used for the transesophageal ones.

Transesophageal Echocardiography

All studies are conducted with conscious patients. The transducer is inserted into the esophagus following the techniques and manouvers commonly used when carrying out a gastroscopy. After patient sedation by intravenous injection of small doses of diazepam, the transducer is inserted with the patient in left lateral decubitus so that excess saliva can easily be got rid of. The gastroscope is carefully put into the mouth and then guided into the esophagus using the left hand to help it pass the proximal esophageal sphincter. Once this has been done, the various echocardiographic planes need to be found by making the gastroscope move in three different ways: (a) downwards; (b) rotating; (c) angling the distal part. The heart is visualized through the left atrium which, being anatomically closest, is the first structure the ultrasound beam crosses. The tomographic planes which can be obtained are obviously different from traditional transthoracic planes because of the different starting point and orientation of the beam.

At the end of a complete examination of the heart (usually lasting no longer than 10−15 min) particular care is paid to the exploration of the coronary arteries (Fig. 1). In order to do this, the transducer is placed at the level of the aortic root. The left main coronary artery usually appears emerging from the corresponding sinus immediately above the aortic leaflets. The ostium of the left main coronary artery is imaged as an echo-free space that interrupts the continuity of the aortic wall borders. Once the ostium is vis-

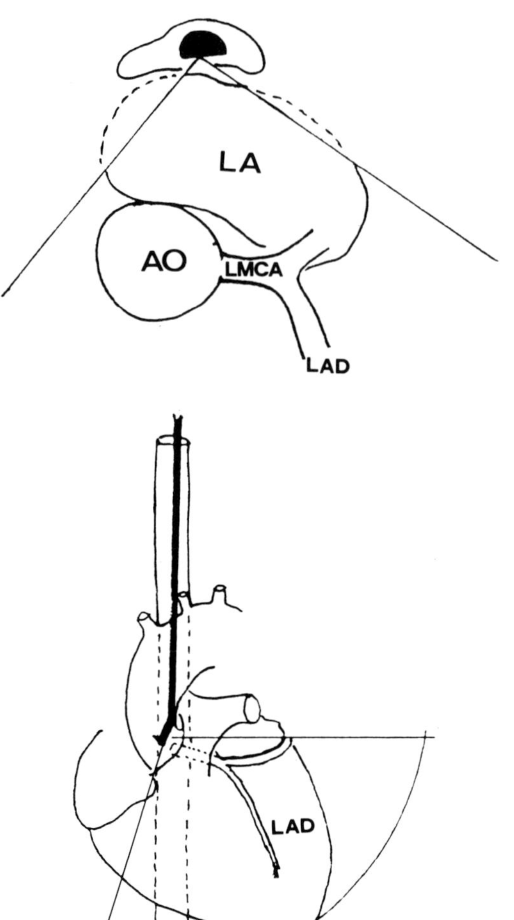

Fig. 1. The cross-sectional transesophageal echocardiographic planes used to visualize the left main coronary artery (*LMCA*), the bifurcation, the circumflex, and the left anterior descending artery (*LAD*). While the left main and the circumflex coronary arteries can be visualized in the majority of instances with horizontal or slightly angulated tomographic planes (*upper panel*), evaluation of the left anterior descending artery very often requires downward angulation of the ultrasonic probe because of its particular orientation. *AO*, aorta; *LA*, left atrium

ualized, slight upwards/downwards and leftwards/rightwards movements of the probe must be made so as to image the left main coronary artery along its full length. This is usually successful in most patients without having to place the probe itself at an angle. On the other hand, in some cases it is necessary to push/pull the probe forwards or backwards in order to cut the left main coronary artery lengthwise. These procedures are necessary since the orientation of the left main coronary artery and consequently its relation to the ultrasound tomographic plane are extremely variable.

The left main coronary artery bifurcation is usually visualized by just slightly changing the probe position and orientation from the position in which the maximum length of the left main coronary artery is imaged (downward direction of ultrasound beam obtained by means of downward angling of the transducer). A decidedly downward angulation of the transducer is often necessary to visualize the left anterior descending artery over a reasonable length because of its typically longitudinal and downward direction. Finally, the circumflex artery can be imaged by rotating leftwards and slightly pulling back the probe from the position in which the ultrasound beam longitudinally intersects the left main coronary artery. Right coronary visualization is decidedly more difficult and only obtained using the tomographic plane best showing the aortic root in its short-axis plane.

Transthoracic Echocardiography

Transthoracic echocardiography imaging of coronary arteries is done using a 3.5-MHz phased array transducer connected to Hewlett-Packard 77020 two-dimensional echocardiographic equipment.

Examinations are performed starting from the short-axis plane of the aortic root with the patients lying supine or in left lateral decubitus. The ostium of the left main coronary artery is identified by very slightly moving the transducer. Once the ostium has been imaged, the angle and rotation of the probe are adjusted to obtain the best image of the left main coronary artery and, when possible, of its bifurcation along with the circumflex and left anterior descending artery.

Reviewing the Transesophageal Echocardiographic Examinations

As previously mentioned, review and interpretation of echocardiographic images is troublesome because of the movement of the coronary arteries due to the motion of the heart itself. To overcome these limitations we use a Microsonics "Prevue" digital reviewing system. A variable number of video fields are automatically acquired by means of the digital system, consecutive fields being acquired every 17 ms. Only consecutive frames clearly showing the lumen of the observed coronary arteries are stored and then reviewed in a continuous cine loop format at a speed that is considerably higher than that of the acquisition phase. Frames in which the coronary vessel is not adequately visualized are eliminated from the acquisition and, consequently, not included in the cine loop. Thus, the number of frames included in the loop does not usually exceed six to eight. All the sequences are permanently stored on a 5.25-in. (13.3-cm) floppy disk.

Coronary Angiography

Coronary angiography was performed in all patients using either the Sones or the Seldinger technique. Coronary angiographic studies were reviewed by an experienced observer. Stenosis of coronary arteries was defined as significant if a narrowing $\geq 75\%$ of the lumen was detected.

Results

Visualization of Coronary Artery by Transesophageal Echocardiography

In Fig. 1 the relationship normally existing between the transesophageal probe and the coronary arteries is shown schematically. While the left main coronary artery and the circumflex artery lie in an approximately horizontal plane (and, therefore, their visualization does not require up— or downwards angling of the probe), the bifurcation and even more so the left anterior descending artery lie in an oblique or decidedly longitudinal plane (and, therefore, perpendicular to the ultrasound tomographic field). Thus, visualization of these two latter portions of the left coronary artery requires the probe angle to be more or less pronounced, depending on the characteristics of the individual cases. Figures 2—5 show different sections of the left coronary artery as visualized by means of slightly different tomographic planes. Due to the curvature of the vessels, it is practically impossible to depict all the different portions of the left coronary artery in just one tomographic plane.

While transthoracic echocardiographic examination was obviously possible in all patients, the transesophageal approach was possible in all but two pa-

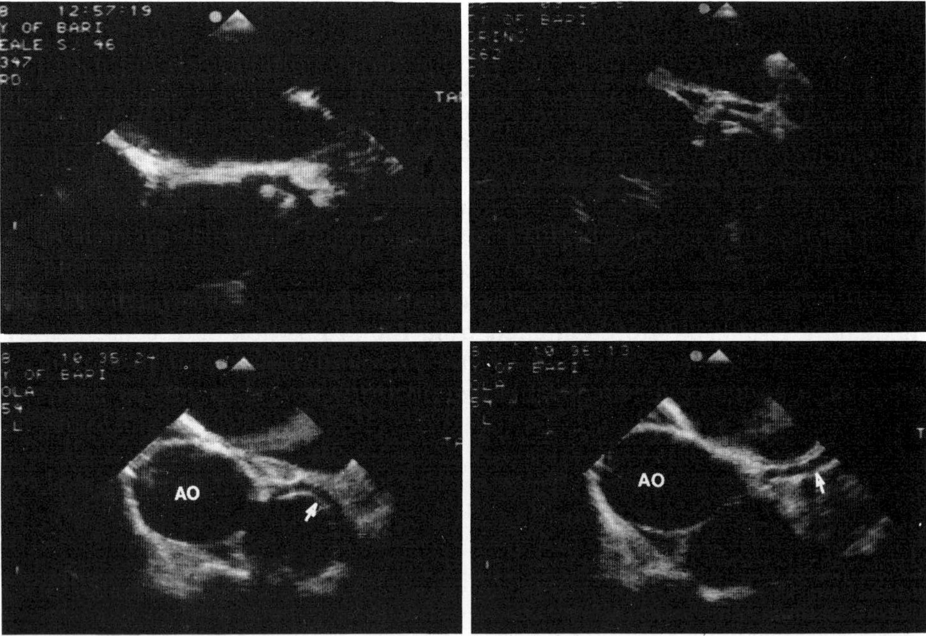

Fig. 2. Different two-dimensional echocardiographic views of left coronary artery obtained by means of the transesophageal approach: left main coronary artery (*upper left panel*), bifurcation (*upper right panel*), circumflex artery (*lower left panel*), left anterior descending artery (*lower right panel*). *AO*, aorta

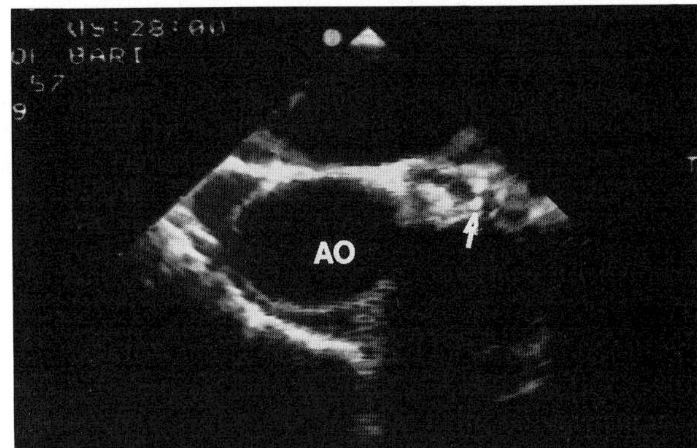

Fig. 3. Left anterior descending artery is imaged along its length by angling the transducer downwards; a smaller vessel (probably the diagonal) arises at a certain distance from the bifurcation

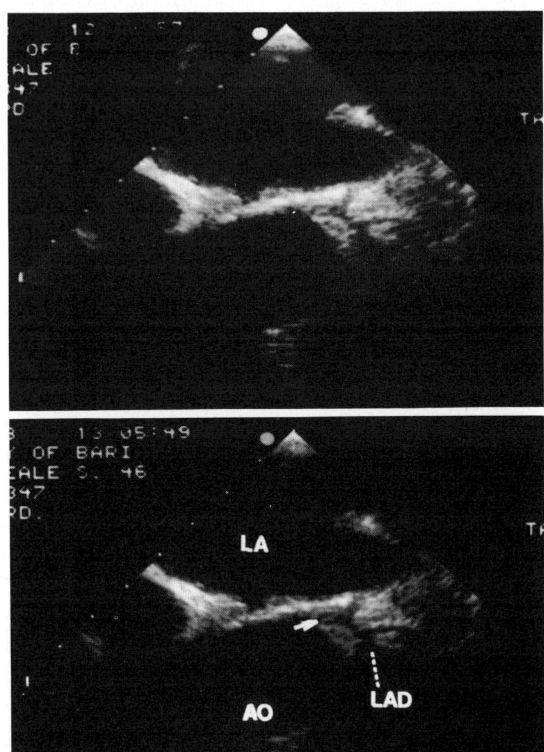

Fig. 4. Significant stenosis of the left main coronary artery shown by angiography (*upper panel*) and by transsesophageal echocardiography (*lower panel*). The *arrows* indicate the stenosis. Echocardiography clearly shows both the narrowing of the lumen and the calcification (*bright echoes*) of the aterial walls that determines the stenosis. *AO*, aorta; *LA*, left atrium; *LAD*, left anterior descending artery

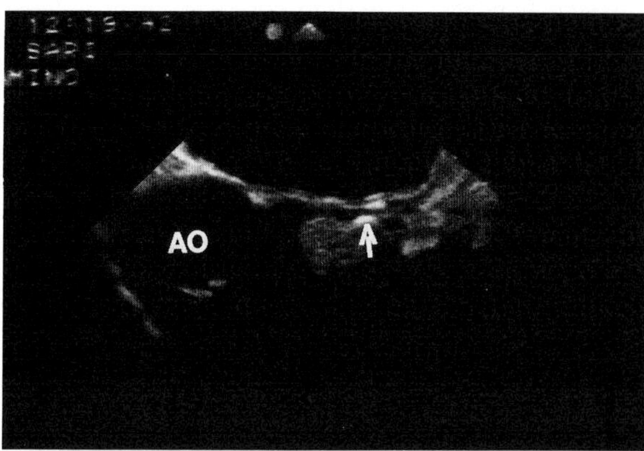

Fig. 5. Stenosis of the circumflex artery. The *arrow* indicates the presence of high-intensity echoes caused by the presence of a calcified narrowing of the vessel. *AO*, aorta

Table 1. Echocardiographic visualization of coronary arteries in 54 patients

	Transthoracic		Transesophageal	
	n	%	*n*	%
Left main coronary artery	40	74	49	90
Bifurcation	20	37	32	59
Circumflex artery	4	7	18	33
Left anterior descending artery	18	33	36	67
Right coronary artery	5	9	4	7

tients. One of these two patients did not tolerate the procedure which, therefore, was prematurely interrupted. In the other patient, it was extremely difficult to pass through the proximal sphincter of the esophagus. Table 1 summarizes the success rate of transthoracic and transesophageal techniques in visualizing the different portions of the coronary arteries in the 54 patients who underwent both examinations. During transesophageal echocardiography the left main coronary artery was visualized in 49 cases (90%), the bifurcation in 32 (59%), the left anterior descending artery in 16 (29%), and the circumflex artery in 18 (33%). All four left coronary artery segments were visualized in a single patient in only eight cases. The initial portion of the right coronary artery was only imaged in four (7%) cases. On the other hand, the success rate for the transthoracic studies was lower.

Detection of Significant Stenosis of the Left Main Coronary Artery

Twenty-four of the 56 patients had significant coronary artery disease as assessed by coronary angiography. Four of these 24 had a significant stenosis of the left main coronary artery. This lesion was correctly diagnosed in all four cases by transesophageal echocardiography but only in two cases by transthoracic examination. Of the 20 cases with significant coronary artery disease but no left main coronary artery disease, a false-positive diagnosis was only made in one case with transesophageal echocardiography but in seven cases with the transthoracic approach.

Discussion

Patients with significant stenosis of the left main coronary artery are at risk of severe cardiac events. Therefore, early identification of these patients is important. Previous studies have shown that stenoses involving this first portion of the left coronary artery can be recognized by two-dimensional echocardiography. Greater diagnostic accuracy is achieved if certain relatively recent technical solutions are used, such as annular phased array transducers and cine loop digital reviewing systems. Adopting these improvements permits more extensive evaluation of the left coronary vessel, including its bifurcation and a variable length of the left anterior descending artery.

Despite these improvements, echocardiographic visualization of the left coronary artery and the identification of possible stenoses has not yet been widely adopted, mainly because of the limited quality of transthoracic echocardiographic images.

Visualization of Coronary Arteries by Transesophageal Echocardiography

The left coronary artery can successfully be visualized by transesophageal echocardiography. In the series of patients we studied, the transesophageal approach allowed us to visualize specific coronary segments with a decidedly higher success rate than the transthoracic approach. Furthermore, the image quality obtained by means of the transesophageal approach was decidedly superior to that obtained traditionally. This superior quality of echocardiographic imaging makes it possible to evaluate each coronary segment in greater detail thanks to the considerably higher resolution of the ultrasonic images obtained. In fact, in the majority of instances, the lumen of the vessel was clearly delineated with an almost complete absence of dropout of echoes at the level of the walls of the vessel itself. This was not the case during transthoracic studies. Using this ultrasound technique, not only was the success rate when visualizing specific coronary segments lower, but also the quality of the images was quite unsatisfactory. The success rate in visualizing the right coronary artery was low because of its peculiar position, which makes it difficult to explore by ultrasonic imaging with either approach.

In our series, a stenosis of the left main coronary artery was correctly identified by transesophageal echocardiography in the four patients with angiographically diagnosed significant narrowing of this portion of the coronary artery. In Fig. 4 an example of a stenosis of the left main coronary artery is shown: ultrasonic imaging not only shows, with excellent resolution, the arterial narrowing, but also the presence of the calcified borders of the stenosis itself. No false-positive results were observed in patients in whom angiography demonstrated a patent coronary vessel.

Therefore, transesophageal echocardiography seems to be useful not only in the visualization of different sections of the left coronary artery, but also in the identification of significant stenoses involving the left main coronary artery. This potential has already been underlined by Taams et al. (1988), who also showed a significant correlation between the degree of narrowing detected with coronary angiography and that observed during transesophageal echocardiography.

Conclusions

Transesophageal echocardiography is a potentially useful technique for exploring the proximal part of the left coronary artery. The superior resolution of echocardiographic images obtainable by means of this approach offers new prospects for ultrasonic noninvasive exploration of coronary vessels. However, studies conducted with larger series of patients are still necessary to definitively assess the feasibility of this approach as well as its sensitivity and specificity in recognizing significant proximal left coronary artery stenoses.

References

Borner N, Erbel R, Braun B, Henkel B, Meyer J, Rumpelt J (1984) Diagnosis of aortic dissection by transesophageal echocardiography. Am J Cardiol 54:1157−1158
Chen CC, Morganroth J, Ogawa S, Mardelli J (1980) Detecting left main coronary artery disease by apical, cross-sectional echocardiography. Circulation 62:288−293
Daniel WG, Nellessen U, Schroder E, Nonnast-Daniel B, Bednarski P, Nikutta P, Lichtlen P (1988) Left atrial spontaneous echo contrast in mitral valve disease: an indicator for an increased thromboembolic risk. J Am Coll Cardiol 11:1204−1211
Douglas PS, Fiolkoski J, Berko B, Reichek N (1988) Echocardiographic visualization of coronary artery anatomy in the adult. J Am Coll Cardiol 11:565−571
Gussenhoven EJ, Taams MA, Roelandt J, Bom K, Honkoop J, de Jong N, Ligtvoet KM (1987) Int J Cardiac Imaging 2:231−239
Presti CF, Feigenbaum H, Armstrong WF, Ryan T, Dillon JC (1987) Digital two-dimensional echocardiographic imaging of the proximal left anterior descending coronary artery. Am J Cardiol 60:1254−1259

Rink LD, Feigenbaum H, Godley RW, Weyman AE, Dillon JC, Phillips JF, Marshall JE (1982) Echocardiographic detection of left main coronary artery obstruction. Circulation 65:719–724

Rogers EW, Feigenbaum H, Weyman AE, Godley RW, Vakili ST (1980a) Evaluation of left coronary artery anatomy in vitro by cross-sectional echocardiography. Circulation 62:782–787

Rogers EW, Feigenbaum H, Weyman AE, Godley RW, Johnston KW, Eggleton RC (1980b) Possible detection of atherosclerotic coronary calcification by two-dimensional echocardiography. Circulation 62:1046–1053

Ryan T, Armstrong WF, Feigenbaum H (1986) Prospective evaluation of the left main coronary artery using digital two-dimensional echocardiography. J Am Coll Cardiol 7:807–812

Shively B, Schiller NB (1987) Transesophageal echocardiography in review. Int J Cardiac Imaging 2:3–19

Taams MA, Gussenhoven WJ, Sutherland GR, von der Brand M, Roelandt J (1988) Detection of proximal left coronary artery stenoses by transesophageal echocardiography (abstract). Eur Heart J 9 (Suppl 1):274

Topol EJ, Weiss JL, Guzman PA, Dorsey-Lima S, Blanck TJJ, Humphrey LS, Baumgartner WA, Flaherty JT, Reitz BA (1984) Immediate improvement of dysfunctional myocardial segments after coronary revascularization: detection by intraoperative transesophageal echocardiography. J Am Coll Cardiol 5:1123–1134

Masses and Vegetation

Sensitivity and Specificity of Transesophageal Echocardiography in the Diagnosis of Vegetations and Abscesses in Infective Endocarditis

B. Maisch, G. Ertl, C. Kleinert, and K. Kochsiek

Introduction

Rivière first described the morphological equivalent of infective endocarditis at the site of the aortic valve in 1646: "In the left ventricle round carunculae were found, the larger of which resembled a cloisture of hazelnuts and filled up the opening of the aorta" (Major 1945).

It becomes clear from the evolution of the full-blown clinical picture of infective endocarditis that different stages in the development of a vegetation must exist, from predisposed, already morphologically altered valves with degenerative, postrheumatic, or myxomatous lesions, to nonthrombotic vegetation and later infected vegetation (Fig. 1). From a clinical point of view this explains why not every vegetation-like structure implies that active endocarditis is present. In this study we therefore wanted to address the following questions:

1. How sensitive and how specific are transthoracic (TTE) and transesophageal echocardiography (TEE) in confirmed infective endocarditis?

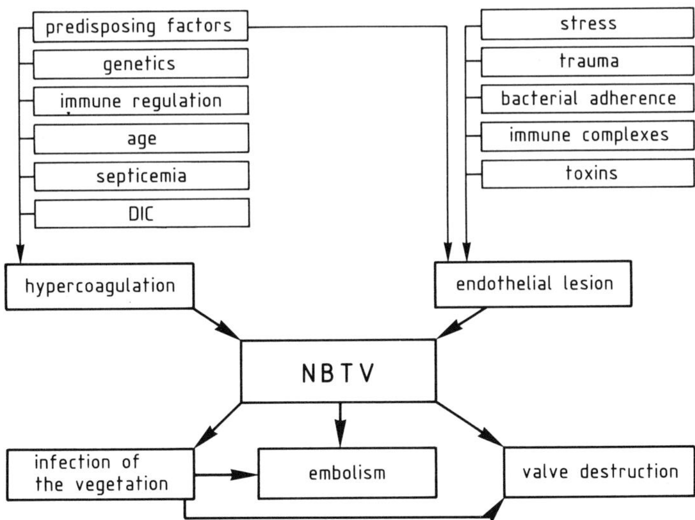

Fig. 1. Evolution of infective endocarditis − pathophysiological aspects (*DIC*, disseminated intravascular coagulopathy; *NBTV*, nonthrombotic vegetation)

Transesophageal Echocardiography
Edited by R. Erbel et al.
© Springer-Verlag Berlin Heidelberg 1989

2. How specific and how sensitive are TTE and TEE in the everyday clinical
   setting where patients are suspected clinically of having endocarditis? This
   patient cohort must not be limited to a predefined group of patients with
   surgically confirmed endocarditis or patients with positive blood cultures
   and valve abnormalities.

Methods

For the transesophageal echocardiographic studies we used a Diasonics echoscope (Diasonics Cardio-Imaging Inc.,Salt Lake City, 3.5 MHz phased array,
distal tip diameter 15.1 and 16 mm).

With the exception of the patients under mechanical ventilation ($n = 7$),
alle investigations were performed with patients in left lateral decubitus after
administering a local pharyngeal anesthetic (lidocaine spray) but no other
premedication and placing a biteguard prior to insertion of the probe. All
patients had fasted for at least 4 h. No complications occurred. Before TEE,
standard TTE was performed. In all patients blood cultures (at least four to
six on two different days) were made and clinical and laboratory examinations
were also done.

Patients

We analyzed prospectively 91 consecutive patients who underwent TEE for
suspected endocarditis. Of these patients, 57 were men (mean age 47.4 + 6.4
years), and 34 were women (mean age 58.4 + 17.3 years). In 70 patients TTE
had been inconclusive or only suggestive. In 21 patients TTE was normal
but the clinical evidence was highly suggestive of endocarditis: 11 patients
suffered from unexplained syncope, three from unexplained fever, and four
from arterial emboli. Only in two patients could this be explained by atrial
myxoma. Additional findings were ventricular or atrial thrombi in nine cases
and a ventricular aneurysm in one case.

Results and Discussion

TTE and TEE in Endocarditis Confirmed at Surgery or Necropsy and
in Blood Culture

The incidence of positive findings with M-mode and two-dimensional echocardiography were recently summarized by Daniel and Lichtlen (1987). Table 1
expands their summary and also includes more recent publications by Daniel
et al. (1988) and Erbel et al. (1988) together with our own data (Maisch et al.
1989).

Table 1. Positive findings with M-mode and two-dimensional echocardiography

Authors	Year	No. of patients	Diseased valves[a]	echocardigraphy positiv		M-mode/2D[b]
				n	%	
Roy et al.	1976	32	36 (A,M)	25	69	M
Thomson et al.	1976	17	20 (A,M,T)	11	55	M
Wann et al.	1976	65	65 (A,M,T)	22	34	M
Andy et al.	1977	25	35 (A,M,T)	26	74	M
Jenzer et al.	1977	36	36 (A,M)	17	47	M
Gura et al.	1978	78	78 (?)	36	46	M
Martin et al.	1978	42	42 (?)	33	79	M,2D
Wann et al.	1979	23	23 (A,M,T,H,Pr)	18	78	M,2D
Mintz et al.	1979	21	22 (A,M,T)	10	45	M,2D
Stewart et al.	1980	87	99 (A,M,T)	59	60	M,2D
Strom et al.	1980	24	32 (A,M,T)	27	84	M,2D
Daniel et al.	1982	134	149 (A,M,T,P,Pr)	104	70	M
Lutas et al.	1983	77	77 (?)	43	56	M,2D
Daniel	1984	62	74 (A,M,T,Pr)	58	78	M,2D
Stafford	1985	62	62 (A,M,T,P)	45	73	M,2D
Daniel et al.	1988	88	88(A,M,T,P)	53	60	M,2D
Erbel et al.	1988	20[c]	(A,M,T)	11	55	M,2D
		39[d]		27	69	M,2D
Maisch et al.	1989	16[e]	(A,M,T)	13	60	M,2D

[a] A, aortic; M, mitral; T, tricuspid; P, pulmonary valve; Pr, prosthetic valve
[b] M, M-mode; 2D, two dimensional
[c] Confirmed endocarditis
[d] Blood culture positive
[e] Confirmed by blood culture and surgery

It can be concluded that in infective endocarditis confirmed either surgically or at necropsy, positive, findings in one- and two-dimensional echocardiography can be expected in 34%−84% of patients. In our own group of patients with endocarditis confirmed at surgery or necropsy or by positive blood cultures, TTE gave either positive or highly suggestive evidence in 13 out of 19 patients (68.4%).

As is shown by recent work by Erbel et al. (1988) and our own experience, the following factors may influence the sensitivity or specificity of TTE in the diagnosis of vegetations:

− The experience of the investigator(s)
− The size of the vegetation (greater or less than 5 mm)
− Whether a patient cohort is chosen where clinical evidence for infective endocarditis is stronger or weaker

In addition, it is obvious that two-dimensional echocardiography has a higher sensitivity and specificity than M-mode. On the basis of surgical confirmation of endocarditis, the sensitivity and specificity of TTE for all of our

Table 2. Positive findings in infective endocarditis by TEE and TTE

Autors	Year	No. of patients	Diseased valves	TTE positive (%)	TEE positive (%)
Daniel et al.	1988	88[b]	A,M,T	60 (16.9)[a]	94 (2)[a]
Erbel et al.	1988	20[b]	A,M,T	55	100
		39[c]	A,M,T	69	82
Maisch et al.	1989	19[b,c]	A,M,T	68	84
		87[d]	A,M,T	15 (85)[a]	60

[a] Questionable findings
[b] Confirmed at surgery or necropsy
[c] positive blood culture: clinical evidence highly indicative of infective endocarditis
[d] Inconclusive TTE clinical symptoms suggestive of infective endocarditis

patients with suspected endocarditis were higher than for patients in whom clinical evidence was less certain (Table 2).

The Value of TEE

The incidence of positive findings on TEE in patients where the clinical evidence was strong (surgically confirmed or positive blood culture) or weak can be derived from Table 2, which includes our own data and compares them to previously published work (Daniel and Lichtlen 1987; Daniel et al. 1988; Erbel et al. 1988). It is evident that the frequency of positive findings is much higher when TEE is used, being up to 82%–100% in patients with strong clinical evidence of infective endocarditis. It can be seen, however, from Erbel et al.'s prospective study and our own data that the more highly selected the group of patients with infective endocarditis is, the more often one finds a positive result with TEE. For endocarditis confirmed at surgery or necropsy, in all studies a high proportion of vegetations were found with TEE (up to 100%).

This was also true of the detection of abscesses. In patients with only suggestive clinical evidence (murmur, fever, increased sedimentation rate), the yield is much lower for both TTE and TEE. Under these circumstances only 16% of our patients had positive findings on TTE and only 60% on TEE, for either vegetations or abscesses. Applied to our patient cohort, specificity (true negative/true negative + false positive) was 58% and sensitivity (true positive/true positive + false negative) was 42%.

This lower sensitivity and specificity is a consequence of the everyday clinical situation; the physician is confronted with a patient with symptoms, but has no surgical or necropsy confirmation of a particular disease.

In a clinical setting with inconclusive TTE results (Fig. 2) but strong or weaker clinical evidence of infective endocarditis, positive findings were seen with TEE in 39 out of 74 patients examined. In only 16 of these 39 (41%) was endocarditis confirmed by necropsy, surgery or positive blood cultures. Out

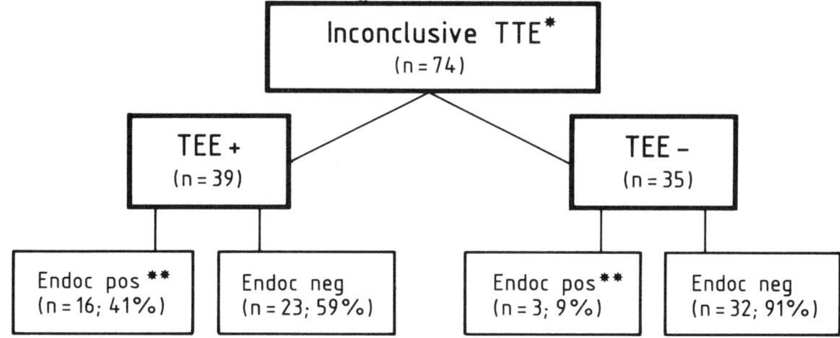

Fig. 2. Findings in patients with inconclusive TTE but an index of suspicion for infective endocarditis. TEE is helpful in sorting out patients with old (sterile) or new (infected) vegetations. *, in pts with target symptoms; **, confirmed at surgery or necropsy or positive BC_s

of 35 TEE-negative patients, only three (9%) turned out in the end to have infective endocarditis.

Representative examples of vegetations observed by TEE only are shown in Figs. 3 and 4. Figure 2 shows a floating vegetation in a febrile patient with mitral valve prolapse that was not detected by TTE. Only the valve prolapse was diagnosed at that time. Surgery confirmed infective endocarditis of the

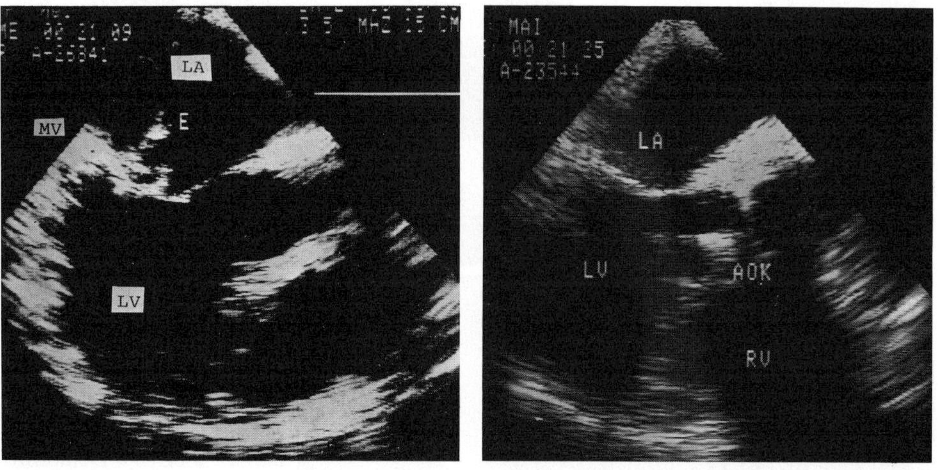

Fig. 3

Fig. 4

Fig. 3. Mitral valve endocarditis of the viridans type in a 36-year-old female patient with mitral valve prolapse, positive TEE findings, mitral incompetence grade 3, and surgically confirmed vegetation. *E*, Endocarditic vegetation; *LA*, left atrium; *LV*, left ventricle; *MV*, mitral valve

Fig. 4. Aortic valve endocarditis (viridans streptococcus) in a 64-year-old male patient. Findings were confirmed at surgery for severe aortic regurgitation and persistent fever. *AOK*, aortic valve; *LA*, left atrium; *LV*, left ventricle; *RV*, right ventricle

lenta type (streptococci). Figure 4 shows a vegetation at the site of the aortic valve due to streptococci, a finding confirmed at surgery.

It has been pointed out that the size of the vegetation may be related to the clinical signs: 63% of small vegetations (< 5 mm) were associated with a positive blood culture and 88%−86% of medium sized (6−10 mm) or large (> 11 mm) ones (Erbel et al. 1988). Similar trends were found with respect to the presence of a cardiac murmur (50% positive for small vegetations, 92% and 93% positive for medium- sized and large vegetations). Our own data showed no difference between medium- sized and large vegetations (6−10 mm vs. > 10 mm) in the number of blood culture-positive patients, but there was a lower proportion of patients (only 38%) who were blood culture-positive (= confirmed endocarditis). The number of patients with vegetations of less than 5 mm was too small to give a data base good enough for comparative analysis.

There are many possible reasons for misdiagnosing infective endocarditis by TEE because of pseudo-vegetations. These false-positive findings may be due to valve thickening or vegetation-like findings in degenerative valve

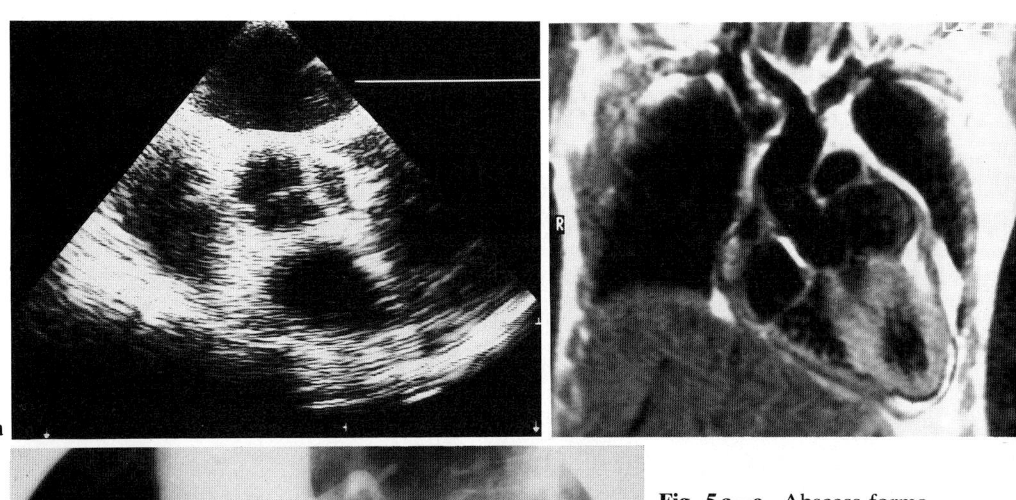

Fig. 5 a−c. Abscess formation in a 31-year-old patient with dramatic aortic regurgitation due to infective endocarditis by *Staphylococcus aureus*. **a** TEE. **b** Demonstration of the huge abscess by nuclear magnetic resonance imaging. Demonstration of the same abscess by angiography of the aorta (left anterior obligue 60°) (**b** Kindly provided by Prof. Lackner, Central Institute of Radiology, Würzburg, using a Philips Gyroscan).

diseases, previous rheumatic valve diseases, congenital valve diseases, Libman-Sacks endocarditis in systemic lupus erythematosus and in myxomatous valve disease (MPS, myxoma), or rupture of cordae through trauma or spontaneously.

Abscesses

In both our patients and in those of Erbel et al. and Daniel et al., surgically confirmed abscesses were detected by TEE in almost all patients with confirmed endocarditis. All four of our patients with abscesses were operated on and the site and number of abscesses assessed by TEE were confirmed. A characteristic example of a large abscess due to staphyloccoccus-induced aortic valve endocarditis is shown in Fig. 5 TEE (Fig. 5 a), magnetic resonance imaging (Fig. 5 b) and aortography (Fig. 5 c) demonstrated the abscess, which had to be operated on immediately after diagnosis. From a clinical point of view, patients with abscesses are suffering from a very severe illness, so it is unlikely that one would not detect a patient with abscesses at all (false negative). False-positive findings of a pseudoabscess could be attributed to a coronary artery or the main stem at the site of the aortic valve, but this has not occurred in Daniel et al.'s, Erbel et al.'s or our study.

Conclusions

1. TEE is extremely helpful in the diagnosis of vegetations and abscesses in infective endocarditis.
2. Bacteriological, clinical and surgical data must, however, complement inconclusive TTE results, or even highly suggestive findings in TEE, before a definitive diagnosis of infective endocarditis can be made.

References

Andy JJ, Sheikh MU, Ali N, Barnes BO, Fox LM, Curry CHL, Roberts WC (1977) Echocardiographic observations in opiate addicts with active infective endocarditis. Am J Cardiol 40:17

Daniel WG (1982) M-mode echokardiographische Untersuchungen bei Patienten mit infektiöser Endokarditis. Thesis, Hannover

Daniel WG, Lichtlen PR (1987) M-mode, transthorakale zweidimensionale und Ösophagusechokardiographie in der Diagnostik der infektiösen Endokarditis. In: Maisch B (ed) Infektiöse Endokarditis. Perimed, Erlangen, pp 119–154

Daniel, WG, Muegge A, Hetzer R., Lichtlen PR, (1983) Prognostische Bedeutung des echokardiographischen Vegetationsnachweises bei Patienten mit infektiöser Endokarditis (abstract). Z Kardiol 72 (Suppl. 1):21

Daniel WG, Schröder E, Muegge A, Lichtlen PR (1988) Transesophageal-echocardiography in infective endocarditis. Am J Cardiac Imaging 2:78–85

Erbel R, Rohmann S, Drexler M, Mohr-Kahaly S, Gerharz CD, Iversen S, Oeler H, Meyer J (1988) Improved diagnostic value of echocardiography in patients with infective endocarditis by transesophageal approach. A prospective study. Eur Hear J 9:43−53

Guray GM, Tajik AJ, Seward JB (1978) Correlation of initial echocardiographic findings with outcome in patients with bacterial endocarditis (abstract). Circulation 58 (Suppl II):232

Jenzer HR, Gollath F, Greaedel E, Amann FW (1977) Die Echokardiographie bei infektiöser Endokarditis. Schweiz Med. Wochenschr. 107:1572

Lutas EM, Roberts RB, Devereux RB, Prieto LM (1983) Predictive value of echocardiography in endokarditis (abstract). Circulation 68 (Suppl III):364

Maisch B (ed) (1987) Infektiöse Endokarditis. In: Beiträge zur Kardiologie, vol 35. Perimed, Erlangen (1989)

Maisch B, Ertl G, Kleinert C, Kochsiek K (1989) The diagnosis of vegetations in patients with suspected endocarditis by TEE and TTE (submitted)

Major RH (1945) Notes on the history of endocarditis. Bull Hist Med. 17:351

Martin RP, Meltzer RS, Chia BL, Popp RL (1978) The clinical utility of two-dimensional echocardiography in bacterial endocarditis (abstract). Circulation 58 (Suppl II):187

Mintz GS, Kotler MN, Segal BL, Parry WR (1979) Comparison of two-dimensional and M-mode echocardiography in the evelution of patients with infective endocarditis. Am J Cardiol 43:738

Roy P, Tajik AJ, Giuliani ER, Schattenberg TT, Gau GT, Frye RL (1976) Spectrum of echocardiographic findings in bacterial endocarditis. Circulation 53:474

Stafford WJ, Petch J, Radford DJ (1985) Vegetations in infective endocarditis: clinical relevance and diagnosis by cross-sectional echocardiography. Br Heart J 53:310

Stewart JA, Silimperi D, Harris P, Wise NK, Fraker TD, Kisslo JA (1980) Echocardiographic documentation of vegetative lessions in infective endocarditis: clinical implications. Circulation 61:374

Strom J, Becker R, Davis R, Matsumoto M, Frishman W, Sonnenblick EH, Frater RWM (1980) Echocardiographic and surgical correlations in bacterial endocarditis (abstract). Circulation 62 (Suppl I):164

Thomson K, Nanda N, Gramiak R (1976) The reliability of echocardiography in the diagnosis of infective endocarditis (abstract). Circulation 54 (Suppl II):112

Wann LS, Hallam CC, Dillon JC, Weyman AE, Feigenbaum H (1979) Comparison of M-mode and cross-sectional echocardiography in infective endocarditis. Circulation 60:728

Assessment of Anatomical Abnormalities in Prosthetic Valve Malfunction by Transesophageal Echocardiography

A. Mügge, W. G. Daniel, J. Grote, G. Frank, and P. R. Lichtlen

Introduction

The assessment of anatomical abnormalities of prosthetic valves by trans-thoracic echocardiography (TTE) is known to be difficult. In particular, mechanical devices which are composed of highly echoreflecting material create considerable artifacts, preventing imaging quality from being high enough to establish a correct diagnosis. In some of these cases, the combined use of M-mode and phonoechocardiography has been shown to be helpful (Brodie et al. 1976; Cunha et al. 1980; Assanelli et al. 1986). In contrast, the leaflets of bioprostheses show an echoreflectivity and motion pattern similar to native valves and can therefore be more easily evaluated by cross-sectional echocardiography, as long as the transthoracic examination allows clear imaging (Schapira et al. 1979; Forman et al. 1985).

In patients in whom imaging quality is low (e.g., patients after cardiac surgery or patients with obesity, emphysema, or chest deformities) TTE does not usually allow a reliable evaluation of prosthetic valve funtion. Trans-esophageal echocardiography (TEE), which provides an unobstructed view to the heart and uses higher transducer frequencies, resulting in an improved resolution, may overcome at least some of the problems associated with the transthoracic examination of prosthetic valves (Nellessen et al. 1985; Erbel et al. 1987; Daniel et al. 1988 a).

We therefore compared the morphological findings obtained by TTE and TEE with the anatomical results obtained during reoperation or necropsy in 73 unselected patients with prosthetic valves.

Methods

The study includes 73 consecutive patients (50 men, 23 women, aged 19−76 years) with 82 prosthetic heart valves (PV) who underwent either cardiac reoperation ($n = 68$) or died ($n = 5$). The reasons for reoperation were PV malfunction and/or replacement of another diseased native heart valve ($n = 16$ patients). Surgery or autopsy provided detailed anatomical description of all PV. Based on the anatomical examination, 63 PV were classified as diseased and 19 PV as normal. The types of PV malfunction found on surgery or autopsy are listed in Table 1. Fifty-two PV were bioprostheses and 30 were

Transesophageal Echocardiography
Edited by R. Erbel et al.
© Springer-Verlag Berlin Heidelberg 1989

Table 1. Types of prosthetic valve abnormalities based on surgical or autopsy findings in 73 patients

	Valves (n)	Patients (n)
Endocarditis	19	18
Degeneration	32	28
Paravalvular leak	7	6
Thrombi	5	5
Normal	19	16
Total	82	73

mechanical devices (44 aortic, 37 mitral, one tricuspid). Patients were studied by echocardiography 60 ± 16 days before reoperation or death. Echocardiographic studies included a conventional transthoracic (TTE) as well as a transesophageal examination (TEE) (M-mode and two dimensional). TTE studies were performed under standard conditions using 2.25- and 3.5-MHz phased array transducers. For TEE studies, we used 3.5- and 5.0-MHz phased array transducers mounted at the tip of a modified gastroscope (Diasonics, Toshiba, Hewlett Packard). All TEE studies were performed after administration of local pharyngeal anesthesia without additional premedication. Patients had

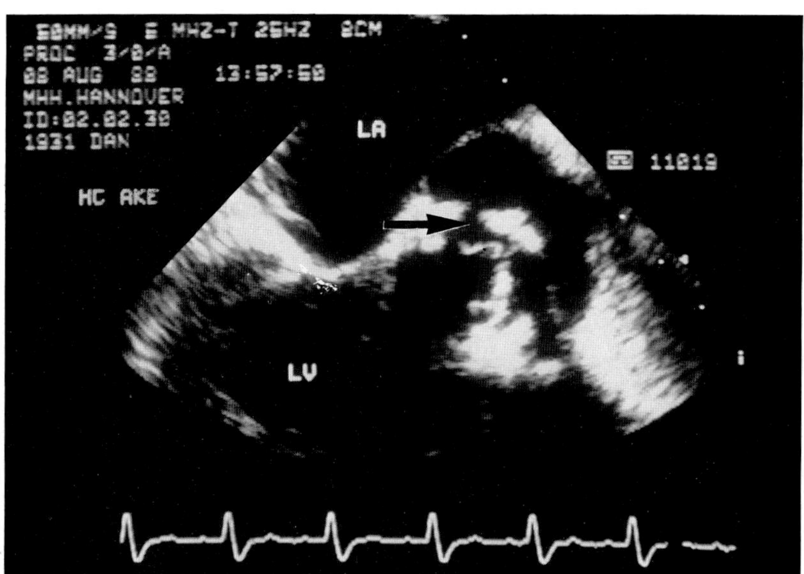

Fig. 1. Transesophageal echocardiogram of a patient with a degenerated Hanckock bioprosthesis in the aortic position. Note the thickening of the leaflets (*arrows*). *LA/LV*, left atrium/ventricle

fasted for at least 4 h and were examined in a left lateral decubitus position; all examinations were carried out without any complications.

Echocardiograms were evaluated by two independent observers. The PV were rated as "normal," "abnormal," or "questionable"; "questionable" was used in cases in which no differentiation between "normal" and "abnormal" was possible due to an inadequate imaging quality or some other cause.

The following echocardiographic criteria for the various PV diseases were used:

1. *Bioprosthesis degeneration:* Thickening of the leaflets ≥ 3 mm (Alam et al. 1981, 1987) (Fig. 1) as well as frail or fractured leaflets associated with restricted or other abnormal valve motion (prolapse into the left atrium or left ventricle)
2. *Endocarditis:* Sessile or pendulating valve-attached masses, not inhibiting the motion of the leaflets or occluder of PV (Fig. 2)
3. *Thrombi:* Sessile valve-attached masses localized within the cage and usually associated with restricted leaflet or occluder motion (Fig. 3)
4. *Paravalvular leak:* Exaggerated rocking of the stent and/or protodiastolic hump of the occluder (Cunha et al. 1980; Bernal-Ramirez and Phillips 1977); occasionally associated with a clearly visible valve ring dehiscence (Fig. 4)

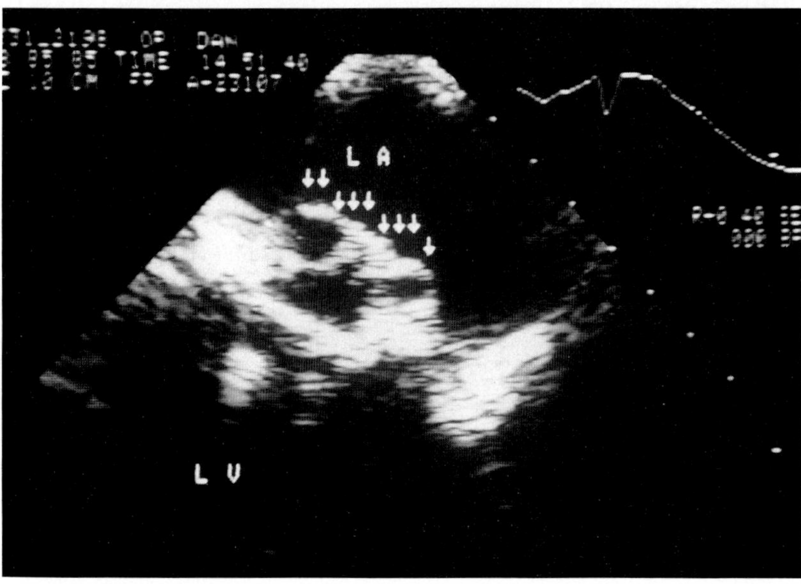

Fig. 2. Transesophageal echocardiogram of a patient with pendulating vegetations at the atrial side of a mechanical prosthesis in the mitral position (*arrows*). *LA/LV,* left atrium/ventricle

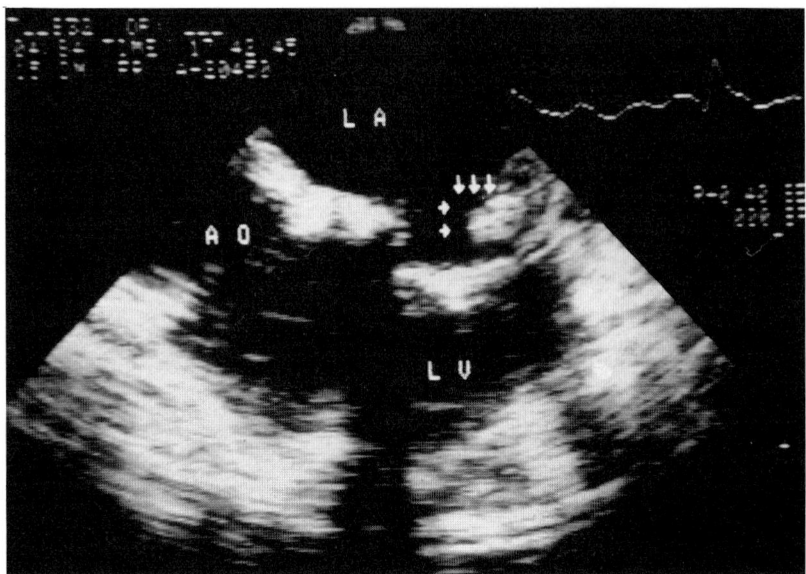

Fig. 3. Transesophageal echocardiogram of a patient with a thrombus within the cage of a Starr Edwards disc prosthesis (*arrows*). *LA/LV*, left atrium/ventricle; *AO* aorta

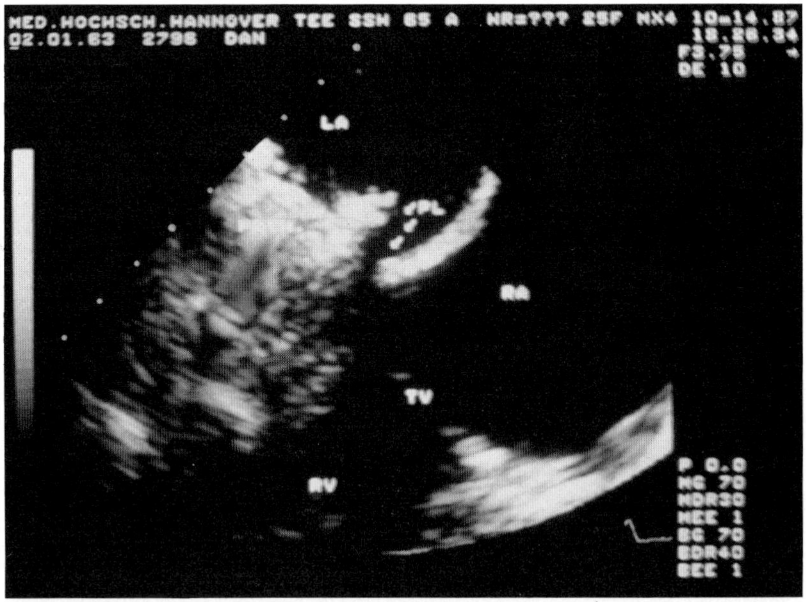

Fig. 4. Transesophageal echocardiogram of a patient with a paravalvular leak (*arrows, PL*) of a mechanical device in the mitral position. *LA/RA*, left/right atrium, *TV*, tricuspid valve, *RV*, right ventricle

Statistics

For statistical analysis the χ^2 test was used. A p value < 0.05 was considered as indicating a significant difference. The detection of PV malfunction by echocardiography as compared to the anatomical findings was determined by calculating sensitivity, specificity, and positive and negative predictive values as follows:

$$\text{sensitivity} = \frac{\text{true diseased PV detected by echocardiography}}{\text{all diseased PV found by anatomical examination}}$$

$$\text{specificity} = \frac{\text{true normal PV detected by echocardiography}}{\text{all normal PV found by anatomical examination}}$$

$$\text{positive predictive value} = \frac{\text{true diseased PV detected by echocardiography}}{\text{true and false diseased PV detected by echocard.}}$$

$$\text{negative predictive value} = \frac{\text{true normal PV detected by echocardiography}}{\text{true and false normal PV detected by echocard.}}$$

Results

The interobserver variations were 12.2% and 7.3% for the transthoracic and transesophageal approaches, respectively.

The detection rates of TTE and TEE for the various PV abnormalities are listed in Table 2. TEE had a significantly higher detection rate than TTE in the assessment of diseased PV; in particular, TEE was superior concerning the identification of vegetations or thrombi attached to the PV. Including all PV, TEE identified PV abnormalities with a sensitivity and specificity of 75% and 79%, respectively; these values were markedly lower for the precordial examination (41% and 58%; Table 3). A significantly higher detection rate of PV abnormalities occurred in bioprostheses and mechanical devices when the

Table 2. Detection of prosthetic valve abnormalities by transthoracic and transesophageal echocardiography

	Correct diagnoses										
	Endocarditis ($n = 19$)		Degeneration ($n = 32$)		Paravalvular leak ($n = 7$)		Thrombi ($n = 5$)		Normal ($n = 19$)		Total ($n = 82$)	
	n	%	n	%	n	%	n	%	n	%	n	%
TTE	5	26	19	59	1	14	1	20	11	58	37	45
TEE	15	79	25	78	2	28	5	100	15	79	62	76

TTE vs. TEE: $\chi^2 = 14.7$, $p < 0.001$.

Table 3. Sensitivity, specificity, and positive and negative predictive values of transthoracic and transesophageal echocardiography for the detection of prosthetic valve abnormalities

	TTE	TEE
Sensitivity (%)	41	75
Specificity (%)	58	79
Positive predictive value (%)	76	92
Negative predictive value (%)	23	47

73 patients with 19 normal and 63 diseased prosthetic valves.

Table 4. Detection of prosthetic valve abnormalities by transthoracic and transesophageal echocardiography: dependency on the type of prosthesis

	Abnormal		Questionable		Normal	
	n	%	n	%	n	%
Bioprosthesis ($n = 45$)						
TTE	23	51	9	20	13	29
TEE	35	78	2	4	8	18
Mechanical device ($n = 18$)						
TTE	3	17	4	22	11	61
TEE	12	67	2	11	4	22

57 patients with anatomically proven prosthetic valve malfunction (63 prosthetic valves, 31 mitral, 32 aortic). TEE vs. TTE bioprosthesis, p < 0.01, mechanical device, p < 0.005.

Table 5. Detection of prosthetic valve abnormalities by transthoracic and transesophageal echocardiography: dependency on prosthetic valve position

	Abnormal		Questionable		Normal	
	n	%	n	%	n	%
Mitral ($n = 31$)						
TTE	11	35	7	23	13	42
TEE	26	84	1	3	4	13
Aortic ($n = 32$)						
TTE	15	47	6	19	11	34
TEE	21	66	3	9	8	25

57 patients with anatomically proven prosthetic valve malfunction (63 prosthetic valves, 45 bioprostheses, 18 mechanical devices). TEE vs. TTE mitral, p < 0.001; aortic, p = n.s.

TEE approach was used; for mechanical devices, however, the difference between TEE and TTE was more pronounced (Table 4). When aortic and mitral PV were analyzed separately, however, a significant difference, was only found for mitral devices (Table 5).

Comments

The close relationship between the esophagus and the heart allows the use of higher transducer frequencies in TEE. Furthermore, in contrast to the transthoracic approach, the ultrasound beam does not have to penetrate lung tissue and the chest wall, resulting in improved resolution and a more detailed imaging of cardiac morphology (Schlüter et al. 1982; Daniel et al. 1988 b; Seward et al. 1988). In addition, TEE allows clear visualization of the left atrium, including the region behind a mitral PV which is − at least in mechanical devices − usually obscured by heavy artifacts when studied from the precordial view. Although TEE is associated with some minor discomfort, this technique has been shown to be a safe procedure with almost no risk in more than 1800 patients studied in our laboratory (Daniel et al. 1988 c).

The present study shows that the various anatomical abnormalities associated with PV malfunction can be evaluated with higher sensitivity and specificity by TEE than by the precordial examination. This is particulary true for the detection of vegetations and PV-attached thrombi, for the evaluation of mechanical devices, and for mitral PV. The detection rate of a paravalvular leakage, however, is low even when TEE is used; it should be noted, though, that in this sudy only anatomical abnormalities were evaluated and Doppler investigations allowing the detection of regurgitant jets were not included. The combined use of Doppler and TEE will further increase the sensitivity for the detection of PV malfunction, especially trans- and paravalvular leakages. This has been shown recently in patients with mitral PV (Daniel et al. 1988 d; Nellessen et al. 1988).

TEE cannot overcome all the problems associated with TTE concerning the assessment of PV. In particular, the evaluation of mechanical devices in the aortic position remains unsatisfactory, since the view into the PV cage is often obscured by shadowing created by the posterior ring circumference. This problem will be solved as soon as TEE probes with additional imaging planes become available. Furthermore, reliable differentiation between infectious vegetations and noninfectious thrombotic material attached to PV is difficult or even impossible in many cases studied by TEE; the combination of information about clinical signs and other laboratory data is usually necessary for the final diagnosis.

In conclusion, TEE is clearly superior to the TTE in detecting anatomical abnormalities of PV; this technique should be used when insufficient information is obtained from the precordial examination.

Acknowledgements. We appreciate the excellent technical assistence of Mrs. R. Schützenmeister and the careful preparation of the figures by Mrs. A. Schafft.

References

Alam M, Goldstein S, Lakier JB (1981) Echocardiographic changes in the thickness of porcine valves with time. Chest 79:663–668

Alam M, Rosman HS, Lakier JB, Kemp S, Khaja F, Hautamaki K, Magilligan DJ, Stein PD (1987) Doppler and echocardiographic features of normal and dysfunctioning bioprosthetic valves. J Am Coll Cardiol 10:851–858

Assanelli D, Aquilina M, Marangoni S, Morgagni GL, Visiolo O (1986) Echophonocardiographic evaluation of the Björk-Shiley mitral prosthesis. Am J Cardiol 57:165–170

Bernal-Ramirez JA, Phillips JH (1977) Echocardiographic study of malfunction of the Bjork-Shiley prosthetic heart valve in the mitral position. Am J Cardiol 40:449–453

Brodie BR, Grossman W, McLaurin L, Starek PJK, Craige E (1976) Diagnosis of prosthetic mitral valve malfunction with combined echo-phonocardiography. Circulation 53:93–100

Cunha CLP, Guiliani ER, Callahan JA, Pluth JR (1980) Echophonocardiographic findings in patients with prosthetic heart valve malfunction. Mayo Clin Proc 55:231–242

Daniel WG, Mügge A, Frank G (1988a) Improved diagnosis of prosthetic valve malfunction by transesophageal echocardiography. Circulation 78 [Suppl II]:II–606

Daniel WG, Schröder E, Mügge A, Lichtlen PR (1988b) Transesophageal echocardiography in infective endocarditis. Am J Cardiac Imaging 2:78–85

Daniel WG, Mügge A, Schröder E, Wenzlaff P, Grote J (1988c) Transesophageal echocardiography in clinical cardiology – indications, practicability and risk (abstract). Circulation 78 [Suppl II]:II–297

Daniel WG, Hanrath P, Mügge A, Langenstein B, Engel H, Grote J (1988d) Assessment of mitral prosthetic valve dysfunction by transesophageal color coded Doppler echocardiography. Circulation 78 [Suppl II]:II–607

Erbel R, Mohr-Kahaly S, Rohmann S, Schuster S, Drexler M, Wittlich N, Pfeiffer C, Schreiner G, Meyer J (1987) Diagnostische Wertigkeit der transösophagealen Doppler-Echokardiographie. Herz 12:177–186

Forman MB, Phelan BK, Robertson RM, Virmani R (1985) Correlation of two-dimensional echocardiography and pathologic findings in porcine valve dysfunction. J Am Coll Cardiol 5:224–230

Nellessen U, Daniel WG, Hecker H, Hetzer R, Schleberger J, Lichtlen PR (1985) Nachweis einer Malfunktion von Herzklappenprothesen mittels zweidimensionaler transösophagealer Echokardiographie. In: Erbel R, Meyer J, Brennecke R (eds) Fortschritte der Echokardiographie. Springer Berlin Heidelberg New York pp 203–210

Nellessen U, Schnittger I, Appelton CP, Masuyama T, Bolger A, Fischell TA, Tye T, Popp RL (1988) Transesophageal two-dimensional echocardiography and color Doppler flow velocity mapping in the evaluation of cardiac valve prostheses. Circulation 78:848–855

Schapira JN, Martin RP, Fowles RE, Rakowski H, Stinson EB, French JW, Shumway NE, Popp RL (1979) Two dimensional echocardiographic assessment of patients with bioprosthetic valves. Am J Cardiol 43:510–519

Schlüter M, Langenstein BA, Polster J, Kremer P, Souquet J, Engel S, Hanrath P (1982) Transoesophageal cross-sectional echocardiography with a phased array transducer system. Br Heart J 48:67–72

Seward JB, Khandheria BK, OH JK, Abel MD, Hughes RW, Edwards WD, Nichols BA, Freeman WK, Tajik AJ (1988) Transesophageal echocardiography: technique, anatomic correlations, implementation, and clinical applications. Mayo Clin Proc 63:649–680

Intracardiac Source of Embolism

J. M. CURTIUS

Introduction

The search for an intracardiac source of embolism is a frequent indication
for daily routine echocardiography. Unless there is a predisposing cardiac
condition such as a mitral valve defect or an appreciable restriction of left
ventricular contraction, the result is mostly negative. However, even if such a
preexisting disease involving the left atrium is known, transthoracic echocardiography (TTE) is often disappointing in its low sensitivity.

In 1983, Shrestha et al. [1] published a study on this in which 293 patients
with a rheumatic mitral valvular defect were investigated with regard to the
detection of left atrial thrombi by means of TTE. The subsequent open-heart
mitral valve surgery served as reference method. There was a high specificity
of 99% but a sensitivity of only 59% with regard to the detection of thrombi
either in the left atrium or in the left atrial appendage. The exclusion of
thrombi merely present in the left atrial appendage led to an increase of the
sensitivity to 75%, but exclusion of this group would not be meaningful in
clinical terms.

Daniel et al. discussed a European multicenter study on the sensitivity of
transesophageal echocardiography (TEE) in detecting the source of an arterial embolism (unpublished). This study involved 375 patients with one or
several embolic episodes in various organs. An abnormal finding was shown
in TTE in only about one-third of the patients (143/375), whereas an abnormal
finding was shown in about two-thirds of the patients (238/375) in TEE. The
abnormal findings detected by means of TEE were above all thrombi in the
left atrium or atrial appendage (79 patients), spontaneous echo contrast (70
patients), a mitral valve prolapse, or vegetations (53 patients each). TEE thus
proved to be very much more sensitive. This study involved a mixed patient
population with embolization in various organs and included patients with
previously known heart disease.

We carried out a small study on a specially selected patient population,
namely patients without previously known heart disease and with exclusively
cerebral embolizations. The aim of the study was to establish how frequently
echocardiographic findings indicate that an intracardiac source of embolism is
possible or probable in this specific patient population, how often this is correct, and the degree of superiority of TEE over TTE.

Transesophageal Echocardiography
Edited by R. Erbel et al.
© Springer-Verlag Berlin Heidelberg 1989

Patients and Methods

The study involved 18 patients (mean age 51 ± 16 years, range 24−75 years: ten men and eight women) who had recently had a cerebral ischemic event. Three cases involved transitory ischemic attacks which had occurred several times, and the remaining 15 cases had cerebral or cerebellar insults with a pronounced clinical picture. In neurological terms, a possible cause of the event had not been found in any case by investigation of the blood vessels supplying the brain using Doppler echocardiography, raising the question of the possible source of embolism.

Cardiac disease was not known in any of these patients. In consequence of this: (1) The history was void in this regard, e.g., patients with stenocardia, arrhythmias, or fever (which might have indicated endocarditis) were excluded. (2) The clinical examination had not provided any indication of heart disease, for example a cardiac murmur was a reason for exclusion. (3) The ECG in these patients did not show any abnormalities such as signs of completed myocardial infarction or of atrial fibrillation.

All patients were initially investigated by means of TTE and immediately afterwards by TEE. Written consent to TEE was given in all cases. Local pharyngeal anesthesia (lydocaine spray) was given, and in nine out the 18 patients additional sedation by intravenous administration of 5−10 mg diazepam.

The TTE investigation was carried out in two parasternal and two apical standard views, in some cases by means of a subxiphoidal view. Doppler investigation of the mitral valve with regard to a possible mitral regurgitation (pulsed, continuous, and color-coded Doppler) was also carried out in all cases. When relevant indications were found, further Doppler investigations were also performed.

The transesophageal investigation was also carried out including pulsed as well as color-coded Doppler. All parts of the heart including the left atrial appendage were imaged. Contrast medium was not administered. In addition, the descending aorta was investigated. Representative images from both methods of investigation were recorded on video cassette. This recording was appraised separately by two experienced persons after the investigation.

Results

In nine cases (see Table 1), the transthoracic investigation revealed normal findings. In five of these patients, this was confirmed by means of TEE. However, in the remaining four patients, an abnormal finding was found with TEE: in one case, a 1.5-cm-long floating deposit on the anterior mitral valve of doubtful age; in the second case, a mitral valve prolapse which could only be detected by means of TEE; in the third case, an aneurysm of the atrial septum (see Fig. 1) associated with a slight left-to-right shunt which could be

Table 1. Results of TTE and TEE in 18 patients

Patient	TTE	TEE
1	Suspected LA tumor	Normal
2	No examination possible	Aneurysm of the IAS
3	Normal	Normal
4	Normal	Normal
5	No examination possible	Normal
6	No examination possible	Normal
7	MVP	MVP
8	LA enlargement	Spontaneous echo contrast
9	Normal	Normal
10	Normal	Floating tumor on the AML
11	Normal	MVP
12	No examination possible	Normal
13	Normal	Aneurysm of the IAS, ASD
14	LV function depressed	Spontaneous echo contrast
15	Normal	Spontaneous echo contrast
16	LV function depressed	Thrombus left atrial appendage
17	Normal	Normal
18	Normal	Normal

AML, anterior mitral valve leaflet; ASD, atrial septal defect; IAS, intraatrial septum; LA, left atrium; LV left ventricle; MVP, mitral valve prolapse

imaged by color-coded Doppler; in the fourth case, spontaneous echo contrast in terms of slow cloudy structures rotating in the left atrium, passing the mitral valve, but which could not longer be imaged in the left ventricle.

An abnormal result was found with TTE in three cases. However, this was not necessarily associated with a cerebral embolization (diffuse moderately reduced left ventricular function in two cases, enlargement of the left atrium in one case). In two of these patients, the TEE showed spontaneous echo contrast. A floating thrombus 1.5−2 cm in size was found in the left atrial appen-

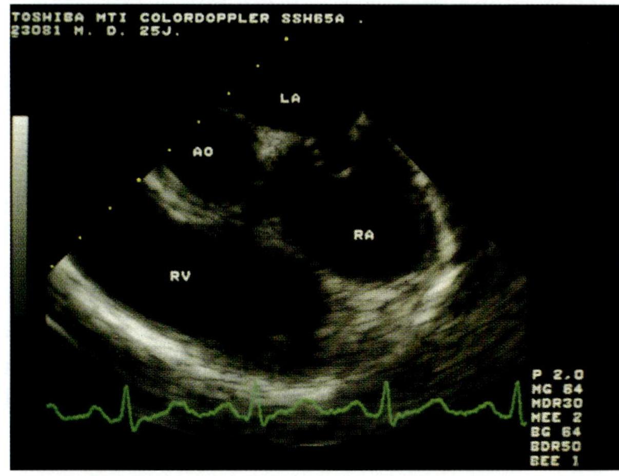

Fig. 1. TEE image of patient 13: aneurysm of the atrial septum

Table 2. Results of TTE

1 × MVP	1 × true positive	33%
9 × normal	5 × true negative 4 × false negative	
4 × no examination possible	4 × no information	
2 × depressed LV function 1 × LA enlargement	3 × incomplete information	66%
1 × suspected LA tumor	1 × false positive	

dage in one of the patients with reduced left ventricular contractions. In the transthoracic investigation of one patient, result suggested an intracavity lesion in the left atrium; this suggestion was clearly refuted by means of TEE, where findings were normal. In one further patient, a mitral valve prolapse was shown both by TTE and by TEE. Finally, the transthoracic investigation could not be evaluated in four patients because the quality of imaging was poor for anatomical reasons. In three of these four patients, the TEE showed normal findings, and in the fourth patient an aneurysm of the atrial septum without atrial septum defect was found.

Thus, TTE and TEE findings were consistent or there was no additional findings with TEE in only one-third of the patients (see Table 2). However, in two-thirds either no information could be found by means of TTE, or it was incorrect, incomplete or false negative.

With TEE abnormalities in the left atrium which may have been associated with an embolic event were found in 9/18 patients (50%) with cerebral embolism but no known previous cardiac disease. Spontaneous echo contrast could be demonstrated in the left atrium in three cases, a mitral valve prolapse in two cases, an atrial septum aneurysm in two cases (a small atrial septal defect in one of these cases), a deposit on the anterior mitral valve leaflet in one case, and a thrombus in the left atrium in one case.

Final Appraisal

The present investigation once more confirms that TEE is far superior to TTE in the search for an intracardiac source of embolism. TTE produced correct and complete results in only 33% of cases, and only one out of a total of nine abnormal findings on TEE could also be detected by means of TTE.

The clinically interesting aspect of our study is the strikingly high percentage (50%) of intracardiac abnormalities which could be detected by means of TEE, although no previous cardiac disease was known in the patients. Incidentally, these findings were all made in the left atrium, and not in the left ventricle.

It must be stated in this regard that the pathological relevance of these results, in particular of spontaneous echo contrast and of an atrial septum aneurysm, is at present uncertain. A relationship with an arterial embolization may be suspected, but cannot by any means be proved. However, studies done so far [2, 3] show a clear statistical correlation between such findings and a raised incidence of embolism. Furthermore, it is completely open at present as to what therapeutic inferences are to be drawn from the findings obtained.

References

1. Shrestha NK, Moreno FL, Narciso FV, Torres L, Calleja HB (1983) Two-dimensional echocardiographic diagnosis of left atrial thrombus in rheumatic heart disease. A clinopathologic study. Circulation 67:341−347
2. Geeren M, Erbel R, Mohr-Kahaly S, Drexler M, Wittlich N, Darius H, Geissert U, Kern A, Meyer J (1987) Embolierate bei spontanem Echokontrast und Thromben im linken Vorhof. Z Kardiol 76 (Suppl II):48
3. Daniel WG, Nellessen U, Schroeder E, Nonnast-Daniel B, Bednarski P, Nikutta P, Lichtlen PR (1988) Left atrial spontaneous echo contrast in mitral valve disease: an indicator for an increased thromboembolic risk. J Am Coll Cardiol 11:1204−1211

Cardiac Tumors and Thrombus: Transesophageal Echocardiographic Experience

J. B. SEWARD

Introduction

Precordial echocardiography has revolutionized the examination of the heart for tumors and thrombus. Most benign and malignant tumors, as well as intracardiac thrombus of all etiologies, have been described in the two-dimensional (2-D) echocardiographic literature. As with any technology, there are limitations and improvements in technology which define and continuously change the diagnostic capabilities. Limitations of transthoracic echocardiography (TTE) include an inability consistently to image targets in the far field, small embedded or mural masses, and certain structures, including the atrial appendages and pulmonary veins. Pedunculated masses, such as cavitary myxomas or thrombus, are usually accurately diagnosed by precordial echocardiography. However, these easily diagnosed masses may appear atypical and require further characterization in order to establish a proper diagnosis or determine pertinent associations.

Transesophageal echocardiography (TEE) has received increasing interest as a superior technology for visualizing certain cardiac structures, including the atria, atrial appendages, pulmonary veins, and atrioventricular valves. This new ultrasonic window often allows better delineation of cardiac structures and is now considered a logical extension of a complete standard transthoracic examination. TEE has been shown to have a particularly unique ability to image the left atrial appendage, as well as masses impining or migrating into the atria.

This retrospective review describes our initial experience utilizing TEE in the awake patient for delineation of cardiac tumors and thrombus, emphasizing the characteristic features, diagnostic strengths and limitations, and clinical utility of the TEE technique.

Experiences

Between October 1987 and October 1988, we studied 552 awake patients utilizing TEE (Table 1). All examinations reporting visualization of a tumor or thrombus were reviewed. Investigation of a mass or thromboembolism accounted for 21% of all examinations. Patients with endocarditis and masses of vegetation or abscess were not included. Each patient had undergone a

Transesophageal Echocardiography
Edited by R. Erbel et al.
© Springer-Verlag Berlin Heidelberg 1989

Table 1. Indications for TEE in 552 patients studied during a 1-year period

	n	%
Prosthetic dysfunction	130	24
Mass/thromboembolism	114	21
Valve dysfunction	79	14
Endocarditis	70	12
Thoracic aortic pathology	50	9
Critically ill	50	9
Coronary heart disease	20	4
Miscellaneons	39	7

comprehensive standard precordial echocardiographic examination prior to the TEE examination.

Because this is a retrospective review of initial experience, only rough estimates of incidence could be ascertained. Sensitivity, specificity, and diagnostic superiority cannot be accurately estimated and must await ongoing prospective studies.

Details of the TEE technique have been previously reported from this laboratory [1]. All examinations were clinically indicated and requested by a cardiologist. Examinations utilized a Hewlett-Packard, Acuson or Aloka TEE instrument. A 5-MHz ultrasonic transducer is mounted on a standard adult sized endoscope. Fiberoptics and suction are not utilized. All patients received local pharyngeal anesthesia and a systemic drying agent (glycopyrrolate). The majority (73%) also received a variable dosage of systemic sedation (midazolam, a benzodiazepine). No adverse effects or reactions to the TEE examination were noted. The average examination lasted 17 min (range 5−25).

Indications for TEE

Following a complete precordial examination, there were generally two clinical indications for further TEE evaluation in patients suspected of having a cardiac mass. *First*, 28 patients (60%) had a probable or definite mass identified by TTE, but the clinical or echocardiographic features were atypical or not adequately explained. In these patients, TEE was requested to better define attachment, location, intracardiac versus extracardiac, size and texture, as well as pertinent associations such as tumor with thrombus. Overall, 21% of examination were performed to determine the source of embolism or tumor mass.

The *second* indication for TEE was inability to visualize a clinically suspected source for embolism. This group (19 patients, 40%) was exclusively confined to thrombus visualization. Patients with mitral valve disease or prostheses make up the majority of these patients. Search for source of embolism, evaluation of a suspect prosthetic valve and anticipated mitral balloon valvuloplasty are frequent clinical requests. Precordial 2-D/Doppler echocardiography was known to be very insensitive for the assessment of left atrial or atrial appendage thrombus while TEE was known to provided excellent visualization of atrial anatomy. Echogenic prostheses also precluded a complete TTE assessment and a complete examination was improved by TEE.

From our previous work and that of others [1–4], superior indications for TEE include (1) visualization of left atrium and atrial appendage for thrombus and (2) better characterization of tumor location, extent, and associations (malignant versus benign and contained versus extracardiac or malignant migration of a mass into the heart).

Thrombus (Table 2)

Left atrium and atrial appendage thrombus was totally inaccessible or inadequately visualized by TTE in each instance (Fig. 1). Clinical suspicion was the only helpful indication for proceeding with TEE. Patients with mitral stenosis or prosthesis associated with systemic embolism, suspected prosthesis malfunction or planned percutaneous balloon mitral valvuloplasty were common referrals most likely to have atrial or atrial appendage thrombus. Recog-

Table 2. Masses found by TEE in 47 patients

	n	%
Thrombus	26	55
Left atrium/left atrial appendage	13	28
Prosthesis	8	17
Other	5	11
Tumor	21	45
Myxoma	7	15
Malignant	4	8
Papilloma, fibroma, miscellaneous	10	21

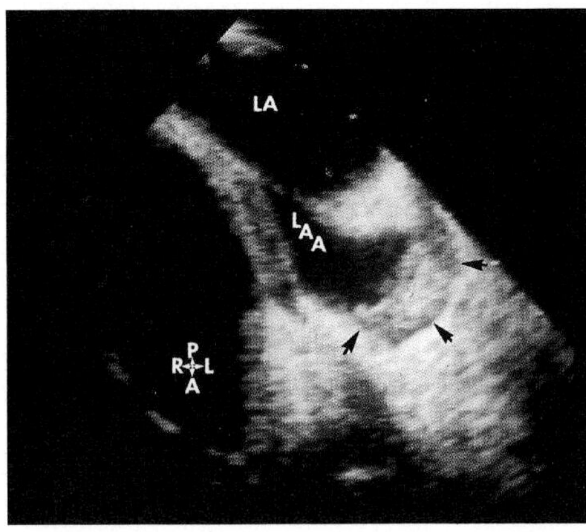

Fig. 1. Thrombus (*arrows*) within the left atrial appendage (*LAA*) in an elderly patient with mitral valve disease. TEE was performed while investigating the source of an embolic event. The thrombus laminated the apex of the LAA. No other left atrial (*LA*) thrombus was noted. (*P*, posterior; *A*, anterior; *R*, right; *L*, left)

nition of thrombus is usually easy by TEE. However, moderate amounts of fluid in the pericardial sac surrounding the left atrial appendage can make the appendage mobile and appear masslike, which could be misinterpreted as a mobile atrial mass. Occasionally the pectinate muscles of the atrial appendage or a bulbous common wall between the left atrial appendage and left upper pulmonary vein can be confused with thrombus.

Prosthetic valve thrombus was second most common (Fig. 2). Occasionally, gross accumulations of thrombus were visible. However, more often pendunculated or filamentous thrombus strands were visualized on the left atrial surface. These undulating strands were easiest to appreciate at the sewing ring or attached to the valve support apparatus. It is presumed that laminated or small thrombus may be missed because of hyperrefractile valve struts or prosthetic valve material. However, when compared to any other imaging technique, including TTE, TEE is superior.

Other instances of visualized thrombus included (1) thrombus attached to pacing wires, (2) thrombus in atrial recess, usually within the fossa ovalis, and (3) ventricular mural thrombus. Of the five patients in this group, only in one was left ventricular thrombus suspected by TTE.

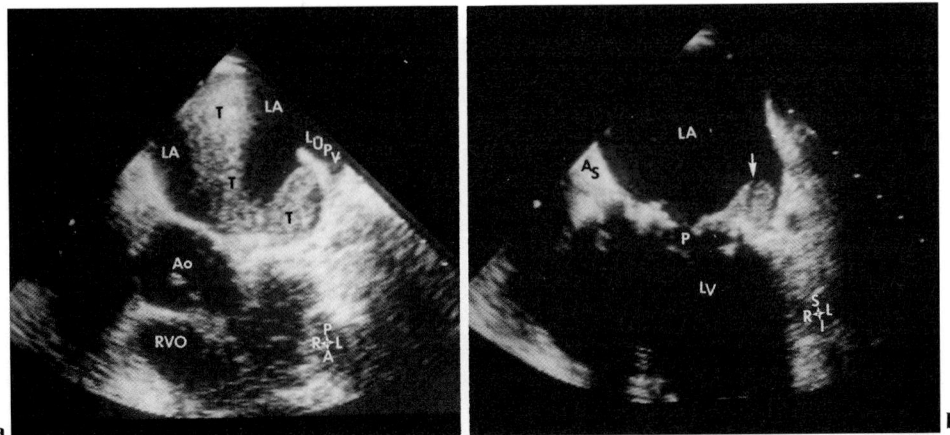

Fig. 2a, b. Left atrial thrombus (*T* and *arrow*) in a patient with mitral bioprosthesis. A left atrial thrombus had not been suspected by a detailed transthoracic examination. Transvalvular inflow velocity and deceleration time had increased, suggesting possible valve obstruction. **a** TEE. Within the left atrium (*LA*) there was a large accumulation of thrombus (*T*) which extended into the site of a previously ligated atrial appendage and beneath the left upper pulmonary vein (*LUPV*). **b** The prosthesis (*P*) was well seated. However, thrombus (*arrow*) at the lateral serving ring extended into the orifice partially obstructed the inflow. (*AS*, atrial septum; *LV*, left ventricle; *RVO*, right ventricular outflow; *Ao*, aorta; *P*, posterior; *A*, anteriour; *L*, left; *R* right)

Tumors (Table 2)

Benign Tumors

Myxomas comprised the single most commonly encountered tumor (seven patients). The location was right atrium in three patients, left atrium in three, and mitral valve in one. Five patients were studied because of clinical presentation and/or atypical tumor appearance or site of attachment. One patient with a history of "syndrome myxoma" had a suspected right atrial recurrence and was found on TEE to have a moderate sized pedunculated myxoma on the free wall of right atrium (Fig. 3). Atypical locations included attachment to the Eustachian valve (one patient) (Fig. 4) or mitral valve (one patient) and biatrial extension through the foramen ovale (one patient). The remaining three patients had incomplete or inconclusive transthoracic examinations and were found to have a more typical myxoma attachment to the fossa ovalis (Fig. 5).

Papillomas are small frondlike ovoid tumors usually attached to the valve leaflets or support apparatus (Fig. 6). A detailed TEE examination allowed confident diagnosis of papilloma in three patients. Two were attached to the mitral valve and one attached to the tricuspid valve leaflet. An ovoid frondlike mass in the absence of a recent infectious history is quite diagnostic of a benign papilloma.

Other tumors with benign appearance and clinical presentation make up a diverse group of clinical and echocardiographic tumor types. Two locations, intramyocardial (three patients) (Fig. 7) and extracardiac (four patients),

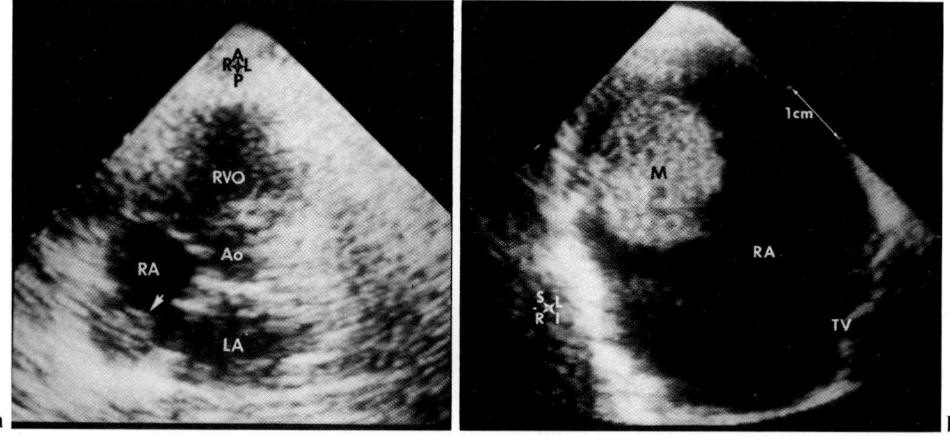

Fig. 3a, b. Atypical right atrial myxoma in a 45-year-old woman with recurrent atrial myxomas. **a** Transthoracic short-axis view at the aortic valve (*AV*) level. Within the right atrium (*RA*) there appeared an ill-defined ovoid mass (*arrow*) near the orifice of the inferior vena cava. A TEE was performed to better define a possible recurrent atrial myxoma. **b** TEE. On the free wall of the RA there was a distinct pedunculated mass (*M*) (2 cm in diameter) consistent with a myxoma. Note the enhanced clarity of the TEE image. (*RVO*, right ventricular outflow; *TV*, tricuspid valve; *LA*, left atrium; *S*, superior; *I*, inferior; *L*, left; *R*, right)

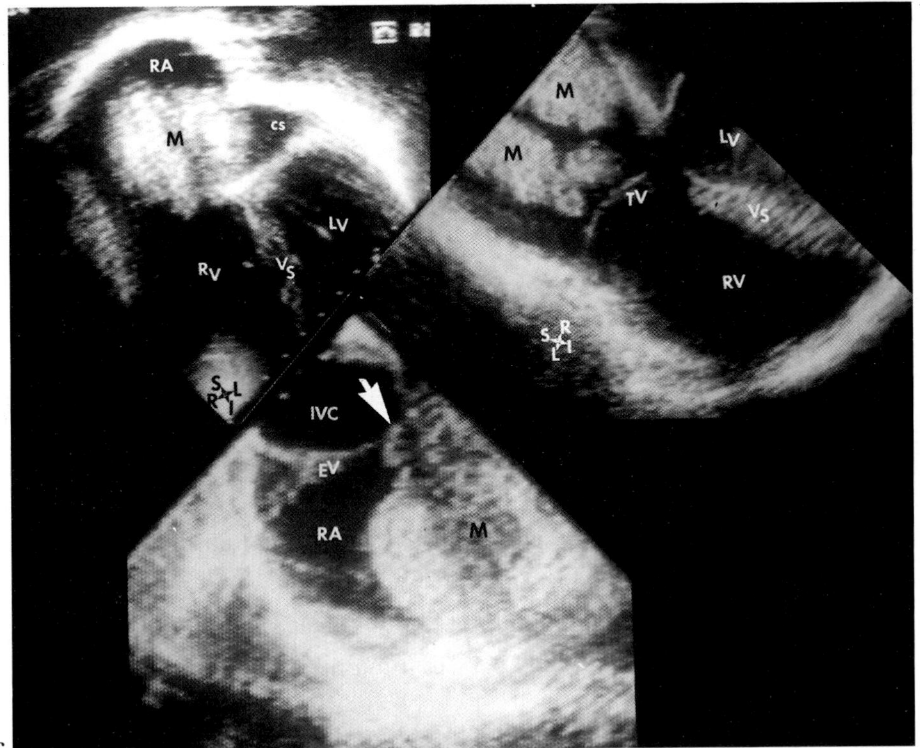

Fig. 4 a–c. Atypical insertion of a right atrial myxoma (*M*). **a** Transthoracic apex-down four-chamber view showing a mobile right atrial (*RA*) mass consistent with myxoma. However, the attachment of the tumor could not be delineated. TEE was performed to better assess attachment and assure operability. **b** A comparable TEE four-chamber view which confirms *lack* of atrial septal attachment. **c** Attachment was localized to the rim of the Eustachian valve (*EV*) (*arrow*) at the orifice of the inferior vena cava (*IVC*). A large atypical right atrial myxoma was found at surgery. (*RV*, right ventricle; *VS*, ventricular septum; *LV*, left ventricle; *TV*, tricuspid valve; *S*, superior; *I*, inferior; *L*, left; *R*, right)

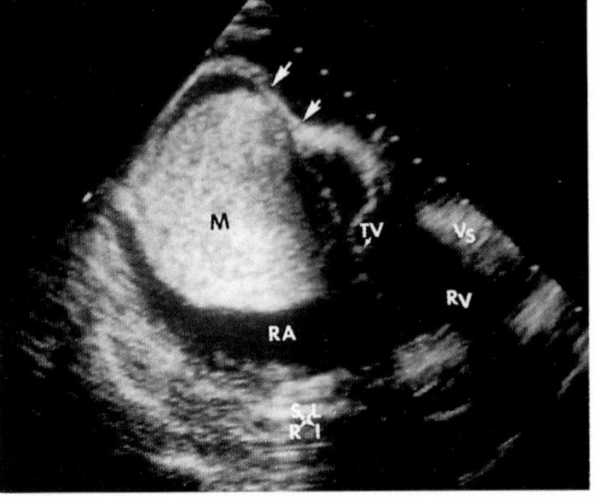

Fig. 5. Typical large right atrial myxoma (*M*) inserting at the fossa ovalis (*arrows*) of the atrial septum. This extremely obese man underwent TEE to better visualize a suspected right atrial (*RA*) myxoma. (*TV*, tricuspid valve; *RV*, right ventricle; *VS*, ventricular septum; *R*, right; *L*, left; *S*, superior; *I*, inferior)

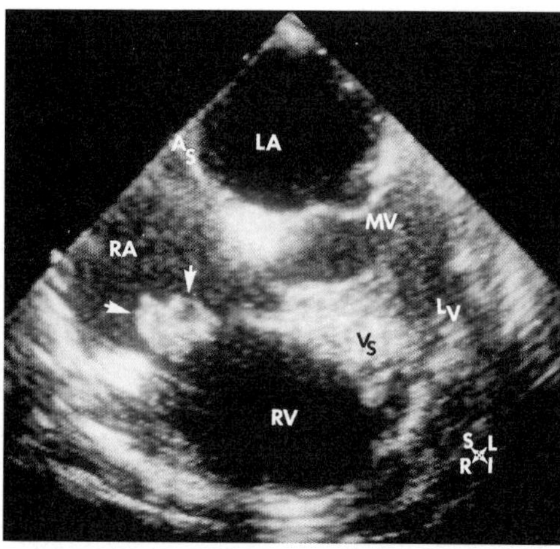

Fig. 6. Papilloma (*arrows*) (1 × 1.5 cm) attached to the tricuspid valve leaflet. This benign tumor has a charcteristic undulating motion to its fronds. (*LA*, left atrium; *RA*, right atrium; *MV*, mitral valve; *LV*, left ventricle; *VS*, ventricular septum)

prompted further assessment for tumor extent, myocardial involvement, and exclusion of infiltration suggesting malignancy. Intramyocardial masses consisted of small embedded fibroma (two patients) and a large atrial septal lymphoma (one patient). Extracardiac masses (four patients) were an atypical pericardial cyst (one patient) and solid tumors, assessed to be benign, recognized as adjacent to the heart and not involving the myocardium (three patients).

Malignant Tumors

Three patients had infiltrating tumor masses within the right (one patient) or left (two patients) atrium (Fig. 8). Tumor types were breast carcinoma (one patient) and melanoma (two patients). The right atrial tumor extended from the superior vena cava and surrounding mediastinum and was not visible on

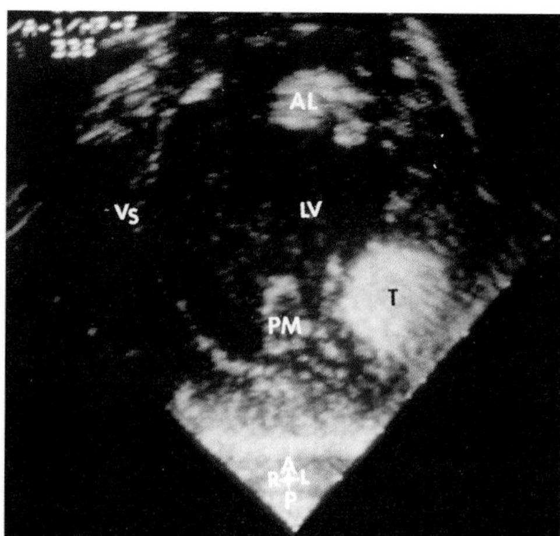

Fig. 7. Fibroma (*T*) (1.5 × 1.5 cm) embedded in the free wall of the left ventricle (*LV*). This ovoid tumor was investigated by TEE to better delineate tumor position, size, and extent. The tumor was located between the anterolateral (*AL*) and posteriomedial (*PM*) papillary muscles on the posterolateral free wall of LV. (*VS*, ventricular septum; *A*, anterior; *P*, posterior; *L*, left, *R*, right)

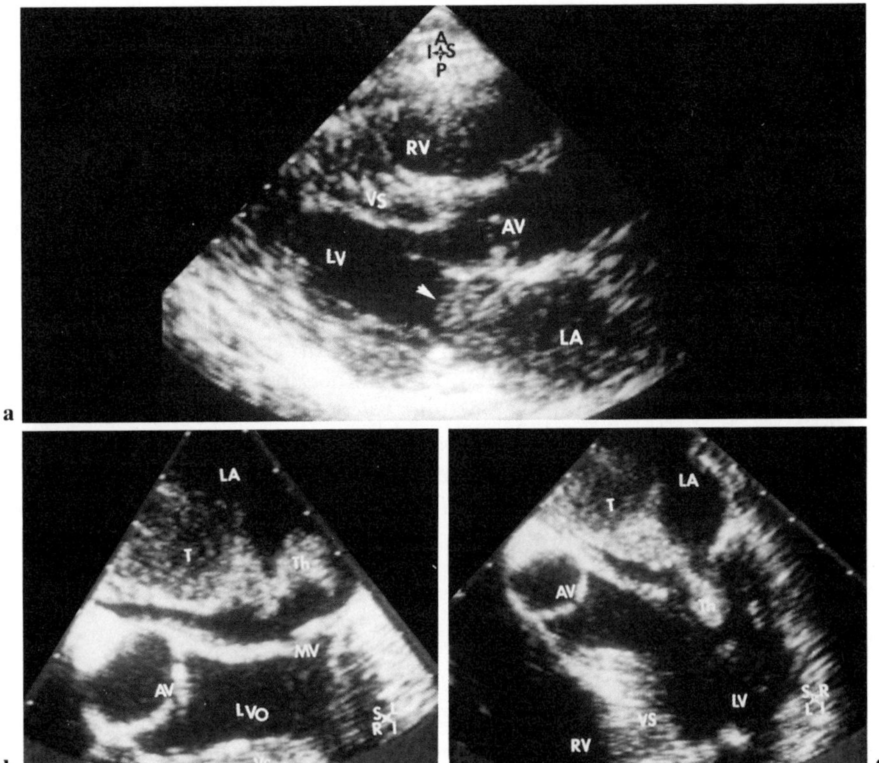

Fig. 8a–c. Left atrial melanoma (*T*). **a** Parasternal (transthoracic) long-axis view of left ventricle (*LV*) and left atrium (*LA*). Within the LA, within the mitral orifice (*arrow*) there appeared to be a mass. TEE was performed to better assess the possibility of a LA mass. **b** (systole), **c** (diastole) A large LA mass (*T*) with an attached penduculated extension (probably an attached thrombus, *Th* prolapsing through the mitral valve (*MV*) orifice. A detailed TEE revealed the tumor to be arising from the right upper pulmonary vein (not shown) consistent with a malignant tumor (subsequently proven to be a malignant melanoma). (*RV*, right ventricle; *AV*, aortic valve; *LA*, left atrium; *S*, superior; *I*, inferior; *R*, right; *L*, left)

detailed precordial echocardiographic examination. Clinical suspicion of caval syndrome had prompted TEE. In two patients with metastatic melanoma, precordial delineation of extent and cavitary impingement was poor. The fourth patient had an anterior mediastinal mass (lymphoma) with poor precordial delineation of myocardial compression. TEE clearly showed severe right ventricular and right ventricular outflow tract compression.

Conclusions

TEE is an extension of a comprehensive TTE examination. Two mass lesions, namely thrombus and atypical intracardiac or extracardiac tumors, comprised the common indications for TEE. Thrombus within the atria or atrial appendage and adjacent to refractile prostheses or endocardial wires is commonly missed or poorly delineated by a standard echocardiographic examination. Clinical suspicion is the primary referral mechanism.

Atypical, poorly delineated, infrequently encountered, infiltrating/extending, and extracardiac tumors deserve further delineation. In most circumstances, significant additional information can be obtained with TEE, often obviating further more elaborate and expensive testing. Clinical decision-making was consistently clarified by detailed TEE examination. Important advantages of TEE over TTE are the high-resolution images of cardiac cavities for tumor location and the visualization of the myocardial wall and great veins for recognition of impingement, containment, migration, and infiltration of diverse tumor types.

References

1. Seward JB, Khandheria BK, Oh JK, Hughes RW, Edward WD, Nichols BA, Freeman WK, Tajik AJ (1988) Transesophageal echocardiography: technique, anatomic correlations, implementation, and clinical applications. Mayo Clin Proc 63:649–680
2. Aschenberg W, Schuter M, Kremer P, Schroder E, Siglow V, Bleifeld W (1986) Transesophageal two-dimensional echocardiography for the detection of left atrial appendage thrombus. J Am Coll Cardiol 7:163–166
3. Hofmann T, Behroz A, Koster W, Kasper W (1987) Detection of intracardial masses by two-dimensional transesophageal echocardiography (abstract). Circulation 76 (Suppl 4):IV37
4. Daniel WG, Schroder E, Nellessen U, Hausmann D (1987) Diagnosis of intra- and extracardiac masses by echocardiography – comparison between the transthoracic and transesophageal approach (abstract). Circulation 76 (Suppl 4):IV38, 1987.

Aortic Dissection

Transesophageal Imaging of the Thoracic Aorta in Aortic Dissection*

European Cooperative Study Group for Echocardiography (R. ERBEL, H. RENNOLLET, R. ENGBERDING, C. A. VISSER, J. J. KOOLEN, W. G. DANIEL, M. TAAMS, W. JAARSMA, S. MOHR-KAHALY, W. J. GUSSENHOVEN, G. R. SUTHERLAND, J. R. T. C. ROELANDT, and J. MEYER)

Introduction

Only the combination of rapid medical and surgical therapy can improve the prognosis of aortic dissection [1]. Therefore, it is necessary that the diagnosis be established with high accuracy. In type I and II dissection (dissection of the ascending aorta) surgical treatment and in type III dissection (dissection of the descending aorta) medical treatment are recommended [1, 2].

Symptoms

In patients with aortic dissection, acute chest pain is a leading symptom. Quite often a pulse difference between the left and right arm can be detected. In about 10% of patients, neurological symptoms are most prominent. Aortic insufficiency is present in 70% of patients with type A dissection and in 10% of patients with type B. Pericardial effusion can be found in 10%, pleural effusion in 10%, and hypotension in 20% [1].

Chest X-Ray Examination

In up to 18% of patients, results of chest X ray are negative [2]. Specific signs of aortic dissection are a disparity in size between the ascending and descending aorta, a double aortic shadow, varying radiolucency, irregular contours, loss of sharpness, and displaced intimal calcification, as well as cardiac dilation and signs of pericardial effusion.

* Presented in part at the Meeting of the European Society of Cardiology, Santiago di Campostela, Spain, 1987. Supported by the Robert Müller Stiftung. In part published in [31]

Transesophageal Echocardiography
Edited by R. Erbel et al.
© Springer-Verlag Berlin Heidelberg 1989

Computed Tomography

After the first report of the detection of aortic dissection by computed tomography, published by Harris et al. [3], other authors confirmed these results [4−7]. The most important sign is the detection of an intimal flap. Contrast material injections are necessary to differentiate between true and false lumen because of different densities of the two lumina and compression deformity of the true lumen by the false lumen and delayed flow in the false lumen by dynamic scanning [6−11]. Differentiation is possible in 50% and in 50% a displaced intimal calcification can be detected [6, 9]. In most cases an aortic dilation is present. Computed tomography is able to detect pericardial effusion as well as pleural effusion. Aortic insufficiency cannot be identified. Only rarely can the location of rupture be imaged.

Echocardiography

As early as 1973, Nanda et al. [12] described the diagnosis of aortic dissection by M-mode echocardiography. In six patients dilation of the aortic root and a

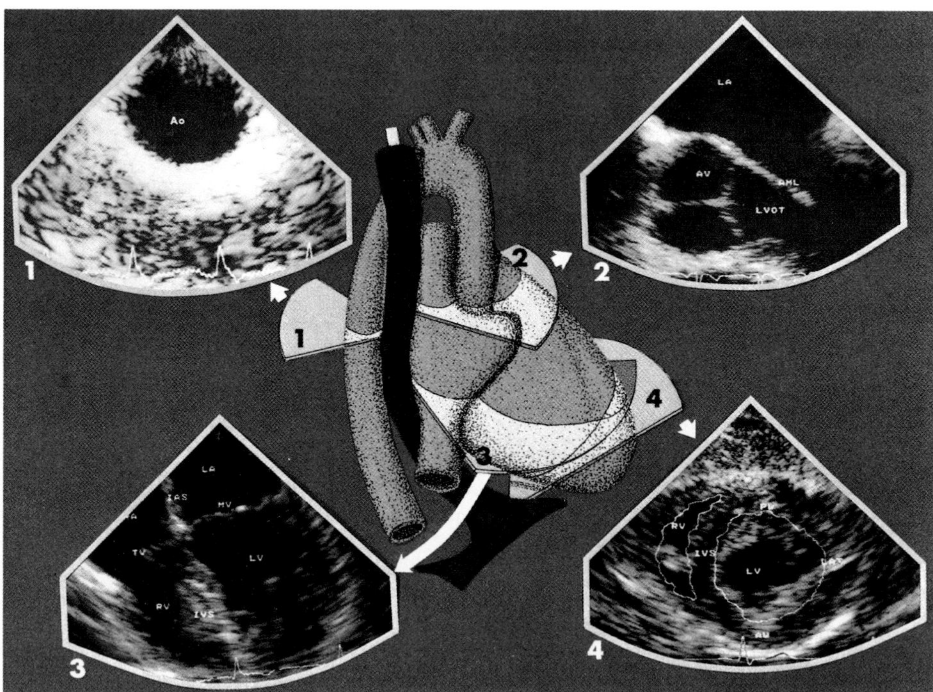

Fig. 1. Schematic drawing of the four typical transesophageal and transgastrial echocardiography scan planes for imaging the heart and the descending aorta. *Ao*, aorta descendens; *AV*, aortic valve; *LA/LV*, left atrium/ventricle; *RA/RV*, right atrium/ventricle; *MV/TV*, mitral/tricuspidal valve; *LVOT*, left ventricular outflow tract; *IVS/IAS*, intervertricular/interatrial septum

double contour of the posterior wall of the aorta were visualized. Very soon, false-positive diagnoses involving extasia of the sinus of Valsalva were published [13, 14]. Suprasternal imaging became particularly important in evaluating the aortic arch [15]. The introduction of two-dimensional echocardiography has improved the sensitivity and specificity of the method. To be able to image the whole thoracic aorta, not only parasternal and apical but also right parasternal and suprasternal subcostal views are necessary [16−23]. Specific signs of aortic dissection are aortic dilation and imaging of an intimal flap [21−23]. The limitation of transthoracic echocardiography is the reduced image quality in patients with pulmonary emphysema, obesity, and thorax deformation or on mechanical ventilation. Only in 70% of patients can the whole thoracic aorta be visualized [17, 19].

The limitations of transthoracic echocardiography were overcome by transesophageal echocardiography [24, 25] (Fig. 1). After local anesthesia, a flexible echoscope is introduced with the patient in the left lateral supine position. To avoid severe adverse gastric reactions, sedation with 10 mg diazepam or even better analgesia with 0.5 mg buprenorphin is necessary. Of course, in all patients with suspected aortic dissection antihypertensive therapy must be started immediately. The best control can be achieved by intravenous administration of nitroprusside or nifedipine.

Echotomographically the whole thoracic aorta, particularly the descending part, can be visualized similarly to computed tomographic images (Figs. 2, 3). The aortic root can also be imaged. Limitations are related to interposition of the trachea when imaging the aortic arch (Fig. 4).

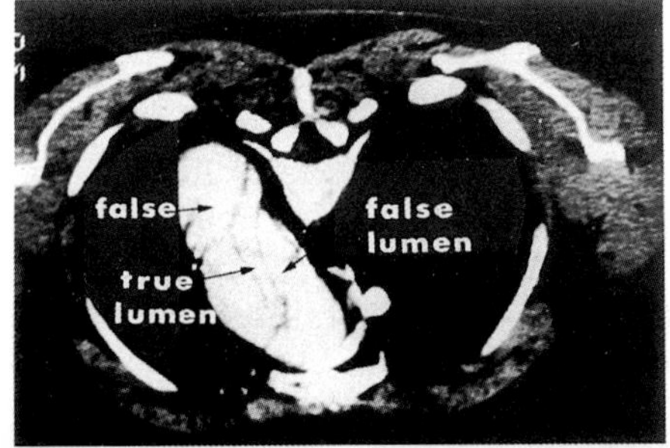

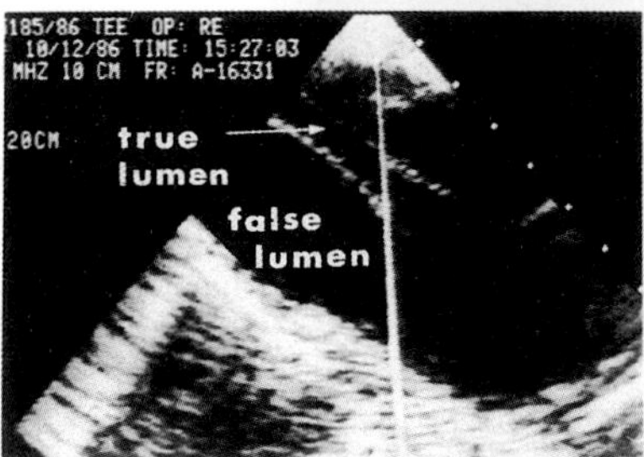

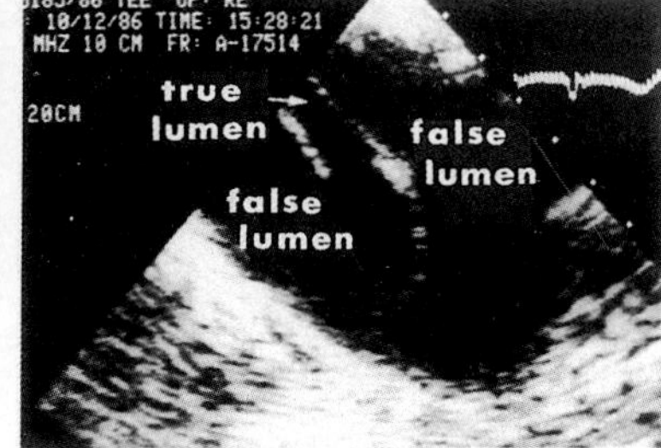

Fig. 2. Computed tomographic image (*top*) and transesophageal echocardiographic imaging (*bottom*) of type I dissection with a compressed lumen and a large false lumen. Comparison of the two techniques demonstrates the similarity in imaging the structures of the aortic arch

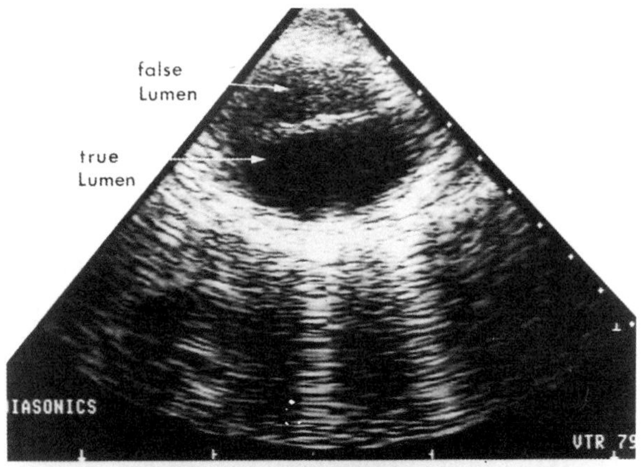

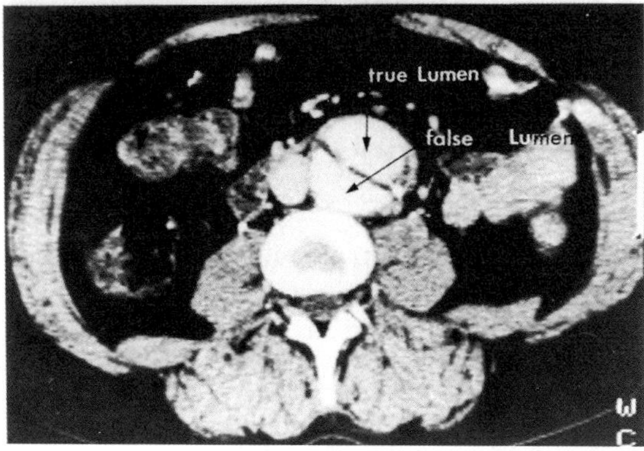

Fig. 3. Transesophageal echocardiographic image (*top*) and computed tomographic image (*bottom*) of the descending aorta illustrated in Fig. 2. With both techniques, true lumen and the false lumen are illustrated in the same way. The false lumen is close to the transducer at the esophagus

The intimal flap separates the true and false lumina. In most cases the true lumen is compressed by the false lumen. They can be differentiated: (a) The systolic enlargement of the true lumen can be detected by M-mode scanning (Fig. 5), (b) by the presence of spontaneous echocardiographic contrast in the false lumen (Fig. 6) with thrombus formation related to the reduced blood flow [26]: (c) with pulsed Doppler echocardiography by demonstration

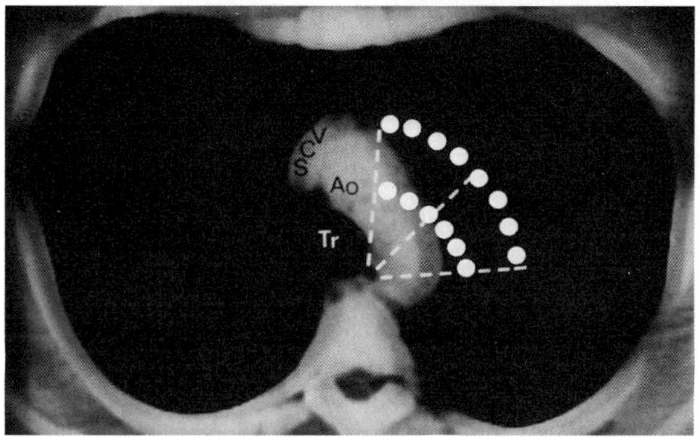

Fig. 4. Computed tomographic image with illustration of the sector scan from an transesophageal echocardiographic transducer near the air-filled trachea (T). The imaging of the entire ascending aorta and aortic arch is prevented by the air filled trachea (*Tr*). *Ao*, aorta; *SVC*, superior vena cava [25].

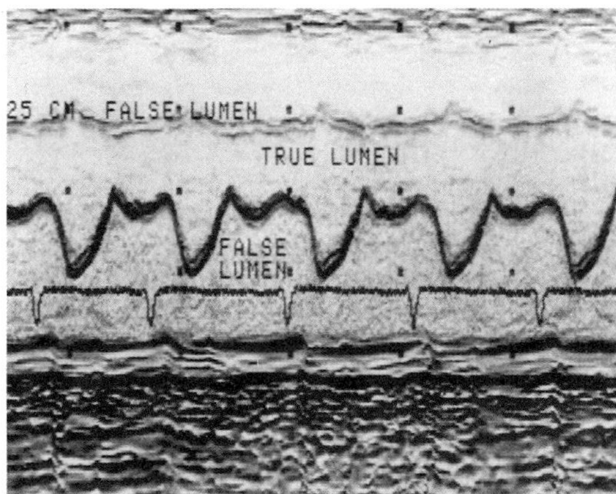

Fig. 5. Transesophageal echocardiographic scanning of the compressed true lumen with the false lumen. They can be differentiated by diameter increase during systole of the true lumen and decrease during diastole

of systolic forward flow in the true lumen and delayed flow or no flow in the false lumen (Fig. 6); and by demonstrating entry jets using color Doppler during systole at the entry tear.

It is important to determine the type of aortic dissection. Type I and II involves the ascending aorta and type III the descending aorta (Figs. 7/8). Entry tears have been detected (Fig. 7).

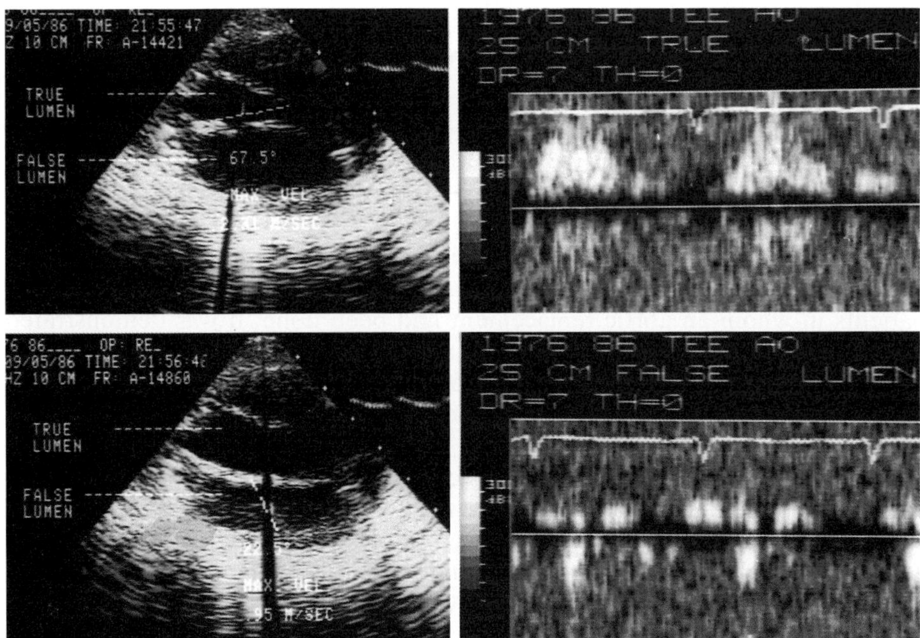

Fig. 6. Compression of the true lumen by the false lumen, which is filled with dense spontaneous echocardiographic contrast and lacks pulsed Doppler flow signals (*bottom right*), in contrast to the true lumen where there is normal systolic flow (*top right*)

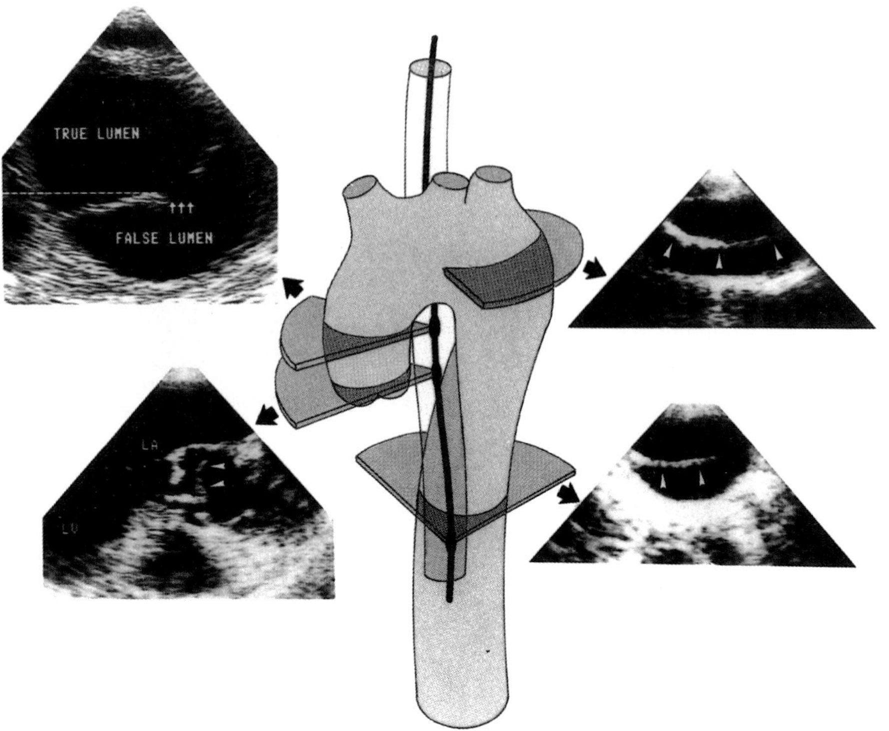

Fig. 7. Aortic dissection type I with entry tear ($\uparrow\,\uparrow\,\uparrow$) and an intimal flap (◄) in the ascending and descending aorta. *LA*, left atrium; *LV*, left ventricle [31]

Aortic dissection must be differentiated from ectasia of the aorta with or without mural thrombus formation (Fig. 9). As for computed tomography, central displacement of intimal calcification is helpful in differentiating between the two clinical entities (Fig. 10).

It is important to differentiate artifacts in the ascending aorta from true aortic dissection (Fig. 11) in order to avoid false-positive diagnoses. In five patients in whom an aortic replacement had been done, it was demonstrated that images such as that in Fig. 11 are not related to true intimal flaps. They may be due to slice thickness artifacts or reverberation. One other important differential diagnosis is aortic rupture leading to mediastinal hematoma with impression of the left atrium.

The diagnostic possibilities of echocardiography were improved by color-coded Doppler [27]. Transthoracically, the true and false lumina can be differentiated by using blood flow imaging. In particular, using transesophageal echocardiography, not only functional and morphological information but also blood flow information can now be provided for cardiac surgery [28].

Of the 164 patients with suspected aortic dissection studied in six European centers by echocardiography and one other diagnostic modality, the diagnosis was proven in 82 and excluded in 82 [31]. Type I dissection (including the ascending and descending aorta) was found in 26 patients (32%), type

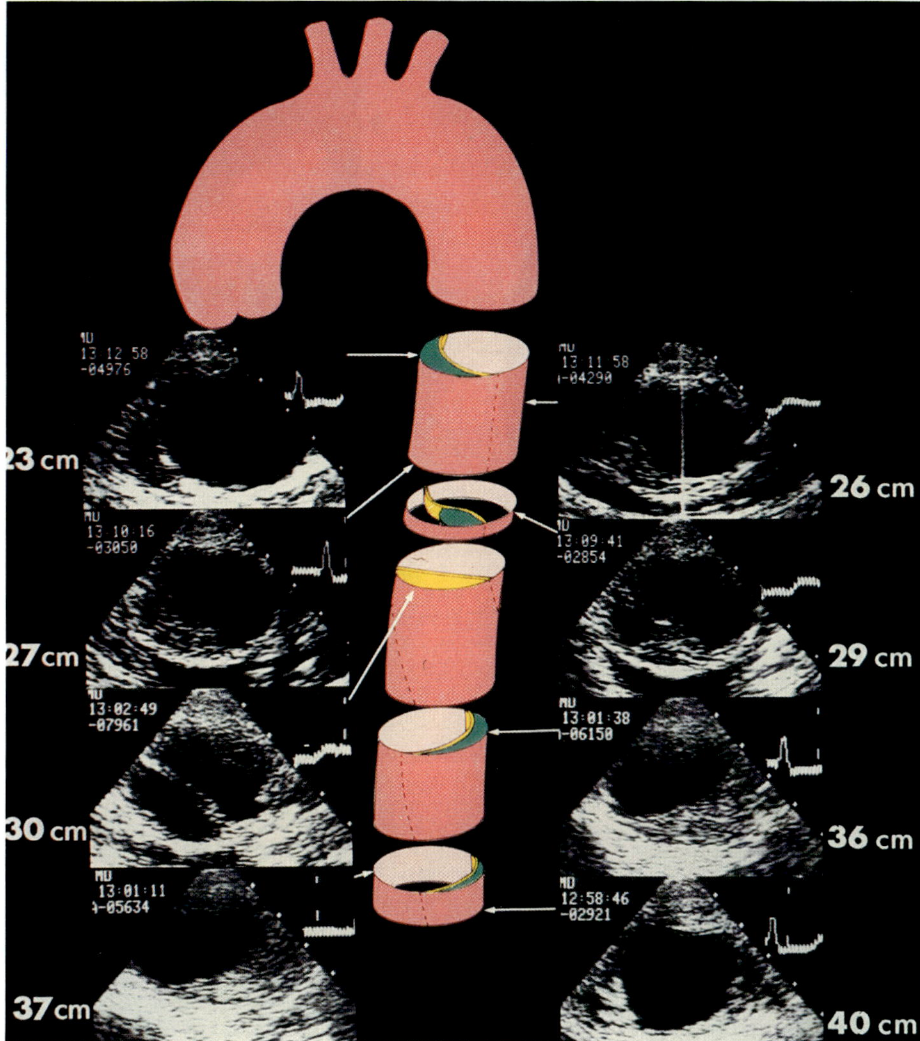

Fig. 8. Start of aortic dissection in the aortic arch in type III dissection imaged by transesophageal echocardiography. The false lumen is partly free and at 36 cm filled with thrombus

II dissection (limited to the ascending aorta) in 21 (25%), and type III dissection (including only the descending aorta) in 35 (43%). Surgery was performed in 23 of the 26 (88%) patients with type I dissection, 20 of the 21 (95%) patients with type II dissection, and 16 of the 35 (46%) patients with type III dissection. Autopsy was performed on three of 26 patients with type I dissection (9%), four of the 21 patients with type II (17%), and five of the 35 patients with type III (15%) (Fig. 12).

Emergency surgery was performed in 16 additional patients with aortic dissection type I, and in one patient with aortic ectasia for whom diagnostic pro-

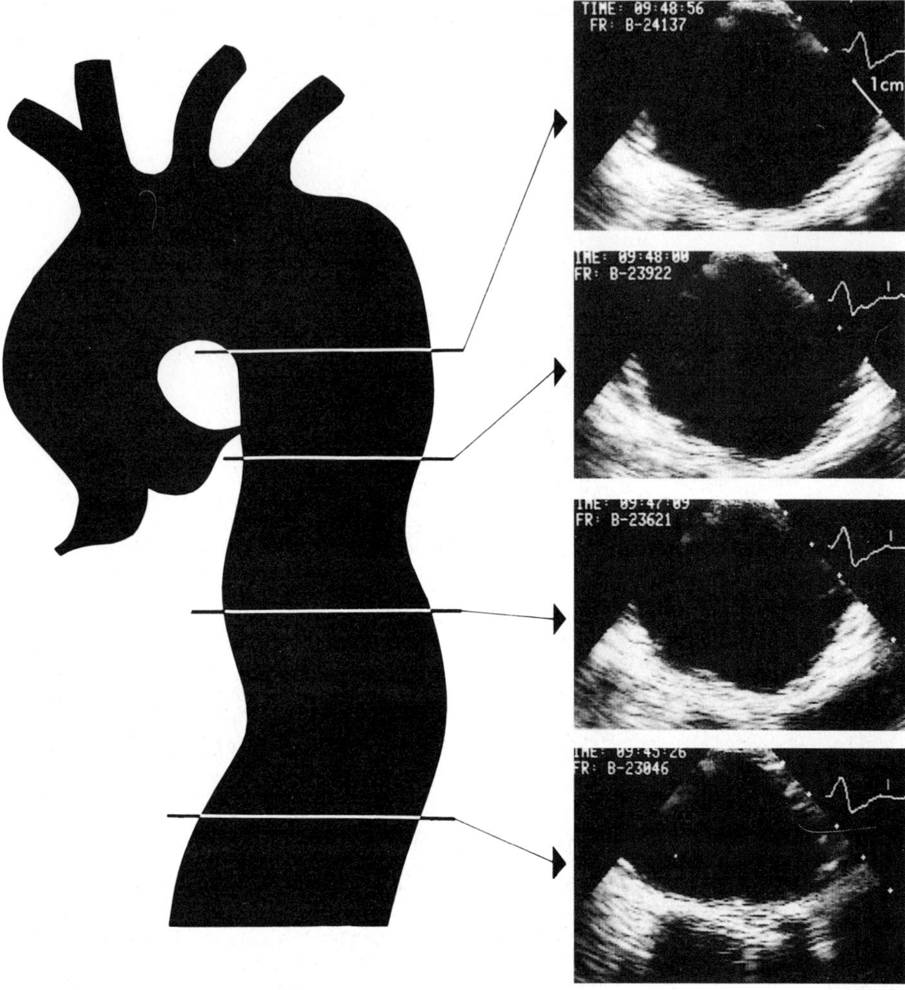

Fig. 9. Ectasia of the aorta without aortic dissection demonstrated by transesophageal echocardiography. Even plaque formations on the aortic wall are visualized

cedures other than ultrasound studies had not been carried out due to the emergency. In 11 of these 16 patients type I dissection was found, in four patients type II dissection, and in one patient type III dissection.

The results of echocardiography, computed tomography, and aortography are given in Table 1. They are listed separately where confirmed by surgery or at autopsy, and where surgery and autopsy were not performed but at least two methods were used, as well as for the whole study group. The 17 patients sent directly to surgery as a result of echocardiographic studies were excluded because computed tomography and/or angiography analyses were not performed.

Table 1. Positive and negative results of transesophageal echocardiography, computed tomography, and angiography in patients diagnosed for aortic dissection with surgery or autopsy, without surgery or autopsy, and in the total patient group

		Transesophageal echocardiography			Computed tomography			Angiography		
		+	−		+	−		+	−	
Surgery/autopsy	+	58	1		20	6		50	6	
	−	2	14		0	3		2	13	
				75			29			71
Without surgery/autopsy	+	23	0		14	1		17	3	
	−	0	66		0	41		1	34	
				89			56			55
Total study group	+	81	1		34	7		67	9	
	−	2	80		0	44		3	47	
				164			85			126

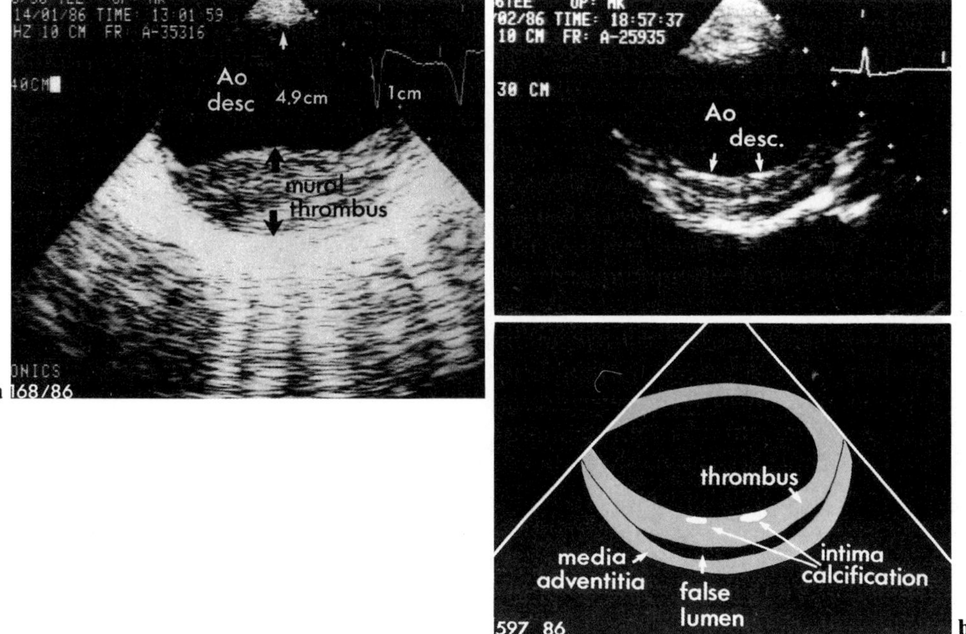

Fig. 10. a Ectasia of the aorta with thrombus formation of the lumen of the aorta. No intimal membrane, no displacement of calcification. **b** Aortic dissection type III with thrombus-filled false lumen and central displacement of calcification. During systole dividing of the different aortic wall layers can be seen. *Ao desc*, descending aorta

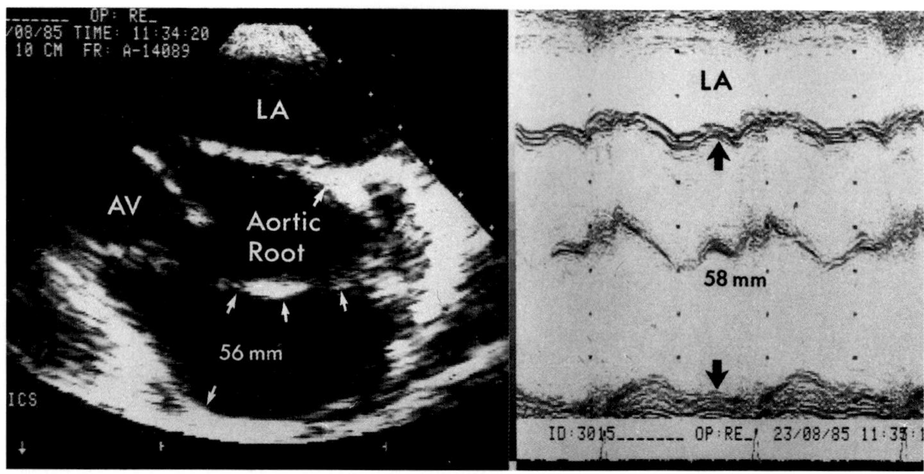

Fig. 11. Transesophageal echocardiographic image in a patient with suspected aortic dissection. In this patient ectasia of the aortic root with a free-moving structure was seen (*arrows*); this was an artifact suggesting an intimal flap, which was excluded at surgery performed because of severe regurgitation *AV*, aortic valve; *LA*, left atrium

Table 2. Results of transthoracic and transesophageal echocardiography, computed tomography, and aortography in patients with aortic dissection. Sensitivity and specificity are given for patients with surgery or autopsy, without surgery or autopsy, and in the whole study group

	Transesophageal echocardiography	Computed tomography	Angiography
Surgery/Autopsy			
Sensitivity (%)	98	77	89
Specificity (%)	88	100	87
Positive predictive accuracy (%)	97	100	96
Negative predictive accuracy (%)	93	33	68
Without surgery/autopsy			
Sensitivity (%)	100	93	85
Specificity (%)	100	100	97
Positive predictive accuracy (%)	100	100	94
Negative predictive accuracy (%)	100	98	92
Total study group			
Sensitivity (%)	99	83	88
Specificity (%)	98	100	94
Positive predictive accuracy (%)	98	100	96
Negative predictive accuracy (%)	99	86	84

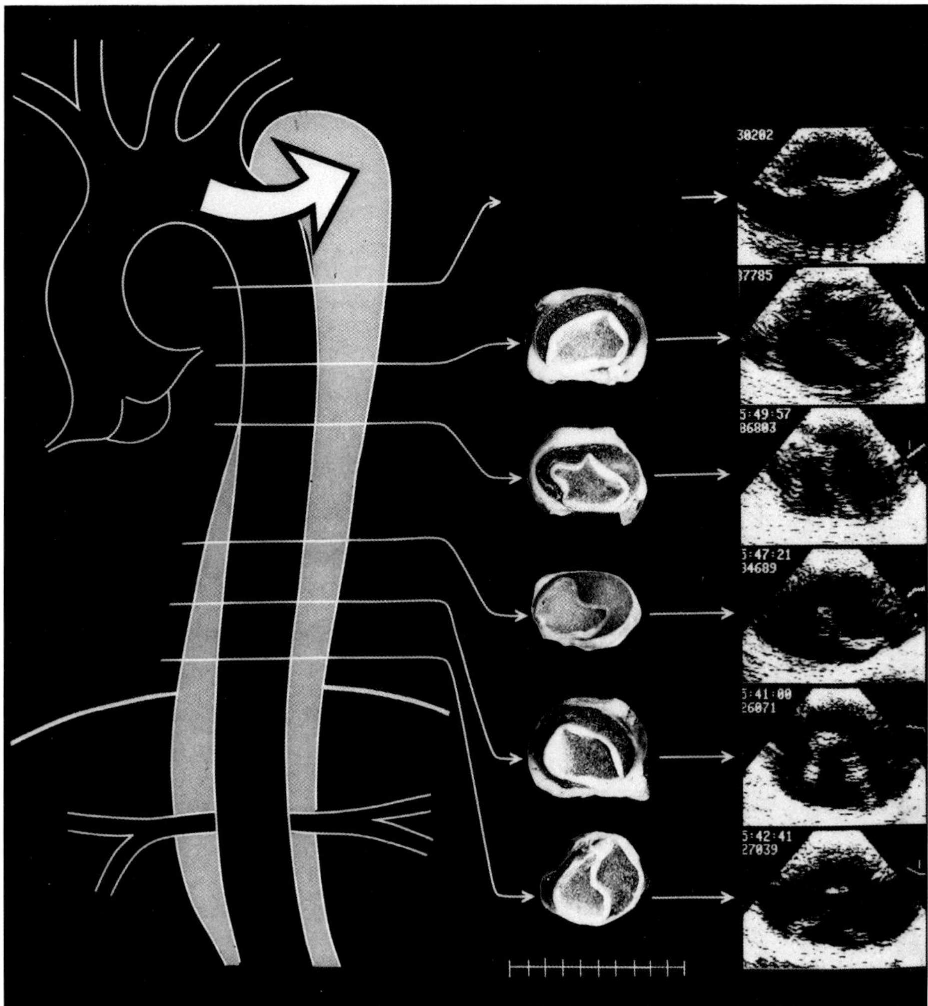

Fig. 12. Transesophageal echocardiographic imaging of the descending aorta, demonstrating an intimal flap in the lumen of the aorta also seen at necropsy. Surgery was not possible

With echocardiography, only one false − negative result occurred; this was in a patient with type II dissection which, retrospectively, was correctly recognized on the scan. Angiography also failed to identify the dissection in this case. The localized dissection of the aortic root was identified during surgery for severe aortic insufficiency and ectasin of aorta.

Computed tomography was performed in 85 patients, of whom 29 underwent surgery. There were seven false − negative diagnoses, in four cases of type I dissection and in three cases of type II dissection.

Angiography was performed in 126 patients, of whom 71 underwent surgery. The method did not demonstrate the dissection in one patient with

Table 3. Detection of intimal tears, intraluminal thrombus formation, pericardial effusion, and aortic insufficiency in patients with aortic dissections of types I, II, and III for transesophageal echocardiography (echo), computed tomography (CT), and aortography (angio)

	Type I						Type II						Type III					
	Echo ($n = 26$)		CT ($n = 12$)		Angio ($n = 25$)		Echo ($n = 21$)		CT ($n = 20$)		Angio ($n = 11$)		Echo ($n = 35$)		CT ($n = 31$)		Angio ($n = 18$)	
	n	%	n	%	n	%	n	%	n	%	n	%	n	%	n	%	n	%
Intimal tear	14	54	–		10	40	9	43	–		10	90	10	29	–		1	3
Intraluminal thrombus	7	27	0		0		6	29	4	36	0		26	74	13	42	5	28
Pericardial effusion	3	12	2	17	–		6	29	2	18	–		1	3	1	6	–	
Aortic insufficiency	12	46	–		10	40	14	67	–		10	90	2	6	–		1	3

Table 4. Comparison of transesophageal echocardiography in angiography in regard to the success in detecting entry tears and aortic insufficiency and with computed tomography with regard to the success in demonstrating intraluminal thrombus formation and pericardial effusion

		Angiography					Computed Tomography				
		Entry tear			Aortic; insufficiency			Intraluminal thrombus			Pericardial effusion		
		+	−		+	−		+	−		+	−	
Transesophageal echocardiography	+	19	16	35	20	8	28	15	2	17	4	6	10
	−	6	35	41	1	47	48	10	14	24	1	30	31
		25	51	76	21	55	76	25	16	41	5	36	41

type I dissection, in four patients with type II, and in four patients with type III. In three patients a false − positive diagnosis of type II dissection was made by angiography.

For the diagnoses before surgery, which were only regarded accurate if positive results were obtained with at least two methods, the overall negative sensitivity measured 96%, specificity 93%, and positive and negative predictive accuracy 98% and 87% respectively. Aortic dissection was not detected by computed tomography or angiography in any patient in whom results of echocardiography were negative. Analysis of the results for the total patient group shows the sensitivity of echocardiography, when the transesophageal approach is used, to be 99%, with a specificity of 98%, a positive predictive accuracy of 98%, and a negative predictive accuracy of 99% (Table 2).

Results concerning the detection of intimal tears, intraluminal thrombus formation, pericardial effusion, and aortic insufficiency are given in Tables 3 and 4. Aortic insufficiency was present in 84 patients. Wall motion abnormalities were found in three of the 82 (4%) patients with aortic dissection, but only in cases of type I dissection. No serious complications of transesophageal echocardiography were noted.

The accuracy of echocardiography, completed by transesophageal echocardiography and sonography, has reached such a level that nowadays surgery can be performed based only on this method [29, 30−32]. In all cases where a diagnosis is not established and in patients where coronary artery disease is suspected, angiography and coronary angiography are performed.

References

1. Doroghazi RM, Slater EE (1983) Aortic dissection. McGraw-Hill, New York
2. Earnest F, Muhm JR, Sheedy PF (1979) Roentgenographic findings in thoracic aortic dissection. Mayo Clin Proc 54:43−50
3. Harris RD, Usselman JA, Vint VC, Warmath MA (1979) Computerized tomographic diagnosis of aneurysms of the thoracic aorta. J Comput Assist Tomogr 3:81−91

4. Sanders JH, Malave S, Nieman HL, Moran JM, Roberts AJ, Michaelis LL (1979) Thoracic aortic imaging without angiography. Arch Surg 114:1326−1329
5. Suchato C, Pekanan P, Singjaroen T, Sereerat P (1980) Indication of dissecting aortic aneurysm on noncontrast computed tomography. J Comput Assist Tomogr 4:115−116
6. Heiberg E, Wolverson M, Sundaram M, Conners J, Susman N (1981) CT findings in thoracic aortic dissection. AJR 136:13−17
7. Lardé D, Bellor C, Vasile N, Frija J, Ferrané J (1980) Computed tomography in dissection of the thoracic aorta. Radiology 136:147−151
8. Godwin JD, Herfkens RL, Skiöldebrand CG, Ferderle MP. Lipton MJ (1980) Evaluation of dissections and aneurysms of the thoracic aorta by conventional and dynamic CT scanning. Radiology 136:125−133
9. Gross SC, Barr I, Eyler WR, Khaja F, Goldstein S (1980) Computed tomography in dissection of the thoracic aorta. Radiology 136:135−141
10. Moncada R, Churchill R, Reynes C, Gunnar RM, Salines M, Love L, Demos TC, Pifarre R (1981) Diagnosis of dissecting aortic aneurysm by computed tomography. Lancet 1:238−241
11. Egan TJ, Nieman H, Herman RJ, Malve SR, Sanders JH (1980) Computed tomography in the diagnosis of aortic aneurysm, dissection or traumatic injury. Radiology 136:141−146
12. Nanda NC, Gramiak R, Shah P (1973) Diagnosis of aortic root dissection by echocardiography. Circulation 48:506−513
13. Krueger SK, Starke H, Forker AD, Eliot RS (1975) Echocardiographic mimics of aortic root dissection. Chest 67:441−444
14. Hirschfeld DS, Rodriguez HJ, Schiller NB (1976) Duplication of aortic wall seen by echocardiography. Br Heart J 38:949−950
15. Kasper W, Meinertz T, Kersting F, Lang K, Just H (1978) Diagnosis of dissecting aortic aneurysm with suprasternal echocardiography. Am J Cardiol 42:291−294
16. Schweizer P, Erbel R, Lambertz H, Effert S (1981) Two-dimensional suprasternal echocardiography in dissection of the thoracic aorta. In: Rijsterburgh H (ed) Echocardiology. Nijhoff, The Hague, pp 55−60
17. Iliceto S, Ettorre G, Francioso G, Antonelli G, Biasco G, Rizzon P (1984) Diagnosis of aneurysm of the thoracic aorta. Comparison between two noninvasive techniques: two-dimensional echocardiography and computed tomography. Eur Heart J 5:545−555
18. Mintz GS, Kotler MN, Segal BL, Parry WR (1979) Two-dimensional echocardiographic recognition of the descending thoracic aorta. Am J Cardiol 44:232−238
19. Bubenheimer P, Schmuziger M, Roskamm H (1980) Ein- und zweidimensionale Echokardiographie bei Aneurysmen und Dissektionen der Aorta. Herz 5:226−240
20. Victor MF, Mintz GS, Kotler MN, Wilson AR, Segal BL (1981) Two-dimensional echocardiographic diagnosis of aortic dissection. Am J Cardiol 48:1155−1159
21. Roudaut R, Billes MA, Gateau P, Besse P, Dallocchio M (1981) Two-dimensional echocardiography in the diagnosis of aortic dissection in 41 patients (Abstr). Circulation [Suppl 4] 64:314
22. Nakamura K, Suzuki S, Satomi G, Adachi F, Hirosawa K, Takao A, Hashimoto A, Toluyasu Y, Kusakabe K, Yamazaki T, Shigeta A (1981) Two-dimensional echocardiographic and angiographic features of aneurysm of the ascending aorta in patients with annuloaortic ectasia. J Cardiogr 11:239−252
23. Bubenheimer P (1981) Fortschritte in der Diagnose der Aortendissektion durch TM- und 2D-Echokardiographie. Cardiology [Suppl 1] 68:66−74
24. Börner N, Erbel R, Braun B, Henkel B, Meyer J, Rumpelt J (1984) Diagnosis of aortic dissection by transesophageal echocardiography. Am J Cardiol 54:1157−1158
25. Erbel R, Börner N, Steller D, Brunier J, Thelen M, Pfeiffer C, Mohr-Kahaly S, Meyer J (1987) Detection of aortic dissection by transoesophageal echocardiography. Br Heart J 58:45−51
26. Stern H, Erbel R, Börner N, Schreiner G, Meyer J (1985) Spontaner Echokontrast. registriert mittels transösophagealer Echokardiographie bei Aortendissektion Typ III. Z Kardiol 74:480−481

27. Mohr-Kahaly S, Erbel R, Börner N, Drexler M, Wittlich N, Iversen S, Oelert H, Meyer J (1986) Kombination von Farb-Doppler und transösophagealer Echokardiographie in der Notfalldiagnostik bei Aortendissektionen vom Typ I. Z Kardiol 75:616−620
28. Takamoto S, Kyo S, Matsumara M, Hojo H, Yokote Y, Omoto R (1986) Total visualization of thoracic dissecting aortic aneurysm by transesophageal Doppler color flow mapping. Circulation [Suppl 2] 74:132
29. Erbel R, Mohr-Kahaly S, Brunier J, Rennollet H, Wittlich N, Drexler M, Iversen S, Oelert H, Thelen M, Meyer J (1987) Stellenwert der transthorakalen und transösophagealen Echokardiographie in der präoperativen Diagnostik der Aortendissektion. Thorac Cardiovasc Surg [Suppl 1] 1:23
30. Lass J, Schlüter G, Haverist A, Daniel W, Hendricks P, Borst HG (1987) Präoperative Diagnostik bei akuter Aortendissektion Typ A. Thorac Cardiovasc Surg [Suppl 1] 35:22
31. Erbel R, Rennollet H, Engberding R, Visser C, Daniel W, Roelandt J (European Cooperative Study Group for Echocardiography) (1989) Complementary role of echocardiography in the diagnosis of aortic dissection including transesophageal echocardiography. Lancet I:457−461
32. Taams MA, Gussenhoven WJ, Schippers LA, Roelandt J, van Herwerden LA, Bos E, de Jong N, Bom N (1988) The value of transesophageal echocardiography for diagnosis of thoracic aorta pathology. Eur Heart 29:1308−1316

Diagnosis of Dissecting Aortic Aneurysm by Transesophageal Color Flow Mapping: Comparison with CT Scanning*

S. Takamoto, H. Hojo, H. Adachi, K. Neya, S. Kyo, Y. Yokote, and R. Omoto

Introduction

Dissecting aortic aneurysm is a severe disease which involves a wide region of the aorta and its branches. Although several echocardiographic approaches have been tried and reported [1−3], due to limited echo beam penetration through the chest or abdominal wall only a part of the lesion is visualized. In 1984 Börner et al. [4] first reported a transesophageal approach to aortic dissection. In 1986 we [5] first reported the use of transesophageal echo (TEE) color flow mapping for this complex disorder and its chinical usefulness in accurately diagnosing it. Although computer tomography (CT) is a major noninvasive diagnostic measure in this disease [6], precise comparisons between these two modalities as yet have not been made. In this study we evaluated the clinical significance of transesophageal color flow mapping in diagnosis of dissecting aortic aneurysm, comparing it with CT.

Materials and Methods

Twenty-six cases, 16 men and 10 women, were examined and diagnosed by both TEE color flow mapping and CT scanning (enhanced, dynamic). The mean age was 57.5 ± 15.2 years. The final diagnoses were made from aortographic or operative findings. There were four cases of DeBakey type I, two of type II, 17 of type III, and three of type III with retrograde extension (III-R).

The color flow mapping systems used were Aloka 860, 870, and 340. Esophageal transducers used were 5 MHz and they were incorporated at the tip of a fiber, the diameter of which was 9 mm. In all cases transverse TEE scanning with a sector-type transducer was performed. In ten cases longitudinal TEE scanning with a convex-type transducer was performed, especially in the aortic arch region. In one of these cases, biplanar TEE was done using a special probe with two sector-type transducers scanning in different direction.

CT scanning was done with a third-generation scanner, usually a Yokokawa CT-8600. Enhanced CT was done in eight cases and dynamic and enhanced CT were done in 18 cases.

---

* This study was supported by grants from the Japan Heart Foundation in 1986, the Mitsui Life Social Welfare Foundation in 1987, and the Japan Medical Association in 1987

Transesophageal Echocardiography
Edited by R. Erbel et al.
© Springer-Verlag Berlin Heidelberg 1989

Results

Diagnosis of Dissection

With TEE, dissection was correctly diagnosed in all cases (100%), but with CT, dissection was diagnosed in 22 out of 26 cases (84.6%). Four cases were diagnosed by CT as true aneurysms (one of type I, two of type II, and one of type III). Two of these cases were not diagnosed correctly even using dynamic CT.

Identification of Initial Entry

Using TEE, the initial entry was identified in 23 cases (88.5%) but in three cases (11.5%) (one each of types I, II, and III-R) it was not identified. On the other hand, CT could not identify a single initial entry (0%).

Differentiation of True and False Lumina

With TEE, differentiation of true and false lumina was possible in 25 cases (96.1%). In 23 cases which were diagnosed as dissection using CT it was possible to differentiate true and false lumina.

Thrombus Formation in the False Lumen

Thrombus formation in the false lumen was evaluated by both methods in all cases. Precise evaluation of the state of thrombus formation in the false lumen was also possible. Five cases had complete thrombus formation in the false lumen, 13 cases had partial thrombus formation, and in eight cases there was no thrombus formation.

Dissection of Aortic Arch Vessels

Longitudinal TEE scanning performed in ten cases was effective in displaying the arch and the arch vessels and in evaluating the extent of dissection in those regions. In particular, the arch vessels were displayed longitudinally at their roots.

In five cases arch vessels were involved in the dissection, and this was visualized by TEE. In another five cases the arch vessels were not involved in the dissection, and this was also correctly interpreted using TEE. CT examination gave no clues regarding arch vessels.

Evaluation of Aortic Regurgitation

TEE was effective in evaluating and grading the severity of aortic regurgitation in all cases of dissection of the aorta. Of twenty-six cases of aortal dissection examined for aortic regurgitation, three had grade III, five had grade II,
two had grade I, and 16 had grade 0 aortic regurgitation. CT gave no clues
about aortic regurgitation.

Identification of Reentry

Reentry was visualized in only four cases using TEE. Of these reentries, two
were in the aortic arch, one was in the descending aorta, and one was in the
upper abdominal aorta. In the other cases, there was either no reentry or one
in the lower abdominal aorta. CT did gave no information on this point.

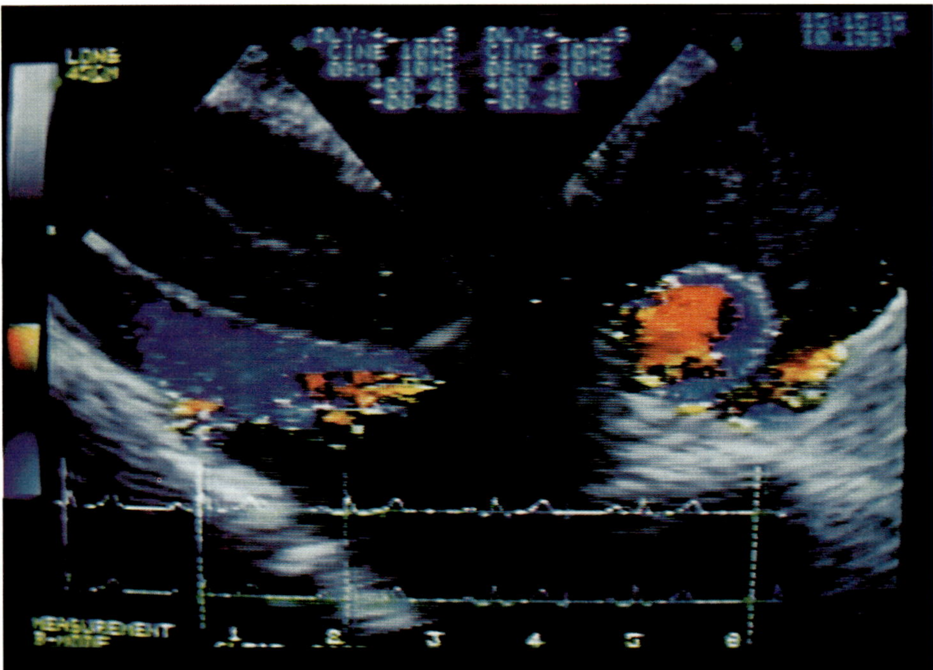

Fig. 1. Biplanar TEE images of the entry at the descending aorta in a case of type III dissecting aortic aneurysm. *Right*, longitudinal scanning; *left*, transverse scanning. The true
lumen is displayed in color and false lumen is displayed in noncolor by a faint white moving
echo. At the bottom of the true lumen is the entry, and the jet flow through it is displayed.
Thus, biplanar TEE allows three-dimensional understanding of the structure and the flow
dynamics

DeBakey's Type Differentiation

Using TEE, in 25 cases (96.1%), correct diagnosis of DeBakey's type was made and in only one case was there misdiagnosis. This was a case of type III-R (confirmed in the surgery) misdiagnosed as type I because the initial entry was not detected. Upon close examination of the video tape recorded material, we could detect the entry in the proximal descending aorta which we missed in the initial examination.

Using CT, a correct diagnosis was made in 17 cases (65.3%) and nine cases (34.7%) were misdiagnosed. Two cases of type I, two of type II, three of type

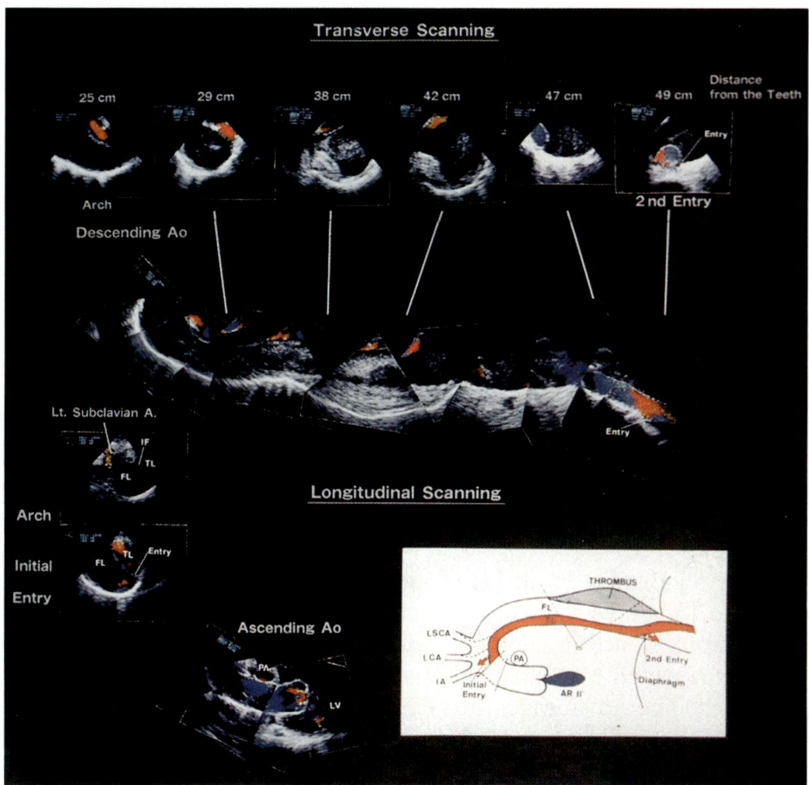

Fig. 2. Serial transverse and longitudinal TEE scans of the same patient as in Fig. 1. The *upper* parts of the figure show serial transverse scans of the descending aorta and the *middle* and the *lower* parts show serial longitudinal scans of the descending aorta (*middle*), the arch (*left part*) and the ascending aorta (*lower part*). The initial entry was at the proximal arch, which is visualized by longitudinal scanning but not by transverse scanning. The arch vessel is displayed in a longitudinal fashion by longitudinal scanning. The ascending and descending aorta are displayed longitudinally, as in aortography. In the descending aorta the true lumen is indicated by colored fast flow, the false lumen is indicated by a slow-moving echo and the thrombus. The second entry is shown at the descending aorta at 49 cm distance from the teeth. *TL*, True lumen; *FL*, false lumen; *IF*, intimal flap

III-R, and two of type III were misdiagnosed by CT examination. Thus, seven cases where there was dissection in the ascending aorta were not diagnosed by CT.

Biplanar TEE

Biplanar TEE displayed the flow through the entry in two scanning directions, transverse and longitudinal, as shown in Fig. 1. The biplanar images allowed three-dimensional understanding of the structure and the flow dynamics. Longitudinal and transverse scans were done separately. Serial images from longitudinal scanning were almost compatible with the aortographical images and transverse images were compatible with those of CT (Fig. 2).

Discussion

Before TEE was available for clinical use, transcutaneous echo studies revealed only parts of the aorta, and magnetic resonance imaging (MRI) was expensive and time consuming [7]. Thus, CT was a major method of noninvasive examination for confirming diagnosis of dissecting aortic aneurysm [6]. CT was found to have advantages in displaying intimal calcification, mural thrombus, and the relationship of the aorta to the adjacent organs. However, it requires contrast medium, scanning planes are limited, especially in dynamic scanning, and precise flow dynamics are not demonstrated. In addition, a strong artifact signal due to the central venous line and other factors may interfere with interpretation. Therefore, despite the earnest desire to avoid invasive aortography in acute dissection of the aorta, CT was not able to replace aortography, which is accepted as the gold standard especially prior to surgery.

In 1984 Börner et al. [4] reported on TEE and its clinical application, and then we [5, 8, 9] reported the clinical significance of transesophageal color flow mapping in thoracic aortic dissection. TEE displayed the whole descending aorta, which had not been visualized using the conventional transthoracic approach. The advantages of TEE are that it is noninvasive, there is no need for contrast medium, and it can display scans in many different sections. TEE color flow mapping can also display the smallest flow through even a tiny entry tear. In this study we evaluated the clinical significance of TEE color flow mapping compared to that of CT.

Our study showed that although CT displays mural thrombus and differentiates true and false lumina well, it cannot display and assess precisely hemodynamic disturbances such as aortic regurgitation, entry, and reentry.

On the other hand TEE color flow mapping can show even the smallest hemodynamic alteration in dissection. Initial entry was detected in 88.5% of the patients. In only three patients (one each with type I, II, and III-R), was the initial entry not identified. The patient with type I had an entry in the upper portion of the ascending aorta which could not be visualized by TEE because of echo beam interruption due to the bronchus intervening between the aorta and the esophagus. This initial entry could be shown using the transthoracic approach. In next patient, with type II, it was also not visualized by TEE for the same reason. Although this initial entry has not visualized by the transthoracic approach either, classification according to DeBakey was possible from the associated findings. The third patient, with type III-R, had an entry in the proximal portion of the descending aorta: TEE had displayes it, but it was overlooked at the time.

Diagnosis of dissection was based on the existence of an intimal flap or double channels in the aorta. With TEE we could accurately diagnose dissection in all cases, whereas CT allowed accurate diagnosis in only 22 out of 26 patients (84.6%). Four patients (one with type I, two with type II, and one with type III) were not diagnosed correctly. In three of the patients, the dissection involved the ascending aorta, where the intimal flap was moving very rapidly. Difficulty in visualizing the moving intimal flap with CT and the limitation of the scanning section in dynamic CT might be the reason that CT failed to diagnose these as dissection, especially in the case where the dissection involved the ascending aorta.

DeBakey's classification was done, based on the site of the entry and the associated findings. With TEE, 25 cases (96.1%) out of 26 were diagnosed correctly. Only one case, of type III-R, was misdiagnosed as type I, because we overlooked the entry. With CT, only 17 cases (65.3%) out of 26 were diagnosed accurately. CT is also not so good in determining the DeBakey classification in dissections of the ascending aorta.

We performed longitudinal TEE scanning with a convex-type transducer and a sector-type biplanar (transverse and longitudinal scanning) transducer. This longitudinal TEE scanning was especially useful in displaying the arch and the arch vessels. Longitudinal TEE scanning displays the cross-sectional view of the arch and the longitudinal view of the arch vessels (Fig. 2). Transverse TEE scanning displays the longitudinal view of the arch and the cross-sectional view of the arch vessels. Comparing the two, longitudinal scanning is far better than transverse scanning for evaluating involvement of the arch vessels in the dissection. The sector-type longitudinal scanning in the biplanar TEE is also useful to display the upper ascending aorta, as this is interrupted by the intervening bronchus in normal transverse scanning, because sector-type longitudinal scanning can display the rear side of the bronchus in the same way that transthoracic sector scanning can display the rear side of ribs.

In one case, the initial entry was thought to exist at the proximal arch but was not displayed by regular transverse scanning (Fig. 2). However, longitudinal scanning using the sector transducer could display the entry. This shows that longitudinal TEE scanning can display a wider area of the asending aorta and the aortic arch, with a much narrower blind spot.

The weak points of TEE were the upper ascending aorta, the arch vessels, the abdominal aorta, and its branches. With the aid of longitudinal TEE scanning the first two were visualized, and transcutaneous color flow mapping could display the ascending aorta, the arch vessels, the abdominal aorta, and its branches. These transcutaneous echography findings may complement TEE diagnosis.

Although transcutaneous color flow mapping supplies echo images of these areas with poor resolution due to the bone or air in the intestine, direct intraoperative scanning is very helpful [10]. In this sense, images of the whole aorta could be obtained by a combination of transesophageal, transcutaneous and intraoperative direct scanning.

Even if Goldman et al. [7] reported that it is possible to avoid aortography in surgical treatment of aortic dissection by using echo Doppler, magnetic resonance imaging (MRI), and CT, we suggested that it is very likely that aortography could be bypassed in acute dissection by using the three modalities of color flow mapping [8]. Imaging of the whole of the aorta should lead to selection of the proper operative procedure and good results. With its three echo modalities, TEE color flow mapping is the most powerful diagnostic tool.

In conclusion: (1) TEE color flow mapping is an accurate and powerful diagnostic measure in dissecting aortic aneurysm which permits precise evaluation of the flow and the structure in the dissected aorta in the thorax. (2) Extension of dissection to the arch vessels can be displayed by longitudinal TEE scanning. (3) Biplanar TEE allows three-dimensional understanding of the dissected aorta. (4) CT scanning is good at displaying thrombus formation in the aorta, but precise evaluation of the hemodynamics and structure of the dissection is not possible.

References

1. Millward DK, et al. (1972) Dissecting aortic aneurysm diagnosed by echocardiography in a patient with rupture of the aneurysm into the right atrium. Am J Cardiol 30:427
2. Nanda NC, et al. (1973) Diagnosis of aortic root dissection by echocardiography. Circulation 48:506
3. Matsumoto M, et al. (1978) A two-dimensional echoaortocardiographic approach to dissecting aneurysm of the aorta to prevent false-positive diagnoses. Radiology 127:491
4. Börner N, et al. (1984) Diagnosis of aortic dissection by transesophageal echocardiography. Am J Cardiol 54:1157
5. Takamoto S (1986) Total visualization of thoracic dissecting aortic aneurysm by transesophageal Doppler color flow mapping. Circulation [Suppl 2] 74:132
6. Moncada R, et al. (1981) Diagnosis of dissecting aortic aneurysm by computed tomography. Lancet 1:238
7. Goldman AP, et al. (1986) The complementary role of magnetic resonance imaging, Doppler echocardiography, and computed tomography in the diagnosis of dissecting thoracic aneurysms. Am Heart J 111:970
8. Takamoto S (1987) Diseases of the aorta and the peripheral vessels. In: Omoto R (ed) Color atlas of real-time two-dimensional Doppler echocardiography, 2nd edn. Shindan-to-Chiryo, Tokyo
9. Takamoto S, Omoto R (1987) Visualization of thoracic dissecting aortic aneurysm by transesophageal Doppler color flow mapping. Herz 12:187
10. Takamoto S, et al. (1985) Intraoperative color flow mapping by real-time two-dimensional Doppler echocardiography for evaluation of valvular and congenital and vascular disease. J Thorac Cardiovasc Surg 90:802

Follow-up of Aortic Dissection by Conventional and Transesophageal Echocardiography: A Cooperative Study

R. ENGBERDING, R. ERBEL, W. G. DANIEL, and S. MOHR-KAHALY

The combination of conventional and transesophageal two-dimensional echocardiography proved a safe and feasible method for diagnosis of thoracic aortic dissection [1−4]. A multicenter study on a total of 164 patients revealed a sensitivity and specificity of the transesophageal technique of 98% and 88% [5]. Especially details such as entry tears, intraluminal thrombus, pericardial effusion, and aortic insufficiency could be better identified by echocardiography than by computed tomography and angiography.

As acute aortic dissection is an emergency, diagnosis is required urgently. The combination of conventional and transesophageal echocardiography may be regarded as the method of choice in the diagnosis of aortic dissection, as it can be performed rapidly at the bedside and it does not require intravenous injection of contrast agent in these patients, who may have compromised renal perfusion [6].

Surgical treatment of this disease can consist in replacement or reconstruction of an aortic segment, with or without aortic valve replacement or reconstruction. Initial echocardiographic observations after the repair of aortic dissection showed persistence of the false lumen postoperatively [7].

This study contains the results of a follow-up study of surgically or medically treated aortic dissection, collected in the centers of Hannover, Mainz, and Münster.

Methods

The study group consisted of 44 patients (31 men, 13 women; mean age 48.1 years) with surgically or angiographically confirmed dissection of the thoracic aorta who underwent a follow-up using conventional and transesophageal echocardiography. Twenty-eight patients received surgical, and 16 patients medical treatment. In 20 of the 28 surgically treated patients a type I dissection was present, in five a type II dissection, and in three a type III dissection. Sixteen patients received medical treatment. In 14 of these patients a type III dissection and in one patient each a type I and a type II dissection were present (Table 1). The follow-up period varied from 12 days to 50 months (mean 12.2 months).

Echocardiography was performed using a Hewlett Packard, Toshiba, or Diasonics conventional and transesophageal device. Transesophageal transducers with 3.5, 3.75, and 5.0 MHz and conventional transducers with 2.25 and

Transesophageal Echocardiography
Edited by R. Erbel et al.
© Springer-Verlag Berlin Heidelberg 1989

Table 1. Classification and echocardiographic identification of persisting false lumen in surgically or medically treated aortic dissections ($n = 44$)

	No. of patients	Persisting false lumen
Surgery	28	
Type I	20	17
Type II	5	0
Type III	3	2
Medical treatment	16	
Type I	1	1
Type II	1	0
Type III	14	12

3.5 MHz were used. Conventional views were attempted from all parasternal, suprasternal, apical, and subcostal transducer positions.

Results

Five of 20 patients treated surgically underwent reconstruction of the ascending aorta and the aortic valve. Three patients received replacement of the ascending aorta and aortic valve reconstruction, whereas 12 patients underwent replacement of the ascending aorta and aortic valve. An intimal flap was detected in the ascending aorta in two cases, and in the descending aorta in 13 patients. In two cases an intimal flap was observed in both the ascending and descending aorta (Table 2).

Six of the 20 surgically treated patients with type I dissection showed thrombus formation. In three patients the thrombus was localized, whereas in another three patients a progressive thrombus formation was revealed (Fig. 1). The one medically treated patient with type I dissection showed no thrombus formation.

Table 2. Surgical management in type I dissection ($n = 20$)

	Reconstruction of ascending aorta + aortic valve	Replacement of ascending aorta + aortic valve reconstruction	Replacement of ascending aorta + aortic valve
No. of patients	5	3	12
Persisting			
False lumen			
Ascending aorta	–	1	1
Descending aorta	5	1	7
Both	–	–	2

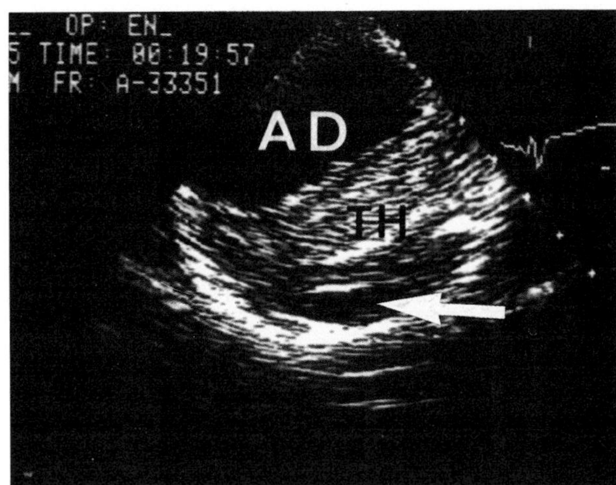

Fig. 1. Transesophageal echocardiogram. Progressive thrombus formation (*TH*) in the false lumen of an aortic dissection. Only a small channel (*arrow*) is not occluded (*AD*, true lumen of the descending aorta)

Five of the 20 surgically treated patients with type I dissections underwent reoperation; this was due to progression of dissection in the descending aorta in three patients and in the ascending aorta in one patient, and to aortic insufficiency in another patient.

In one of three patients with type III dissection who underwent surgery, and in eight of 14 patients who had medical therapy, a persisting false lumen was revealed by transesophageal echocardiography. Eleven of the 14 patients treated medically presented thrombus formation, which was localized in four patients, progressive in four patients, and complete in three patients (Table 3).

One of the 15 patients with type III dissection who were treated medically underwent secondary surgery due to progressive dilatation of the false channel.

In 19 patients treated surgically color flow imaging using the transesophageal approach was performed. In 12 of 15 patients with type I dissection, but in none of the patients with type II and type III dissection, blood flow in the false lumen was detected. In 11 of these patients, one to four entry tears were identified (Table 4, Fig. 2).

Table 3. Persisting intimal flap and thrombus formation in type III dissection (*n* = 17)

	Surgery	Medical treatment
No. of patients	3	14
Persisting intimal flap	2	12
Thrombus formation	0	11
Localized	–	4
Progressive	–	4
Complete	–	3

In the medically treated group, 16 patients were studied by color flow imaging. In 11 of 14 type III dissections, blood flow in the false lumen was revealed. In eight patients, one to three entry tears were detected (Table 5).

Three of six patients with localized thrombus formation showed laminar flow characteristics in the false lumen, whereas in three patients the flow was

Table 4. Color flow imaging in surgically treated patients ($n = 19$)

	Type I	Type II	Type III
No. of patients	15	3	1
Flow in false lumen	12	0	0
Entry tears	11	0	0
1 tear	8	–	–
2 tears	1	–	–
3 tears	1	–	–
4 tears	1	–	–

Table 5. Color flow imaging in medically treated patients ($n = 16$)

	Type I	Type II	Type III
No. of patients	1	1	14
Flow in false lumen	1	0	11
Entry tears	1	0	8
1 tear	–	–	4
2 tears	–	–	2
3 tears	–	–	2

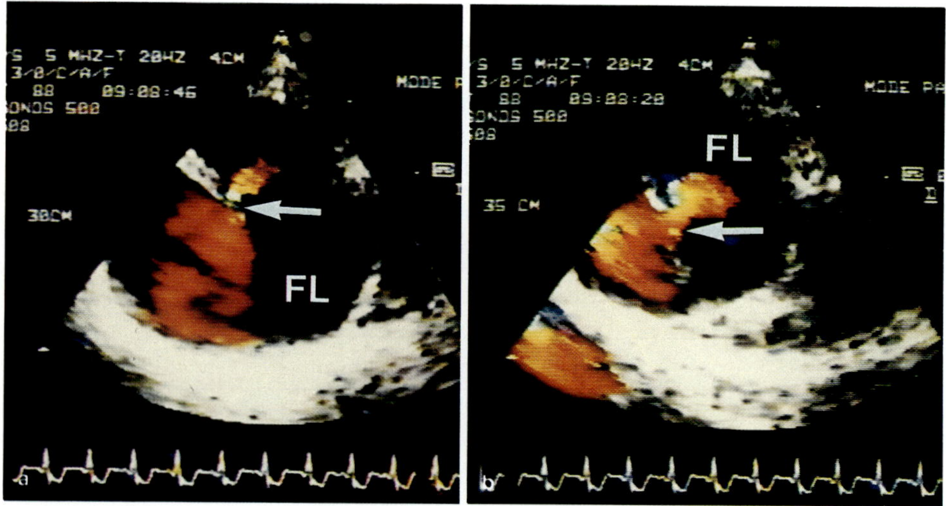

Fig. 2a, b. Blood flow from the true to the false lumen (*FL*) through an entry tear (*arrow*) with the transducer **a** 30 cm and **b** 35 cm from the teeth

swirling. Only in one of six patients with progressive thrombus formation was laminar flow observed; in the other five patients swirling blood flow in the false channel was present.

Discussion

Transesophageal two-dimensional echocardiography allows visualization of the proximal ascending aorta, the aortic arch, and almost the entire descending thoracic aorta. Only the distal ascending aorta appears as a blind region for the transesophageal approach, because of interposition of the trachea between the esophagus and aorta [8]. Entry tears and other aortic pathologies in this segment can be missed. Sometimes the ascending aorta can be better visualized by the conventional approach with parasternal and suprasternal transducer positions [1]. Therefore, the ascending aorta should always be examined by the combined technique of conventional and transesophageal echocardiography.

When the literature is reviewed for data on prognosis after surgery for aortic dissection, a survival rate of 57% after 5 years, 32% after 10 years and 5% after 20 years is found [9—12]. About 30% of all late deaths after surgical repair of aortic dissection are due to rupture of an aneurysmal segment of the aorta [10]. To prevent this complication, detailed analysis of changes of the true and false lumen in patients with surgically treated aortic dissection is required.

In this study, echocardiography revealed a progressive dilatation of the false lumen postoperatively in four of 20 repaired type I dissections, and reoperation was performed. In one of 14 medically treated cases of type III dissection, the echocardiographic observation of progressive dilatation of the false lumen led to secondary surgery. The postoperative persistence of the false lumen was due to one or more persisting or newly developed entry tears, as could be shown by color flow imaging. Thrombus formation in the false lumen was observed in 17 of 38 type I and III dissections, only in three of these cases was a complete thrombotic obstruction of the false channel found.

Thus, echocardiography using conventional and transesophageal approaches, proved a feasible method for follow-up of thoracic aortic dissection. A persisting false lumen due to persisting blood flow is a frequent finding in medically and surgically treated dissections of the thoracic aorta. Progression of the disease can easily be detected by the combination of conventional and transesophageal techniques. Decision-making on reoperation can be based on these observations.

References

1. Engberding R, Bender F, Große-Heitmeyer W, Müller US, Schneider D (1986) Diagnosis of thoracic aortic aneurysms by combined transthoracic and transesophageal 2D-echocardiography. Z Kardiol 75:225–230
2. Engberding R, Bender F, Große-Heitmeyer W, Most E, Müller US, Bramann HU, Schneider D (1987) Identification of dissection or aneurysm of the descending thoracic aorta by conventional and transesophageal two-dimensional echocardiography. Am J Cardiol 59:717–719
3. Erbel R, Börner N, Steller D, Brunier J, Thelen M, Pfeiffer C, Mohr-Kahaly S, Iversen S, Oelert H, Meyer J (1987) Detection of aortic dissection by transesophageal echocardiography. Br Heart J 58:45–51
4. Engberding R, Hasfeld I, Chiladakis I, Dohrmann A, Große-Heitmeyer W, Stoll V (1988) Transesophageal echocardiography: increased risk by rise in arterial blood pressure and cardiac arrhythmias? Herz Kreisl 20:233–236
5. Erbel R, Engberding R, Daniel W et al. (1989) Echocardiography in diagnosis of aortic dissection Lancet 1:457–461
6. Schnittger I, Popp RL (1988) Transesophageal doppler echocardiography. Mayo Clin Proc 63:726–728
7. Engberding R, Schneider D, Bender F (1987) Follow-up study of surgically treated thoracic aortic dissection by conventional and transesophageal echocardiography (Abstract). Abstracts of the 7th symposium on echocardiology. Rotterdam, June 24–26, p 5
8. Seward JB, Khandheria BK, Oh JK, Abel MA, Hughes RW, Edwards WD, Nichols BA, Freeman WK, Tajik AJ (1988) Transesophageal echocardiography: technique, anatomic correlations, implementation , and clinical applications. Mayo Clin Proc 63:649–680
9. Campbell CD (1981) Aortic dissections. In: Campbell CD (ed) Aortic aneurysms: surgical therapy. Futura, Mount Kisco, pp. 47–78
10. Crawford ES, Crawford JL (eds) (1984) Diseases of the aorta. Williams and Wilkins, Baltimore
11. DeBakey ME, McCollum CH, Crawford ES, Morris GC, Howell JF, Noon GP, Lawrie G (1982) Dissection and dissecting aneurysms of the aorta: twenty-year follow up of five hundred twenty-seven patients treated surgically. Surgery 92:118
12. Doroghazy RM, Slater EE (eds) (1983) Aortic dissection. Mc Graw-Hill, New York

Prosthetic Valve Function

Functional Assessment of Polyurethane Valve Prostheses in Calves by Transesophageal Echocardiography

H. LAMBERTZ, H. B. LO, M. HEROLD, F. A. FLACHSKAMPF, H. REUL, S. HANDT, B. J. MESSMER, G. RAU, S. EFFERT, and W. KÜPPER

Introduction

Even 30 years after the first successful heart valve replacement by Harken et al. [7] and shortly afterwards by Starr and Edwards [23], the ideal heart valve prosthesis has not yet been designed [8]. Although mechanical valves are of an acceptable durability, hemolysis and valve thrombosis remain complications to be feared. Therefore, a lifelong anticoagulation therapy is required to prevent thromboembolic events. This introduces a considerable risk of serious bleeding complications, which amount to up to two or three per 100 patient-years [5, 14] but; this is however significantly lower than the risk of thromboembolic complications in patients with mechanical valves with inadequate or without anticoagulation therapy [5].

To overcome the risk of thromboembolism inherent in all mechanical prosthetic valves, porcine heterografts were developed. In bioprostheses, anticoagulation therapy is often no longer necessary after the first three postoperative months while the sewing ring is endothelialized. However, early degeneration represents the main disadvantage of the bioprostheses used today. Several reports indicate that mineralization of the prosthetic leaflets can be observed shortly after implantation in animals as well as during follow-up in patients [1, 3, 4, 6, 18, 22]. After 10 years, only 42-76% of the bioprostheses implanted in patients were still functioning; after 12-15 years, more than 70% of the valves had to be replaced [12]. As a consequence, in certain centers the choice of bioprostheses particularly in the mitral has decreased distinctly [2]. A heart valve prosthesis combining the hemodynamics and the long durability of mechanical valves with the low incidence of thromboembolic complications found in bioprostheses would be an optimal alternative. Therefore, the obvious choice is to develop heart valve prostheses using modern synthetic materials. The polyurethane valve presented here was first tested in vitro [17] and has now been implanted in calves [13]. Transesophageal echocardiography was used to determine after what time interval the first detectable degenerative leaflet alterations, especially calcifications, became visible.

Transesophageal Echocardiography
Edited by R. Erbel et al.
© Springer-Verlag Berlin Heidelberg 1989

Methods

Prosthetic Valve Design and Material

The polyurethane prosthesis implanted is a trileaflet valve; the leaflets consist of polyurethane and the stent material is polyamide (Ultramid B 35G, BASF). It can be implanted in the aortic or in the mitral position. Four different polyurethanes were used as test materials. The materials Cardiomat 610 (Kontron) and Mitrathane M 2007 (Mitral-Medical International) are commercially available polyurethanes. The materials Pampul-3 Ameo (Beiersdorf) and PUR 1025/1 (Enka) are prototypes. The exact manufacturing techniques of the prostheses have already been described in detail [9, 17].

Implantation in Calves

Between 1985 and 1987, polyurethane valves were implanted in eight Jersey calves in the mitral position. At implantation, the calves were 12-18 weeks old (average 15 weeks). Their weights were between 65 and 95 kg (average 70 kg). Two valves of each material were implanted in the calves as a test series basically to evaluate the different materials.

For anesthesia, halothane and tramadol were used. Extracorporal circulation was installed after cannulation of either the aorta or the left carotid artery as well as the pulmonary artery and the left jugular vein. Surgery was performed at moderate hypothermia of 32°C. The mitral valve was removed through left atriotomy, and the prosthesis was sutured into the mitral annulus with 12-14 20 pledgeted sutures. Detailed information about the operation technique and postoperative intensive care has already been published [16]. Anticoagulation therapy was initiated using heparin during surgery and continued using phenprocoumon until therapeutic prothrombin time was reached. This anticoagulation therapy was discontinued after 3 months except in two calves who received a lifelong anticoagulation therapy. During the first postoperative week, aspirin was administered to all animals (2 g on the first day and 1 g from the second day on).

Transesophageal Echocardiography

The echocardiographic examinations with a transesophageal probe were conducted using an electronic phased array sector scanner (Diasonics, Varian 3400 R, 3.5 MHz). M-mode and two-dimensional echocardiograms were recorded on video tape (U-Matic, 25 pictures per second). The vocal chords could be visualized in all animals using a laryngoscope especially developed for this purpose. At the first attempt, an adequate visualization of the heart was not possible at all. Only after filling up the esophagus completely with ultrasound transmission gel (average 113 ml) through a gastric tube, which was then withdrawn, both atria could be visualized after the probe was introduced to 71 ± 6 cm. Problems arose when the animals produced a large amount of gastric juice during surgery and required the placement of a gastric tube during the examination. This in turn interfered with the image quality of echocardiograms in two cases. For topographic orientation, initial contrast echocardiography was performed at the first examination with opacification of the right heart cavities and the superior vena cava. In two animals, echocardiograms were recorded 2 days preoperatively to provide exact knowledge of the anatomy visualized. Adequate determination of atrial size and the relation between right atrial (RA) and left atrial dimensions proved to be difficult and not standardizable. However, the mitral valve or the polyurethane prosthesis implanted could be depicted in all animals with satisactory image quality (Fig. 1). Motion analysis and measurement of leaflet thickening of the prostheses was carried out using the M-mode technique (Fig. 2, 3).

In two calves, the first examination was carried out intraoperatively, and in six animals immediately after valve implantation. In four calves, further echocardiograms were recorded on the third postoperative day, and in all ani-

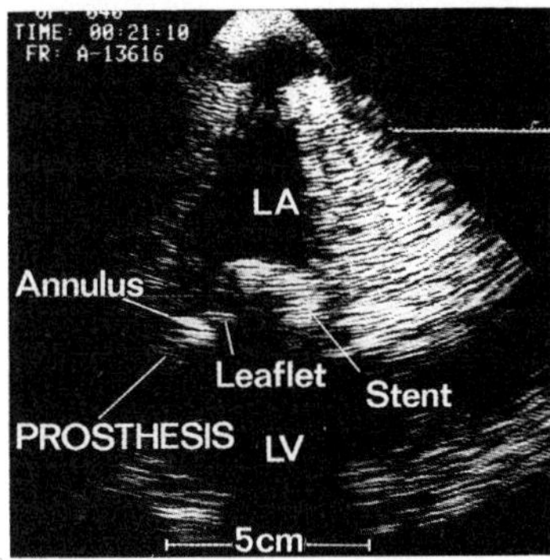

Fig. 1. Transesophageal echocardiogram of the implanted polyurethane prosthesis in the mitral position. On postoperative day 3 the leaflets show normal mobility. *LA*, left atrium, *LV*, left ventricle

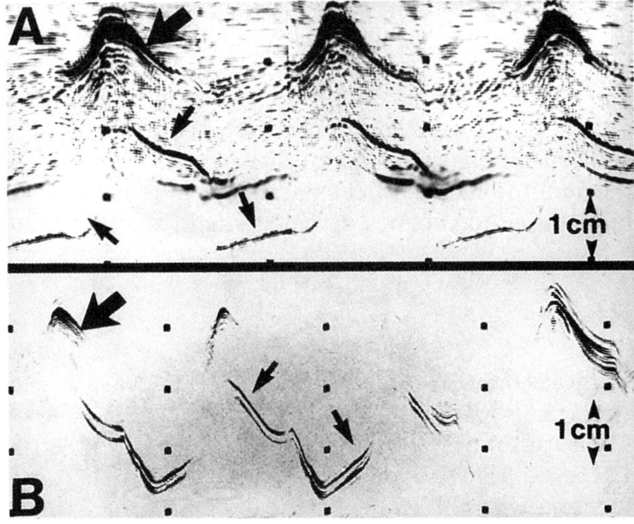

Fig. 2. A Intraoperative transesophageal M-mode echocardiogram showing normal leaflet appeerence and mobility (*small arrows*). *Large arrow*, stent **B** Transesophageal M-mode echocardiogram on postoperative day 3 showing discrete homogeneous thickening of the leaflet. A thin and parallel double echo pattern is seen (*small arrow*)

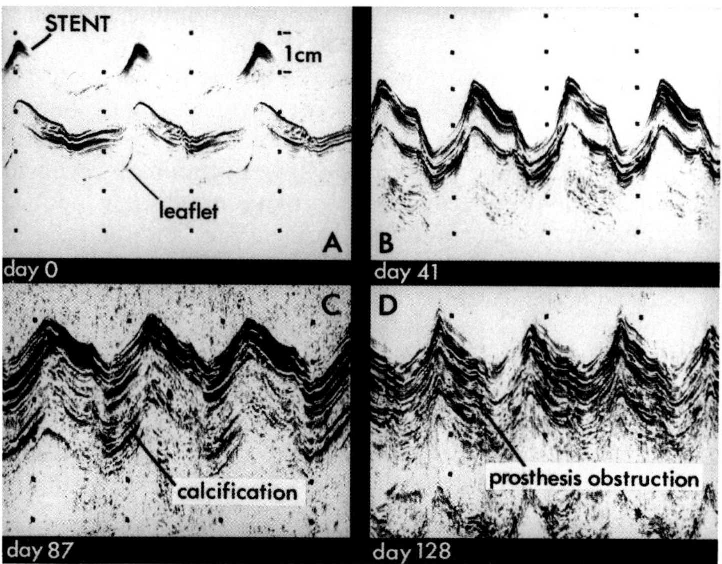

Fig. 3 A—D. Calf Lissy: serial transesophageal M-mode echocardiograms showing the follow- up and progressive calcifications of the leaflets

mals at regular time intervals of 40 ± 3 days. For this purpose, the calves received narcosis of short duration using ketamine HCl. Specific attention was directed to motion abnormalities of the prosthetic leaflets as well as to the degree of leaflet calcification. The following degenerative alterations were noted; leaflet thickening [1], focal calcification [2], leaflet calcification [3], reduced opening motion of the prosthesis [4], and mobile echo structures [5].

Alterations were considered as leaflet thickening when a thin and parallel double echo pattern such as is shown in Fig. 2 became visible.

To differentiate calcification from fibrosis, digital image control (pre- and postprocessing) was used. For all examinations the depth − gain was constant and remained unchanged. The maximum brightness was set to its maximum and the background brightness to its minimum. The relation between the intensity of the echo signal and the gray levels of the scope were varied by gray-scale manipulation using an S-curve [10, 15]. The slope of the curve was set to maximum and the reject parameter was chosen in such a way that only the high-amplitude echoes of the stents of the prostheses were visualized.

Results

Clinical Data

The survival time of the calves is shown in Fig. 4 (average 217 days, minimum 127, maximum 291 days). All animals died because of severe prosthetic dysfunction with the clinical signs of rapid progressive heart failure.

(calf)	SURVIVAL-TIME (days)	VALVE MATERIALS	time after implantation/days					
			40±3	80±9	120±16	160±21	200±24	240±31
Eli	127	CARDIOMAT 610	focal calcification	leaflet calcification	leaflet calcification +			
Gilda	267	CARDIOMAT 610		focal calcification	leaflet calcification	leaflet calcification	valve obstruction	mobile echo structure +
Lissy	130	MITRATHANE M2007	leaflet thickening	focal calcification	leaflet calcification + valve obstruction +			
Nelly	181	MITRATHANE M2007	focal calcification	focal calcification	focal calcification	leaflet calcification + valve obstruction +		
Polly	278	PAMPUL–3 AMEO		leaflet thickening	focal calcification	focal calcification	leaflet calcification	valve obstruction +
Gretchen	291	PAMPUL–3 AMEO	leaflet thickening	leaflet thickening	focal calcification	leaflet calcification	mobile echo structure	valve obstruction +
Esther	215	PUR 1025/1		focal calcification	focal calcification	focal calcification	leaflet calcification +	
Dorothee	251	PUR 1025/1		leaflet thickening	focal calcification	leaflet calcification	valve obstruction	+

Legend: leaflet thikening · focal calcification · leaflet calcification · valve obstruction · mobile echo structure

Fig. 4. Chronology of echocardiographic alterations for the four valve materials investigated. The polyurethane materials Pampul-3 Ameo and PUR 1025/1 had the best long-term results

Echocardiography

The mitral valve prostheses implanted could be visualized in all animals with satisfactory image quality. In the four calves examined on the third postoperative day, M-mode already revealed a discrete but homogeneous thickening of the leaflets. Careful examination of the leaflets showed that these findings were not focally restricted but could also be visualized in the area of attachment of the polyurethane leaflets. The chronology of echocardiographic alterations is summarized in Fig. 3-5. Two calves showed focal leaflet calcifications after 40 days. After 120 days, calcifications were found in all animals. All calves showing no leaflet calcifications at 80 ± 9 days survived longer than 250 days. An influence of anticoagulation therapy on the development of

Fig. 5. Differentiation between leaflet fibrosis and calcium deposition using digital image control [15]. By eliminating weak echoes and accentuating strong reflections, fibrosis and calcification can be differentiated objectively. Calcium deposits were first noted at the free edges (*arrow*) and at the commissures

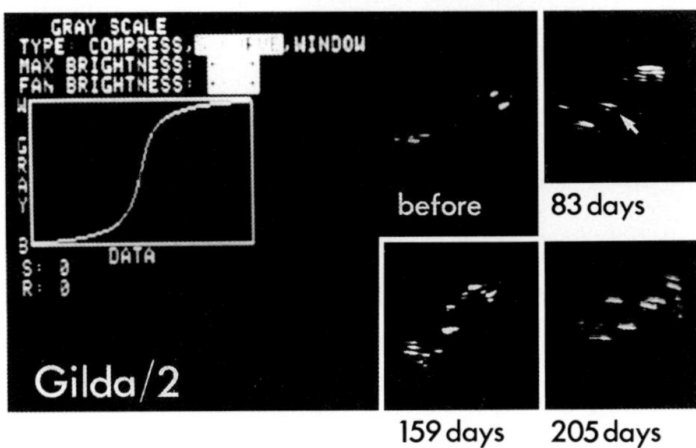

valve degeneration was not noted. Statistical analysis, however, was not possible due to the small number of animals studied. In two calves, mobile echo structures adhering to the prosthesis were seen, which were revealed to be mobile thrombi at autopsy. Left atrial thrombi were found to be present in two additional calves.

Postmortem Findings

The histological examination of the explanted and severely degenerated valve prostheses showed a distinct focal leaflet thickening in all cases; calcium depositis were found on the atrial as well as on the ventricular surface (Fig. 6). By means of Kossa staining and energy dispersive analysis of X-rays (EDAX), we were able to prove that those deposits were in fact focal calcifications (Fig. 7). The deposits were concentrated along the free edges of the leaflets and at the commissures. Adherent thrombi were commonly seen when calcification was prominent on the leaflet surface. Generally, calcification was restricted to the leaflet surface, and did not extend through the cross section. In addition to severely calcified polyurethane prostheses, two calves showed left atrial thrombi with focal calcification.

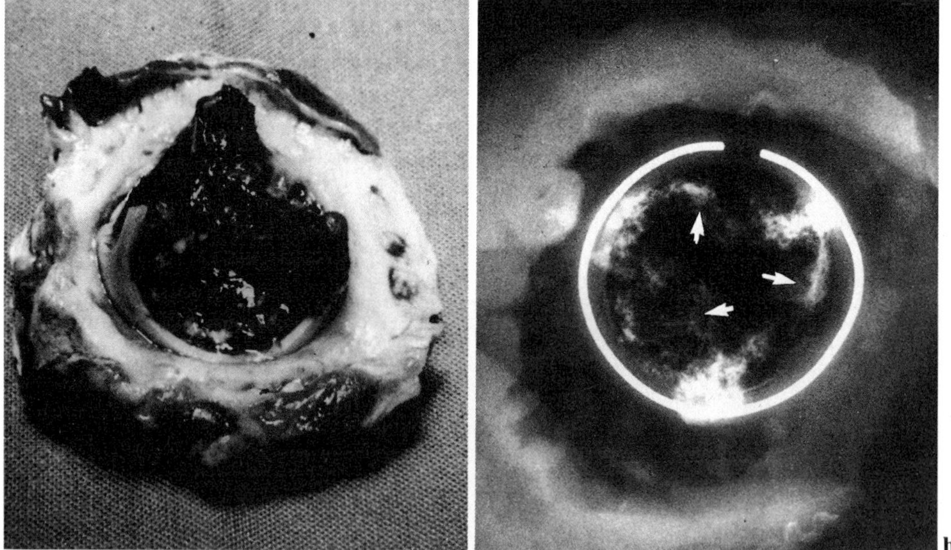

a   b

Fig. 6. a Example of an explanted valve with massive thrombus. **b** X-ray of the same valve showing focal calcium deposits especially at the free edges, which are shrunken, (*arrows*) and at the commissures

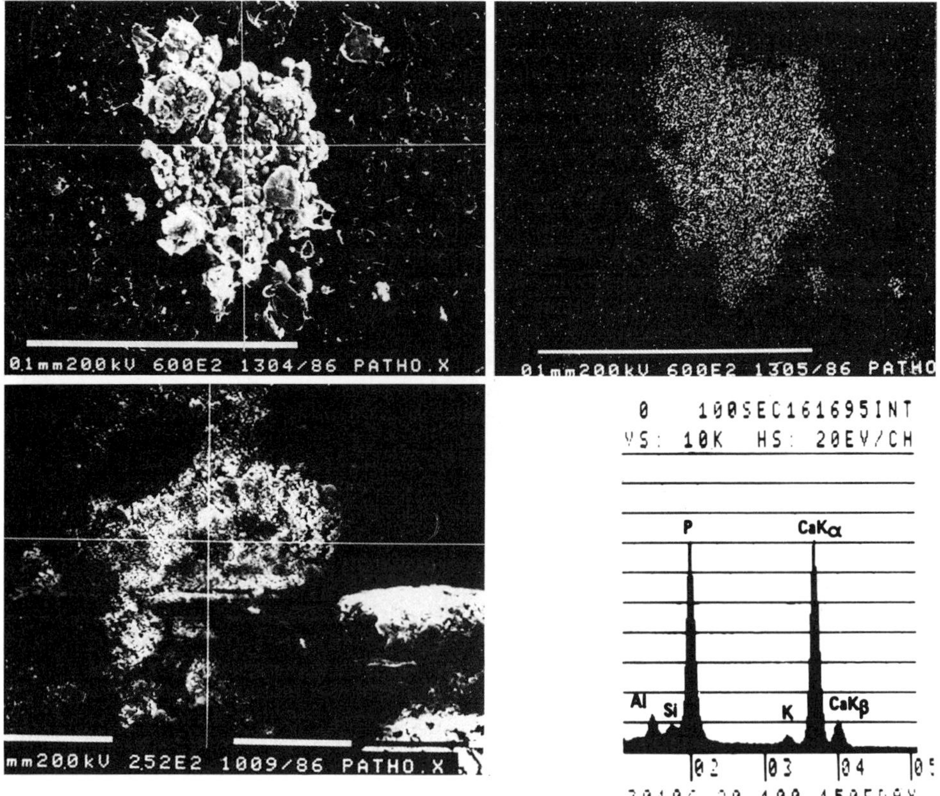

Fig. 7. Scanning electron micrographs of leaflet surface and EDAX analysis at the same location, showing phosphorous and calcium peaks

Discussion

Transesophageal echocardiography is suitable for detecting prosthesis degeneration in calves. Confirming clinical experiences, calcification deposits were first noted at the commissures. The time interval between surgery and detection of the first calcium deposit was of prognostic value regarding life expectancy of animals with polyurethane prostheses. At least two polyurethane materials calcified later than 80 days and resulted in survival times far beyond those with bioprostheses under similar conditions.

Transesophageal Echocardiography

Visualization of the heart by the transesophageal approach has been used in adult cardiology for years. An exact anatomic representation of cardiac structures is guaranteed and the clinical usefulness has been demonstrated in a large number of studies [20, 21]. Transesophageal two-dimensional echocardiography always represents an alternative to the transthoracic approach when insufficient diagnostic information is obtained by precordial transducer positioning such as in patients with pulmonary emphysema, thoracic deformities, or extreme obesity. Evaluation of cardiac function during surgery and in mechanically ventilated patients in the intensive care unit by transesophageal echocardiography has proven to be useful [19].

We applied the technique to the longitudinal examination of a newley developed mitral valve prosthesis implanted in calves. The polyurethane prostheses could be well visualized in all animals, with good image quality. Calcifications of the prosthetic leaflets were diagnosed by digital image control. By eliminating weak echoes and accentuating strong reflections, fibrosis and calcification could be differentiated objectively. Sufficient differentiation between extensive fibrosis and calcium deposits seemed not to be possible using conventional echocardiographic images. This became feasible only when using computer-assisted S-curve analysis. Novak and coworkers [15] reported that calcifications of the mitral valve in patients were found with a sensitivity of 89.5%, a specificity of 91.7%, and a predicitve accuracy of 90.3% when using the digital image control of echocardiograms.

We were able to confirm reports that the heart could be visualized from a right paracardial window in dogs but not in calves. In contrast to human studies, we encountered several methodological and practical problems in our animal studies:

The whole esophagus of the calves had to be filled with ultrasound transmission gel to obtain echo images of good quality. This is partly due to the larger dimension of the esophagus in the calves. Because of incomplete coaptation of the echo probe, either no echocardiogram free of artifacts or no echocardiogram at all could be recorded without using this gel.

A further aspect is the position of the calves. During surgery the calves were positioned on the right side, making echocardiographic visualization of the mitral valve very difficult. Therefore, we examined all animals in a kneeling position during follow-up.

As a third aspect, the alkali pH value of 8.5 of the gastric juice in calves should be mentioned: after examining five calves, we noted that the seal of the transesophageal probe crumbled away and the probe became porous. Repair of the probe was not feasible, so a new transesophageal transducer had to be bought. Improved coating of currently available probes will probably present this problem.

Visualization of the mitral valve or valve prosthesis was highly accurate in all calves. The best visualization of the mitral prosthesis was obtained from slightly different positions in each calf. Consequently, exact determination of the atrial size and the change of size was not possible during follow-up.

Polyurethane Valve Prostheses

Four of the eight calves survived longer than 250 days. As shown in Fig. 4, the polyurethane materials Pampul-3 Ameo and PUR 1025/1 showed the best long-term results. In comparison, bioprostheses implanted under similar conditions showed calcifications after only 30-75 days [26]. Similarly to previously reported studies, the anticoagulation therapy did not influence the degree of calcium deposits on the polyurethane prostheses [11, 26, 27]. Wisman and coworkers reported an average survival rate of about 155 days after implantation of polyurthane valve prostheses in mitral the position [27]. These evaluations were carried out in still growing Holstein calves weighing 90-120 kg. Detailed analysis of our results (Fig. 4) revealed that the time interval in which no calcification appeared was distinctly longer when using Pampul-3 Ameo and PUR 1025/1 than when using valves made from other polyurethane materials. Leaflet thickening noted during the first postoperative days seems not to be useful for predicting the durability of the prostheses. However, the prognostic value of leaflet calcification was different: early focal leaflet calcifications (before 80 days) indicated early valve failure. Reviewing our results however, we were not able to clarify definitely which was the decisive initial factor leading to later complete loss of prosthesis function. Focal leaflet calcification was always preceded by leaflet thickening. Thus, we have to assume that an alteration of the leaflet surface precedes all further changes noted. Comparable findings reported by other authors show that calcification is initiated at the sites of the highest stress and may occur secondary to tissue degeneration resulting from stress [24, 27]. In previous examinations calcification was found in the area of greatest flexion facing the ventricular surface [25]. In our experience however, Kossa staining of the cross sections through explanted valve leaflets emphasizes that there was no difference in the quantity of calcium deposits between atrial and ventricular surfaces of the leaflets.

Unfortunately, we were not equipped with a Doppler device when performing the examinations in the present series. However, we assume that by means of Doppler echocardiography, inflow obstruction through the prosthesis as well as regurgitation jets can be detected early. Early calcifications of the prostheses are due to the increased calcium phosphate turnover in still growing animals. Therefore, further studies of the behavior of this type of prosthesis after implantation in adult sheep or goats are required.

References

1. Barnhart GR, Jones M, Ishihara T, Rose DM, Chavez AM, Ferrans VJ (1982) Degeneration and calcification of bioprosthetic cardiac valves: bioprosthetic tricuspid valve implantations in sheep. AJ Pathol 106:136
2. Borst HG, Frank G, Frimpong-Boateng K, Bednarski P (1986) Herzklappenprothesenwahl − 1985. Z Kardiol 75:311−315
3. Carpentier A, Dubost C, Lane E, Nashef A, Carpentier S, Relland J, Deloche A, Fabiani JN, Chauvand S, Perier P, Maxwell S (1982) Continuing improvements in valvular bioprostheses. J Thorac Cardiovasc Surg 83:27
4. Derck JD, Thubrikar MJ, Nolan SP, Aouad J (1982) The role of mechanical stress in calcification of bioprostheses. In: Cohn LH, Gallucci V (eds) Cardiac bioprostheses. Proceedings of the Second International Symposium. Yorke Medical Books, New York, pp 293−305

5. Duveau D (1986) Anticoagulation is necessary in all patients with mechanical prostheses in sinus rhythm. Z Kardiol 75 (Suppl) 2:326
6. Farrans VJ, Boyce SW, Billingham ME, Jones M, Ishihara T, Roberts WC (1980) Calcific deposits in porcine bioprostheses: structure and pathogenesis. Am J Cardiol 46:721
7. Harken DE, Soroff HS, Taylor WJ (1960) Partial and complete prosthesis in aortic insufficiency. J Thorac Cardiovasc Surg 40:744
8. Heiliger R, Lambertz H, Minale C, Mittermayer C (1988) Bioprothese versus mechanische Herzklappe: ein hydrodynamischer Vergleich von Prothesen gleicher Größe. Herz/Kreisl 20:43−53
9. Herold M, Lo HB, Reul H, Mückter H, Taguchi K, Giersiepen M, Birkle G, Hollweg G, Rau G, Messmer BJ (1987) The Helmholtz-Institute-Tri-Leaflet-Polyurethane-heart valveprosthesis: design, manufacturing and first in-vitro and in-vivo results. In: Plank Hetal (eds), Polyurethanes in biomedical engineering II Amsterdam
10. Hillard W (1982) Basic physics of ultrasound. In: Shapira J, Chamruzi Y, Devidson R (eds) Two-dimensional echocardiography Williams and Wilkins, Baltimore, pp 319−334
11. Hoffacker W (1979) Blood compatibility of elastomers for leaflet heart valves. Plastic in medicine and surgery III. In: Abstracts of the 2nd meeting of the european society of biomechanics. Straßbourg, 13−15 Sept
12. Horstkotte D (1987) In: Erworbene Herzklappenfehler. Horstkotte D, Loogen F (eds) Urban and Schwarzenberg, München p 319
13. Lo HB, Herold M, Reul H, Mückter H, Taguchi K, Surmann M, Hildinger KH, Lambertz H, de Haan H, Handt S, Hollweg G, Messmer BJ, Rau G (1982) A tricuspid polyurethane heart valve as alternative to mechanical- or bioprostheses. Trans Am Soc Artif Intern Organs 34:839−844
14. Loeliger EA (1966) Der holländische Thrombosedienst und seine Probleme. Z Gesamte Inn Med 21:210−212
15. Nowak B, Reifart N, Satter P (1988) Kalknachweis bei Mitralvitien mittels rechnergestützter zweidimensionaler Echokardiographie. Z Kardiol 77:305−309
16. Pierce WS et al. (1980) Calcification inside artificial hearts: inhibition by warfarin sodium. Science 208:601
17. Reul H, Ghista DN (1980) The design, development, in vitro testing and performance of an optimal aortic valve prosthesis. In: Dhanjoo N, Ghista DN (eds), Biomechanics of medical devices. Dekker, New York
18. Sanders SP, Levy RJ, Freed MD, Norwood WI, Castaneda AR (1980) Use of Hancock porcine xenografts in children and adolescents. Am J Cardiol 46:429
19. Schiller NB (1982) Evaluation of cardiac function during surgery by transesophageal 2-dimensional echocardiography. In: Hanrath P, Bleifeld W, Souquet J (eds) Cardiovascular diagnosis by ultrasound. Martinus Nijhoff, The Hague, pp 289−293
20. Schlüter M, Hinrichs A, Thier W, Kremer P, Schröder S, Cahalan MK, Hanrath P, Siglow V (1984) Transesophageal two-diemensional echocardiography comparison of ultrasonic and anatomic sections. Am J Cardiol 53:1173−1178
21. Schüter M, Thier W, Hinrichs A, Kremer P, Siglow V, Hanrath P (1984) Klinischer Einsatz der transösophagealen Echokardiographie. Dtsch med Wochenschr. 109:722−727
22. Silver MM, Pollock J, Silver MD, Williams WG, Trusler GA (1980) Calcification in porcine xenograft valves in children. Am J Cardiol 45:685
23. Starr A, Edwards ML (1961) Mitral valve replacement: clinical experience with a ballvalve prosthesis. Ann Surg 154:726
24. Thubrikar MJ, Deck JD, Aouad J, Nolan SP (1982) The role of mechanical stress in the calcification ofaortic bioprosthetic valves. J Thorac Cardiovasc Surg 83:111
25. Thubrikar MJ, Skinner JR, Eppink RT, Nolan SP (1982) Stress analysis of porcine bioprosthetic heart valves in vivo. J Biomed Mater Res 16:811
26. Thubrikar MJ, Nolan SP, Deck JD, Aouad J, Levitt LC (1983) Intrinsic calcification of T-6 processed and control porcine and bovine bioprostheses in calves. Trans Am Soc Artif Intern Organs 29:245
27. Wisman CB, Pierce WS, Donachy JH, Pae WE, Myers JL, Prophet GA (1982) A polyurethane trifleaflet cardiac valve prosthesis: in vitro and in vivo studies. Trans Am Soc Artif Intern Organs 28:164

Value and Limitations of Transesophageal Echocardiography in Mitral Valvular Prosthesis

B. K. KHANDHERIA

Introduction

Assessment of prosthetic valve function, a frequently encountered challenge to the clinician, is often confounded by superimposed cardiovascular problems such as ventricular dysfunction, multivalvular disease, and ischemic heart disease. Fluoroscopy, phonocardiography, and echocardiography have been tools used in the evaluation of normal and abnormal prosthetic valve function over the past several years [1−4]. The advent of Doppler echocardiography has given a big boost to noninvasive hemodynamic assessment of prosthetic valve function [5]. There are now available normal values for most prosthetic valves [6]. Increased gradients and prolonged half-times with decreasing valve areas are characteristically seen in prosthetic valve stenosis. This hemodynamic assessment is now possible noninvasively by transthoracic Doppler interrogation of the valve. Aortic prosthesis dysfunction due to regurgitation can be detected and semiquantitated both by pulsed/continuous wave Doppler and color flow imaging. The usefulness of transthoracic two-dimensional echocardiography as well as Doppler and color flow imaging in assessment of mitral prosthetic function is limited due to attenuation and flow masking behind the nonbiologic material of the prosthesis [7, 8]. Detection of other potential complications such as mural thrombus in the atrium/atrial appendage, vegetations, and ring abscesses via the transthoracic route is limited due to acoustic shadowing by the prosthetic valve material.

Transesophageal echocardiography provides a clear view of the left atrium, mitral annulus, mitral valve, and its supporting structures. This procedure of transesophageal echocardiography can readily be performed in the awake patient and therefore, is ideally suited for evaluation of the mitral prosthesis [9, 10].

The clinical utility of transesophageal echocardiography is reviewed in this report of 33 patients who underwent transesophageal echocardiography for assessment of the mitral prosthesis in our initial experience with this technique.

Transesophageal Echocardiography
Edited by R. Erbel et al.
© Springer-Verlag Berlin Heidelberg 1989

Material and Method

Study Patients

Between November 1987 and April 1988, 33 patients underwent transesophageal echocardiography for assessment of mitral prosthesis. The mean age of this group was 62 years (range 16—83 years). There were 24 women and 9 men. A comprehensive precordial two-dimensional Doppler evaluation of the mitral prosthesis had been performed prior to the transesophageal echocardiography.

The distribution of different prosthesis was as follows: 18 patients with ball-cage prosthesis, 5 patients with disc prosthesis, and 10 patients with bioprosthesis. The implantation age of the prosthesis ranged from 1 to 222 months (mean 88 months). Eleven of these 33 patients had dual prosthesis: mitral and aortic (10 patients), and mitral and tricuspid (1 patient).

Technique and Instrumentation

Transesophageal Echocardiography. Our technique of transesophageal echocardiography has been described in detail elsewhere [11]. Patients were instructed to abstain from oral intake for 4-6 prior to the examination. Routine questioning for symptoms suggestive of esophageal diseases, drug allergies, glaucoma, and urinary retention was done. A 23-gauge butterfly needle was placed in a peripheral vein for venous access. Bacterial endocarditis prophylaxis was administered as per recommendations laid down by the American Heart Association in 27 patients and was withheld from 6 patients who were being evaluated for bacterial endocarditis. The oropharynx was liberally sprayed with aerosolized lidocaine spray 5-10 min prior to the procedure. All patients received premedication in the form of 0.2 mg intravenous glycopyrrolate to reduce salivary secretions. In addition, 75% of the patients received sedation with midazolam at a dose of 0.04 mg/kg body weight (total dose per patient 1—3 mg intravenously). The patients were sedated to the point of being awake but drowsy. The examination was performed with the patient in the left lateral decubitus position.

A commercially available transesophageal ultrasonic echoscope with a 5.0-MHz transducer was used. This transducer has a 90 degree field of view as well as pulsed and color flow Doppler capability. Imaging planes that were utilized included the basal short axis, four-chamber, and transgastric short axis (Fig. 1). These have been described by us in a previous publication [11].

Transthoracic Examination. A comprehensive two-dimensional echocardiography and Doppler examination utilizing previously described methods was untertaken in all patients [12, 13]. Doppler hemodynamic data that were obtained included peak diastolic antegrade velocity across the mitral prosthesis, maximal and mean resting gradients, and pressure half-time across the mitral

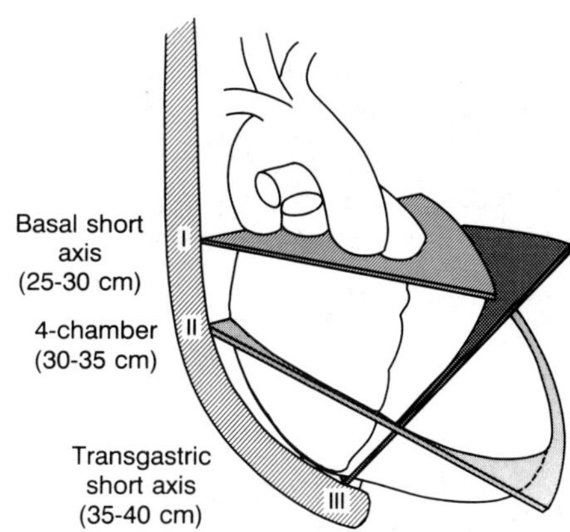

Fig. 1. Schematic diagram showing different scan planes. The distance of the transducer from incisor teeth to obtain different planes is shown

prosthesis [14]. Color flow imaging was performed utilizing multiple transducer positions with a technique that has also been described previously [15].

Clinical Data

Clinical data with regards to history, physical examination findings, date of valve implantation, and indication for transthoracic and transesophageal echocardiography were obtained from review of the patient's records. Cardiac catheterization data and surgical/pathological findings were also recorded from the patient's history.

Results

Doppler echocardiographic examination was carried out in these 33 patients to evaluate a wide variety of clinical problems. These included detection quantitation and localization of mitral prosthetic regurgitation in 24 patients, suspected endocarditis in 6 patients, and unexplained thromboembolism despite good anticoagulation in 3 patients.

Transesophageal Echocardiography

There were 12 patients who were found to have an abnormal functioning prosthesis on transesophageal echocardiographic examination. These included 5 patients with severe perivalvular mitral regurgitation, 4 patients with severe valvular mitral regurgitation (Fig. 2), 2 patients with ring abscess, and 1 patient with an obstructed disc.

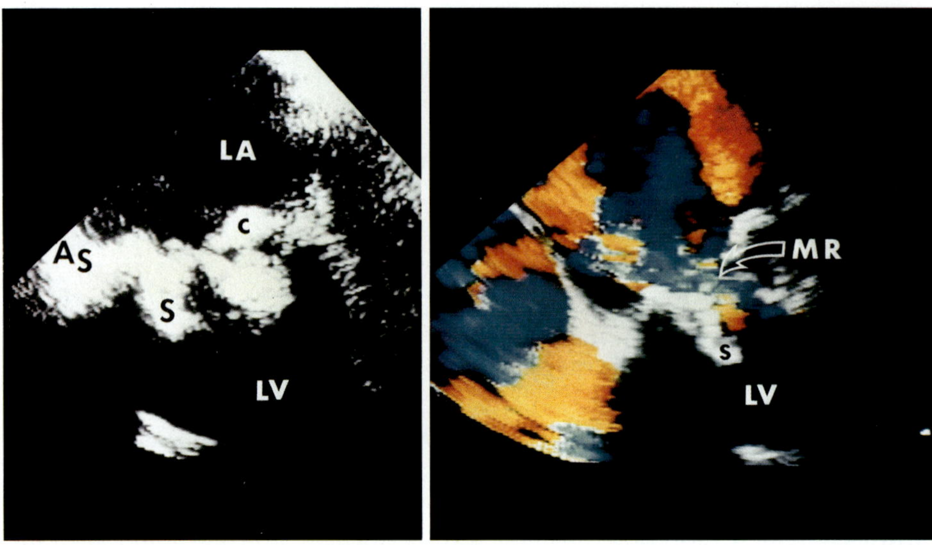

Fig. 2. Still frames from a patient with valvular regurgitation. *Left*, two-dimensional echocardiographic image showing the tissue prosthesis (*C*) and stents (*S*). *LA*, Left atrium; *LV*, left ventricle; *AS*, atrial septum. *Right*, Color flow image showing severe mitral regurgitation (*MR*)

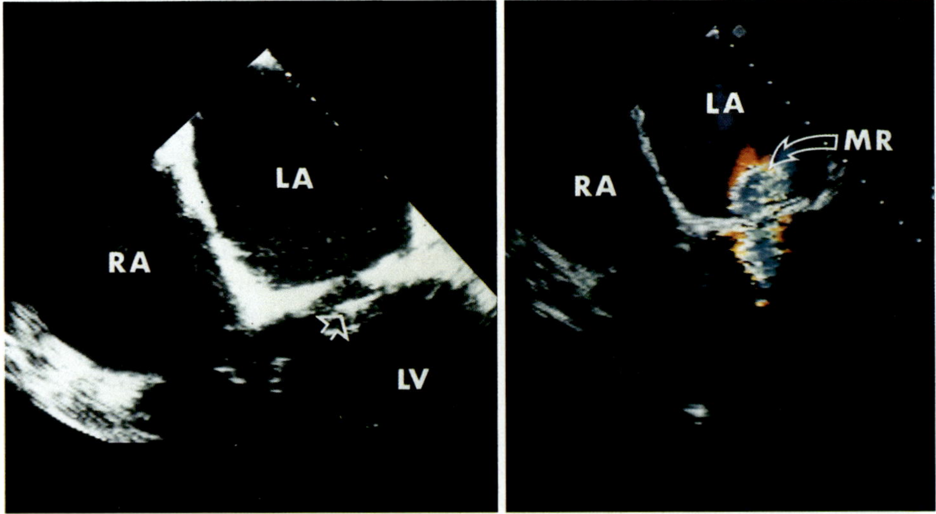

Fig. 3. Still frame showing 'closing volume' ball-cage prosthesis. *Left*, two dimensional echocardiogram showing ball-cage prosthesis (*arrow*). Note the enlarged left atrium (*LA*). *LV*, Left ventricle; *RA*, right atrium. *Right*, 'Closing volume,' trivial mitral regurgitation (*MR*) seen on color flow imaging

Trivial mitral regurgitation with the jet appearing in early systole at the closure of the prosthesis and giving the appearance of a "puff of smoke" was seen in 11 patients (Fig. 3). This finding represents the normal closing volume of the prosthetic valve. These were judged to be normal on the basis of transesophageal echocardiography.

Operation were performed in 12 of 33 patients. Findings seen on transesophageal echocardiography were confirmed in 11 of these 12 (92%). A patient with a ball-cage prosthesis who underwent operation on the basis of strong clinical suspicion of prosthetic dysfunction had normal results on transesophageal examination. At operation, a small thrombus at the sewing ring was detected. This was on the ventricular side of the prosthesis. This, then was a false-negative result. Five patients (42%) underwent operation without cardiac catheterization.

Discussion

Noninvasive assessment of prosthetic valve dysfunction continues to be a challenge since the date of the first human implantation of a prosthetic valve. A variety of noninvasive techniques have met with limited success. Structural abnormalities of the bioprosthetic valves have been evaluated with some degree of success with transthoracic two-dimensional echocardiography [16−19]. Masking by the nonbiologic material and the inability to visualize the left atrial appendage in a large majority of adults are shortcomings of the transthoracic two-dimensional echocardiography in evaluation of mitral prostheses [7]. Mechanical prostheses emanate reverberations and, therefore, also pose a problem in evaluation via the transthoracic approach. However, some of these shortcomings have been alleviated to an extent by the addition of Doppler echocardiography [20, 21]. Doppler echocardiography has provided a nonivasive tool to assess hemodynamics across the mitral prosthesis. However, both pulsed wave and continuous wave Doppler are limited in detection, localization, and semiquantitation of mitral prosthetic regurgitation due to the masking effect of the prosthetic material [7, 8]. It also has been relatively insensitive in detection of perivalvular regurgitation [8]. Color flow imaging has helped overcome this insensitivity to some extent. However, it also suffers from the same limitations, especially in the mechanical mitral prosthesis.

Transesophageal echocardiography provides a unique acoustic window for imaging the mitral valve and its supporting structures. Since the ultrasound beam does not have to traverse the prosthetic material, masking is not a limitation. Transesophageal echocardiography has been shown to be extremely sensitive in detection of mitral regurgitation. Our data substantiates the useful-ness of transesophageal echocardiography in assessment of mitral valve prosthesis. Transesophageal color flow imaging is particularly useful in localizing the site of mitral regurgitation − prosthetic versus periprosthetic regurgitation. Utilizing the color subtraction technique, one can then locate the anatomical defect. Transesophageal color flow imaging also provides a reasonable semiquantitative estimate of the degree of regurgitation and, hence, alleviates the need for left ventriculography even in those patients who may require a subsequent coronary arteriography. In patients with suspected bacterial endocarditis, transesophageal echocardiography not only allows detection of vegetation or abscess but also allows, with the aid of color flow imaging, delineation of the hemodynamic effect of the vegetation or abscess [22].

Potential pitfalls and limitations must be kept in mind when utilizing this technique. It is essential that scanning be carried out in different planes as well as at all tomographic levels when assessing for site and degree of regurgitation. All prosthetic valves have trivial regurgitation which represents the normal closing volume. This should not be misinterpreted as abnormal. Assessment of the ventricular surface of mechanical mitral valve prostheses suffers from limitations due to reverberation and acoustic shadowing. Hence, transesophageal echocardiography should be considered as an adjunct in a complementary procedure to transthoracic Doppler echocardiographic examination.

Transesophageal echocardiography is a promising technique which should be a part of comprehensive Doppler echocardiographic examination in evaluating patients with mitral valve prosthesis.

References

1. Sands MK, Lachman AS, O'Reilly DJ, Leach CN, et al (1982) Diagnostic value of cinefluorscopy in the Evaluation of prosthetic heart valve dysfunction. Am Heart J 104:622−627
2. Kotler MN, Segal BL, Parry WR (1978) Echocardiographic and phonocardiographic evaluation of prosthetic heart valves. Cardiovasc Clin 9:187−207
3. Cunha CL, Giulliani ER, Callahan JA, Pluth J (1980) Echophonocardiographic findings in patients with prosthetic heart valve malfunction. Mayo clin Proc 55:231−242
4. Miller FA, Tajik AJ, Seward JB, et al (1981) Prosthetic valve dysfunction: two-dimensional echocardiographic observations (abstract). Circulation 64 (Suppl IV):315
5. Cooper DM, Stewart WJ, Shiavone WA, Lombardo HP, et al (1987) Evaluation of normal prosthetic valve function by Doppler echocardiography. Am Heart J 114:576−582
6. Reisner SA, Meltzer RS (1988) Normal values of prosthetic valve Doppler echocardiographic parameters: a review. J Am Soc Echocardiogr 1:203−210
7. Sprecher DL, Adamick R, Adams D, Kisslo J (1987) In vitro color flow, pulsed and continuous wave Doppler ultrasound masking of flow by prosthetic valves. J Am Coll cardiol 9:1306−1310
8 . Come PC (1987) Pitfalls in the diagnosis of periprosthetic valvular regurgitation by pulsed Doppler echocardiography. J Am Coll cardiol 9:1176−1179
9. Neuessen U, Schnittger I, Appleton C, et al (1988) Transesophageal two-dimensional echocardiography and color flow velocity mapping in the evaluation of cardiac valve prosthesis. Circulation 78:848−855
10. Khandheria BK, Seward JB, Oh JK, Freeman WK, Tajik AJ (1989) Mitral prosthesis malfunction: utility of transesophageal echocardiography. J Am Coll Cardiol (Suppl A) 13:69
11. Seward JB, Khandheria BK, Oh JK, Abel M, et al (1988) Transesophageal echocardiography: technique, anatomic correlation implementation and clinical applications. Mayo Clinic Proc 63:649−680

12. Tajik AJ, Seward JB, Hagler DJ, Mair DD, Lie JT (1978) Two-dimensional real-time ultrasonic imaging of the heart and great vessels: technique, image orientation, structure identification, and validation. Mayo Clinic Proc 57:271−303
13. Nishimura RA, Miller FA, Callahan MJ, Benassi RC (1985) Doppler echocardiography: theory, instrumentation, technique, and application. Mayo Clinic Proc 60:321−343
14. Hatle L, Angelsen B (1982) Doppler ultrasound in cardiology: physical principles and clinical applications. Lea and Febiger, Philadelphia
15. Khandheria BK, Tajik AJ, Reeder GS, Calahan MJ, et al (1986) Doppler color flow imaging: a new technique for visualization and characterization of the blood flow jet in mitral stenosis. Mayo Clinic Proc 61:623−630
16. Helnstein IR, Marbarger JP, Perez JE (1983) Ultrasonic assessment of the St Jude prosthetic valve: M-mode, two-dimensional and Doppler echocardiography. Circulation 68:879−905
17. Alam M, Lokjer JB, Pickard SD, Goldstein S (1983) Echocardiographic evaluation of porcine bioprosthetic valves: experience with 309 normal and 59 dysfunctioning valves. Am J Cardiol 52:309−315
18. Forman MB, Phelon BK, Robertson RM, Virmani R (1985) Correlation of two-dimensional echocardiography and pathologic findings in porcine valve dysfunction. J Am Coll Cardiol 5:224−230
19. Kotler M, Mintz G, Panidis I, et al (1983) Non-invasive evaluation of normal and abnormal prosthetic valves. J Am Coll Cardiol 2:151−173
20 Panidis IP, Rose J, Mintz GS (1986) Normal and abnormal prosthetic valve function as assessed by Doppler echocardiography. J Am Coll Cardiol 8:317−326
21. Sagar KB, Wann LS, Paulsen WHJ, Romhilt DW (1986) Doppler echocardiographic evaluation of Hancock and Bjork-Shiley prosthetic valves. J Am Coll Cardiol 7:681−687
22. Erbel R, Rohman S, Drexler M, et al (1988) Improved diagnostic value of echocardiography in patients with infective endocarditis by transesophageal approach. A prospective study. Eur Heart J 9:43−53

Evaluation of Mitral Prosthesis
by Transesophageal Echocardiography

M. SCHARTL, S. DREYSE, E. WEIMANN, A. DESIDERI, H. BIAS, D. LOOS,
P. WALKER, and K. AFFELD

There are three primary considerations in the evaluation of mechanical mitral valve prostheses:

1. Is there evidence of an anatomic abnormality suggesting the presence of vegetation, thrombus, or abscess?
2. Is antegrade flow impeded with a resultant functional stenosis?
3. Is there evidence of systolic regurgitation through a valvular or paravalvular leak?

We are especially interested in the problem of systolic regurgitation in patients with mechanical mitral valve prostheses.

Under normal conditions all mechanical prostheses demonstrate a certain degree of regurgitation, which represents the sum of two components — regurgitant flow at the moment of closure of the valve and leakage during the period of closure. This normal regurgitant flow ranges from 3–13 ml — or about 10% of forward flow — in mechanical prostheses and is greatest in the St. Jude medical prosthesis [1].

We have developed a pulsatile flow model to define the normal degree of regurgitant flow in mechanical heart valves using color flow imaging and particle flow visualization with a suspension of glass beads in water as flow markers. The microspheres are suitable as light reflectors and as targets for Doppler color flow imaging.

Figure 1 shows a Björck-Shiley prosthesis with one jet originating at the margin of the valve. Doppler color flow imaging also demonstrates the presence of one lateral regurgitant jet (Fig. 2). When the mitral valve is rotated through 90° two jets of different sizes flow together at approximately 2 cm from the valve prosthesis (Fig. 3). Doppler color flow imaging also documents the presence of two regurgitant jets which flow together in the middle of the atrium (Fig. 4). This means that in Björck-Shiley prostheses, normal regurgitant flow occurs at the rim through the large and small openings and that the number of visible jets will necessarily vary with the imaging plane. In St. Jude Medical prostheses there are three theoretical possibilities for normal regurgitation: through the middle of the two mechanical occluders, and through both sides of the rim of the prosthesis. In our model, we usually found two small jets diverging from the central part of the prothesis. The jets extend to the middle of the atrium. Doppler color flow imaging also documents the presence of two divergent jets with slight turbulence. However, in exceptional cases, up to three jets have been found.

Transesophageal Echocardiography
Edited by R. Erbel et al.
© Springer-Verlag Berlin Heidelberg 1989

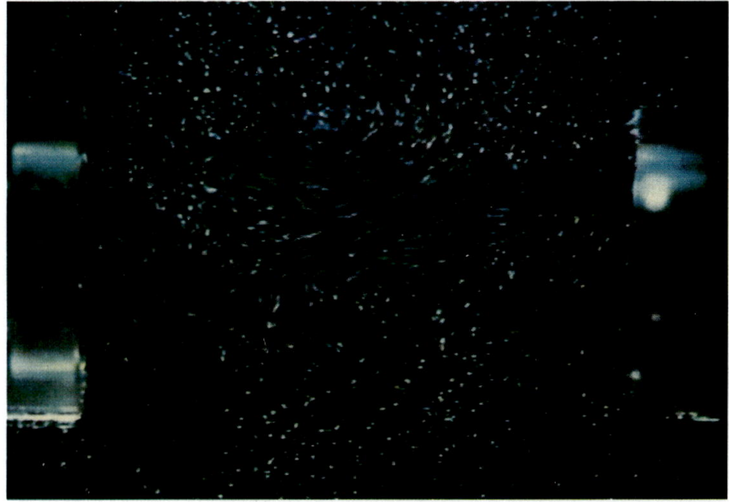

Fig. 1. Pulsatile flow model with a Björk-Shiley prosthesis on the right side. One jet originates at the margin of the valve

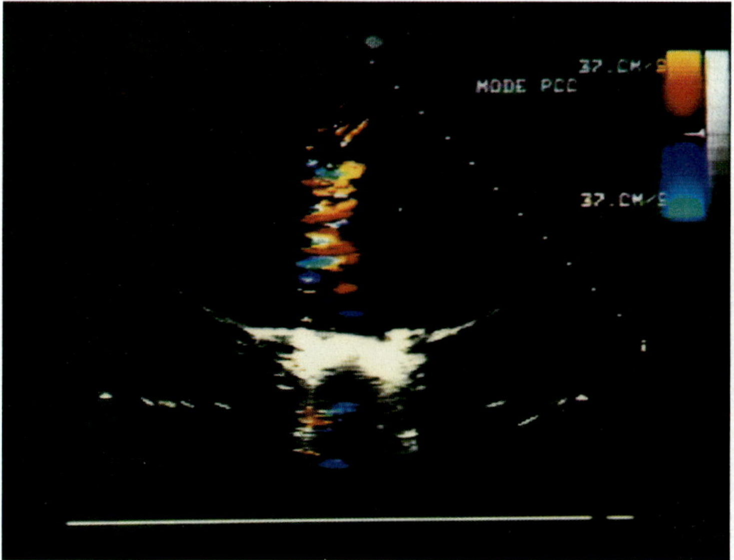

Fig. 2. Doppler color flow imaging in the pulsatile flow model demonstrates the presence of one lateral regurgitant jet

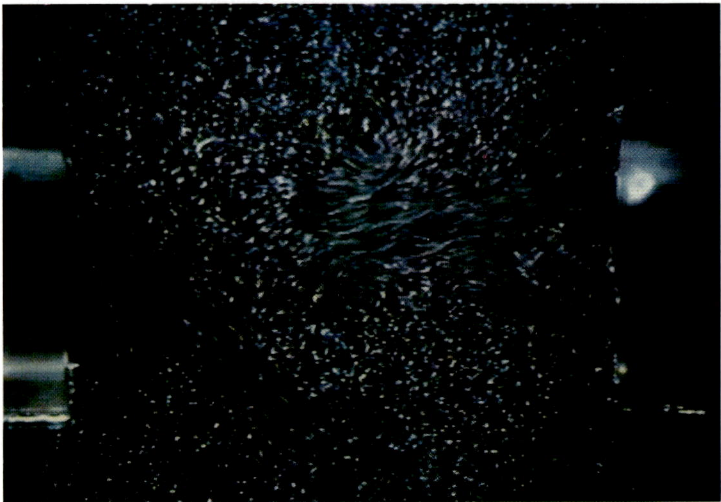

Fig. 3. The Björck-Shiley prosthesis is rotated through 90°. There are two jets of different sizes flowing together at approximately 2 cm from the valve prosthesis

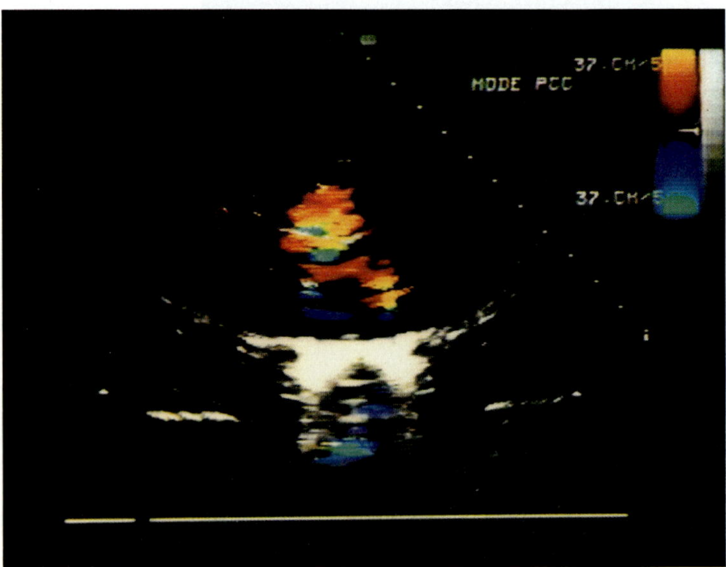

Fig. 4. Doppler flow imaging also documents the presence of two regurgitant jets when the Björk-Shiley prosthesis is rotated through 90°

In Duromedics prostheses there is one central jet from the middle of the prosthesis because of the wide opening between the two occluders. In our experimental model, and in most patients, we found a central, slightly turbulent holosystolic jet extending to the middle of the atrium.

It should be emphasized that there is great variability in jets between patients and from beat to beat in the same patient. We measured the maximum length and area of jets in 40 patients with normal valve function evaluated on the basis of history and clinical examination. Using these findings, we have developed the following preliminary criteria for normal function of mechanical mitral valve prostheses.

All patients with Björck-Shiley, St. Jude medical, and Duromedics prostheses had one to three jets at transesophageal echocardiographic examinations. These jets were holosystolic and slightly turbulent. Only 5% of the jets were detected by the transthoracic approach. Maximum jet length was 4 cm and the maximum area 6 cm^2. Only in a few cases did the jets extend to the roof of the atrium. These measurements must be examined critically, since the variability of these parameters is great, and calibration of color flow measurements is unsatisfactory (Table 1).

Pathological jets are usually characterized by severe turbulence and greater length and larger area than jets associated with normal valve function. Paravalvular leakage can often be recognized on the basis of location, lateral to the valve prosthesis. However, it may be difficult to differentiate between paravalvular and transvalvular leakage in some cases since the paravalvular jet may appear to lie in the plane of the valve.

Comparison of findings with transthoracic and transesophageal echocardiography reveals that the transthoracic approach demonstrated only 44% of 25 pathological jets documented by transesophageal echocardiography. Eight of 25 patients were examined by cardiac catheterization, during surgery, or at autopsy; the echocardiographic diagnosis was confirmed in all eight cases (Table 2).

Qualitative demonstration of normal and pathological jets by transesophageal echocardiography is possible, but the problem of estimating the hemodynamic significance of these lesions remains [2]. We are currently using our in vitro model to address this question, and we hope to report our initial findings in the near future.

Table 1. Systolic color Doppler criteria in "normal" mechanical mitral valve prostheses

	Björk-Shiley ($n = 8$)	St. Jude Med. ($n = 17$)	Duromedics ($n = 15$)
Jets (n)	2	1–3	1–3
Length (cm)	0.5–3.6	0.5–4.3	0.3–3.9
Area (cm^2)	0.2–3.8	0.2–6.4	0.4–4.8
Duration	holosystolic	holosystolic	holosystolic
Turbulence	low	low	low

Table 2. Pathologic regurgitation in mechanical mitral valve prostheses

	TTE (CW, PW, color flow)	TEE (PW, color flow)	Autopsy, surgery, catheterization
Transvalvular	11	5	3/3
Paravalvular		20	5/5
	11/25 (44%)	25/25 (100%)	

TTE, transthoracic echocardiography; TEE, transesophageal echocardiography; CW, Continuous wave; PW, pulse wave

References

1. Mayer YR, Stevenson DM, Allen DT et al. (1986) Flow characteristics of four commonly used mechanical heart valves. Am J Cardiol 58:743–752
2. Vandenberg BF, Dellsperger KC, Chandran KB, Kerber E (1988) Detection, localization and quantitation of bioprosthetic mitral valve regurgitation. Circulation 78:529–538

Transesophageal Evaluation
of Aortic Valve Prostheses

S. Mohr-Kahaly, I. Kupferwasser, R. Erbel, M. Todt, H. Oelert,
and J. Meyer

Introduction

The noninvasive evaluation of prosthetic heart valves in the aortic position
remains a diagnostic challenge. Although numerous studies have established
the diagnostic value of transthoracic two-dimensional (2-D) and Doppler
echocardiography [1−3], image quality is often impaired by emphysema,
obesity, valve artifacts, and shadowing or flow masking due to the artifical
valve materials [4]. Transesophageal echocardiography has overcome these
methodological problems. Due to the proximity of the esophagus and the
heart, the aortic valve can be visualized with a high image quality [5−7].

However, compared to flow across mitral valve prostheses, flow within the
left ventricular outflow tract is visualized from a less advantageous Doppler
angle. The first aim of this study was to analyze forward and regurgitant flow
across normally functioning aortic valve prostheses. In addition, the diagnostic value of the transesophageal approach was compared to that of transthoracic 2-D echocardiography with regard to the detection of complications
in aortic valve prostheses.

Patients and Methods

Patients. From January 1986 to October 1988, 152 patients (94 men, 58
women) aged 16−79 years (mean 63 years) were included in this study. Seven-
ty-nine prostheses (16 Björk-Shiley, 25 St. Jude Medical, 20 Duromedics, and
18 porcine bioprostheses) were considered as normally functioning using
physical examination and conventional echocardiography and Doppler
techniques. In 83 patients (8 Björk-Shiley, 15 St. Jude Medical, 9 Duromedics
and 51 Bioprostheses), 121 complications or dysfunctions were detected.

Echocardiographic Instrumentation. 2-D and color-coded Doppler echocardiographic recordings were made using electronic sector scanners (Toshiba
SSH 65 A, 160 A). For transthoracic examinations a 2.5-MHz transducer was
used and for transesophageal studies a 3.75-MHz endoscopic phased array
probe.

Patient Preparation and Examination Technique. Patients were examined in
the left lateral decubitus position. For transthoracic studies, parasternal long-

Transesophageal Echocardiography
Edited by R. Erbel et al.
© Springer-Verlag Berlin Heidelberg 1989

and short-axis and apical right anterior oblique equivalent views were used. For the transesophageal examination, patients had fasted for a minimum of 4 h and received local anesthesia of the throat. When there was an adverse reaction, mild sedation (diazepam 5–10 mg) was given. The probe was advanced 30–35 cm into the esophagus. From this position the left atrium, mitral and aortic valves, and the left ventricular outflow tract can be scanned by moving the transducer slightly.

Analysis of Normal Valve Prostheses. The timing of forward flow was analyzed for different types of prostheses by determining the percentage of the duration of systole taken up by the preejection and ejection periods. Aortic regurgitation was diagnosed when diastolic turbulent flow originating from the aortic valve was visualized in the left ventricular outflow tract. For determining the flow timing and the duration of regurgitant flow, ECG-triggered 2-D echo and high speed M-mode recordings were used.

Analysis of Dysfunctioning Prostheses or Complications. Transprosthetic regurgitation was differentiated from periprosthetic regurgitation by noting where the regurgitant jet originated. Regurgitation was considered periprosthetic when the origin was outside the valve annulus. Vegetations were diagnosed when additional floting echo structures were visualized and the patient had symptoms of an inflammatory process. Paravalvular abscesses were diagnosed when additional echofree cavities within the aortic ring − with or without flow − were visualized. Futhermore, sinus valsalvae aneurysms, bioprosthetic degeneration, and prosthetic obstructions were searched for.

Results

Normal Prostheses. Forward flow across mechanical prostheses started significantly ($p \leq 0.05$) later than in bioprostheses due to the prolonged preejection period (Figure 1). No significant differences in the relative duration of forward flow were detected between different types of mechanical prostheses.

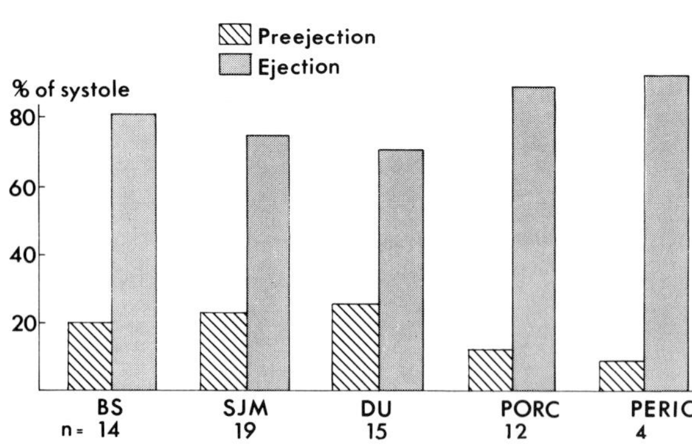

Fig. 1. Relative duration of the preejection (*hatched bars*) and ejection period (*stippled bars*) across different types of aortic valve prostheses analyzed using transesophageal high-speed M-mode color-coded Doppler recordings. *BS*, Björk-Shiley; *SJM*, St. Jude Medical; *DU*, Duromedics; *PORC*, porcine bioprostheses; *PERIC*, pericardial bioprothesis

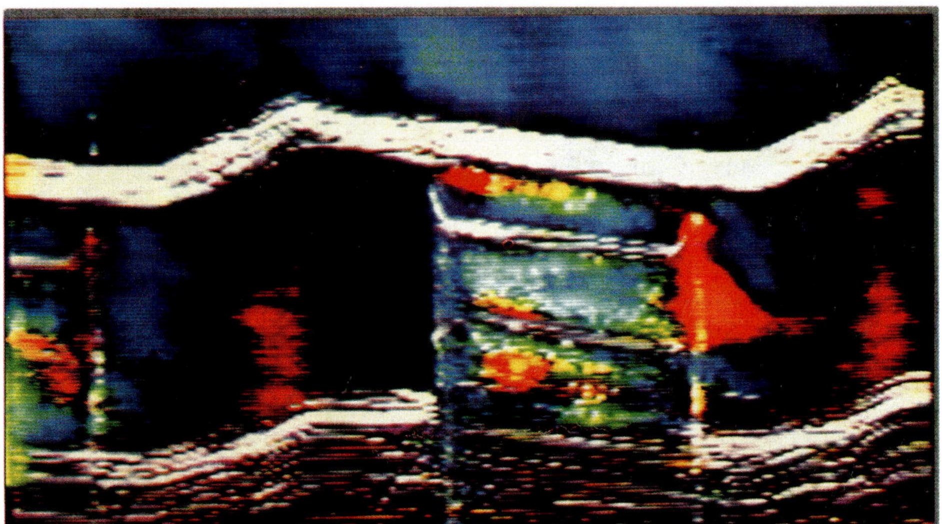

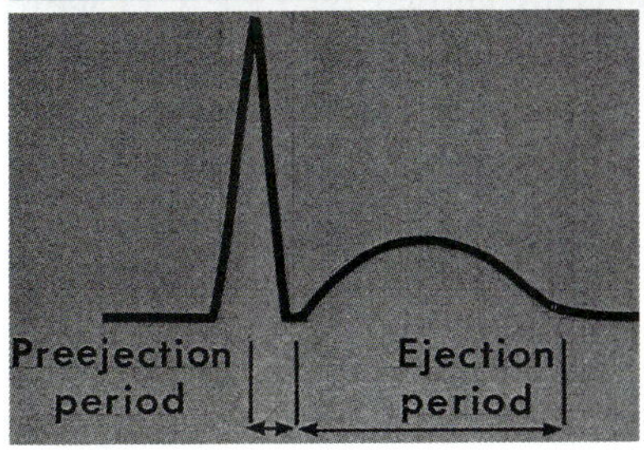

Fig. 2. Typical example of antegrade flow across a Duromedics bileaflet mechanical prosthesis in the aortic position using M-mode TEE-CD

Typical flow patterns were differentiated for the different valve types. In bioprostheses one central inflow jet was noted, whereas in St. Jude prostheses flow was visualized across the three orifices and in Björk-Shiley prostheses across the major and minor orifice (Fig. 2).

Regurgitation of aortic prostheses was noted by transthoracic color-coded Doppler echocardiography (TTE-CD) in 29% of cases (21/73) and transesophageally (TEE-CD) in 44% (35/79) (Table 1). The maximal jet length and area detected by TTE-CD were larger than those visualized by TEE-CD ($p \leq 0.05$) (Fig. 3).

With TTE-CD, regurgitant jets were detected only during early diastole in 88% of cases (18/21) and lasted to mid-diastole in 12% (3/21). Using TEE-CD, early diastolic regurgitant flow was noted in 68% (24/35); it lasted to mid-diastole in 9% (3/35) and was holodiastolic in 23% (8/35).

Prosthetic Dysfunction or Complications. Transprosthetic regurgitation was noted by TEE-CD in 22 patients. Only in 15 cases were regurgitant signals depicted by TEE-CD. Periprosthetic regurgitation was visualized by TEE-CD in 11 patients but could be noted in only three patients by TTE-CD. Degeneration of bioprostheses was detected in 14 patients by TEE-CD compared to

                                                  S. Mohr-Kahaly et al.

Table 1. Regurgitation in Aortic Valve Prostheses

	transthoracic		transesophageal	
	n	%	n	%
BS	6/15	40	5/16	31
SJM	5/22	23	14/25	56
DU	6/18	33	9/20	45
Porc	4/18	22	7/18	39
Total/Mean	21/73	29	35/79	44

BS, Björk-Shiley; SJM, St. Jude Medical; DU, Duromedics; Porc, Porcine valve prosthesis; n, Number.

eight by TTE-CD (Fig. 4). Vegetations were noted in 21 patients by TEE-CD but could be visualized in only five by TTE-CD. Paravalvular abcesses were found in 13 patients by TEE-CD, but only one abcess could be detected using TTE-CD. Three of eight sinus valsalvae aneurysms shown by TEE-CD were noted using the transthoracic approach (Fig. 5). Prosthetic obstruction or

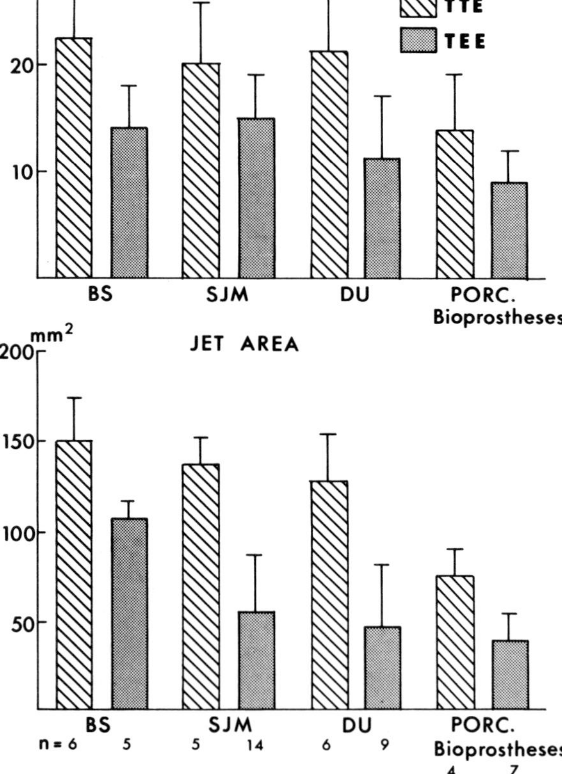

Fig. 3. Maximal jet length and jet area in normally functioning aortic prostheses analyzed by TTE-CD (*hatched bars*) and TEE-CD (*stippled bars*). For abbreviations, see Fig. 1

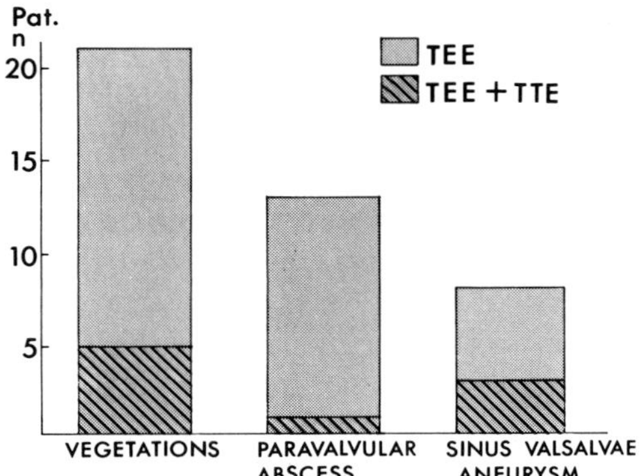

Fig. 4. Detection of complications of aortic valve prostheses using TTE-CD (*hatched areas*) and TEE-CD (*stippled areas*): vegetations, paravalvular abscesses, and sinus valsalvae aneurysms

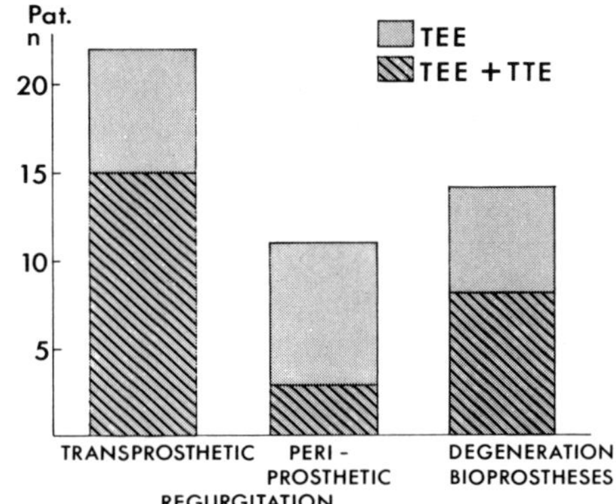

Fig. 5. Detection of complications in aortic valve prostheses using TTE-CD (*hatched areas*) and TEE-CD (*stippled areas*): regurgitations and degeneration of bioprostheses

stenosis were identified using TEE-CD in 15 patients, but TTE-CD and continuous wave Doppler failed to show obstruction in six patients. On the other hand, TEE-CD was negative in four patients where TTE-CD demonstrated pathological flow acceleration.

Discussion

Transesophageal 2-D and color-coded Doppler echocardiography offers new possibilities for the evaluation of prosthetic heart valves. High quality structure and flow information can be obtained in a higher percentage of patients by this method than with the transthoracic approach as has been shown before [8–10].

Especially the left atrial aspect of mitral prostheses can be visualized without interference of valve artifacts and flow masking [4, 9, 11]. Thus, TEE-CD seems to be the method of choice for the evaluating of mitral prostheses. For prostheses in the aortic position, its role had not previously been determined.

For the evaluation of aortic valve morphology, TEE seems to be superior to TTE due to the short distance between the aortic valve and the transducer allowing higher transducer frequencies. This is shown by the higher detection rate of degeneration of bioprostheses as well as of aortic ring abcesses, sinus valsalvae aneurysms, and vegetations. However, in mechanical protheses there may be shadowing of the anteriorly located parts of the aortic ring.

Concerning the evaluation of flow across aortic valve prostheses, it is important to be aware of the less favorable Doppler angle which, in contrast to mitral prostheses, is close to 90° to flow within the left ventricular outflow tract. Nevertheless, forward flow across normally functioning aortic valve prostheses can be visualized at higher spatial and temporal resolution than with TTE-CD. Differences between mechanical and bioprostheses in the relative duration of forward flow during systole were detected. This finding had not previously been reported in vivo. Furthermore, the spatial distribution of antegrade flow across different types of aortic valve prostheses within the aortic root can be determined in the same way as has been shown across mitral prostheses using the transthorac approach [12].

Regurgitant flow could be detected in a higher percentage of normally functioning aortic valve prostheses by TEE-CD than by TTE-CD (44% vs. 29%), but in a significantly lower percentage than in mitral valve prostheses (95%). The former may be due to the close proximity of the aortic valve and the transducer. The latter may be the result of the unfavorable Doppler angle and the limited imaging planes of TEE-CD. The jet length and area were significantly larger with TTE-CD than with TEE-CD. According to our findings, a regurgitant jet area of less than 1 cm^2 and a length of less than 1.5 cm may be considered a normal finding for TEE-CD in the absence of morphological pathology [13]. These results are supported by the in vitro findings of Switzer et. al., who found regurgitant jets of up to 2 cm in length in an aortic flow model in normally functioning mechanical prostheses [14], as well as by TEE-CD studies from Lange [15]. The differentiation between transprosthetic and periprosthetic regurgitation may be easier using TEE-CD because of the higher image quality but it remains a diagnostic problem. Due to restricted imaging planes, partial shadowing of the aortic ring, and the cross-sectional display, the origin of a regurgitant jet may not be visible in all cases. Also, regurgitant jets may be visualized in the central part of the left ventricular outflow tract, giving the impression of transvalvular regurgitation when there is in fact periprosthetic leakage.

Angiography is not better for differentiating between transprosthetic and periprosthetic leakage. Combined transthoracic and transesophageal examination seems to be the method of choice.

For the detection of prosthetic obstruction or stenosis, transthoracic continuous wave Doppler will be the first diagnostic method. Only in patients with no transthoracic acoustic window or in patients with bioprostheses will TEE-CD be superior to the transthoracic approach, as most transesophageal probes are not equipped with continuous wave Doppler.

Conclusion

Because of the high image quality, TEE-CD is the method of choice for the detection of endocarditis-related complications in aortic valve prostheses as well as for the detection of bioprosthetic degeneration.

In about 40% of normal prostheses, regurgitation with a jet area ≤ 1 cm^2 and a jet length ≤ 1.5 cm can be detected. The differentiation of transprosthetic and periprosthetic regurgitation is better with TEE-CD but still not possible in all patients. Its value for the detection of stenosis or prosthetic obstruction is limited mostly to bioprostheses.

References

1. Kottler MN, Mintz GS, Panidis I, Morganroth J, Segal BL, Ross J (1983) Noninvasive evaluation of normal and abnormal prosthetic valve function. J Am Coll Cardiol 2:151–173
2. Alam M, Rosman HS, Lakier JB, Kemp S, Khaja F, Hautamaki K, Magilligan DJ, Stein PD (1987) Doppler and echocardiographic features of normal and dysfunctioning bioprosthetic valves. J Am Coll Cardiol 10:851–858
3. Reisner SA, Meltzer RS (1988) Normal values of prosthetic valve Doppler echocardiographic parameters: review. J Am Soc Echocardiogr 1:201–210
4. Sprecher DL, Adamick A, Adams D, Kisslo J (1987) In vitro color flow and continous wave Doppler ultrasound masking of flow by prosthetic valves. J Am Coll Cardiol 9:1306–1310
5. Schlüter M, Hinrichs A, Thier W, Kremer P, Schröder S, Cahalan K, Hanrath P (1984) Transesophageal two dimensional echocardiography: comparison of ultrasonic and anatomic sections. Am J Cardiol 53:1173–1178
6. Erbel R, Mohr-Kahaly S, Drexler M, Pfeiffer C, Börner N, Schuster S, Zenker G, Meyer J (1987) Diagnostischer Stellenwert der transösophagealen Echokardiographie. Deutsch Med Wochenschr 112:23–29
7. Seward JB, Khandheria BK, Oh JK, Abel MD, Hughes RW, Edwards WD, Nichols BA, Freeman WK, Tajik AJ (1988) Transesophageal echocardiography: technique, anatomic correlations, implementation, and clinical applications. Mayo Clin Proc 63:649–680
8. Nellessen U, Daniel WG, Hecker H, Hetzer R, Schleberger J, Lichtlen PR (1985) Nachweis einer Malfunktion von Herzklappenprothesen mittels zweidimensionaler transösophagealer Echokardiographie. In: Erbel R, Meyer J, Brennecke R (eds) Fortschritte der Echokardiographie. Springer, Berlin Heidelberg New York
9. Nellessen U, Schnittger I, Appleton CP, Masuyama T, Bolger A, Fischell TA, Tye T, Pop Rl (1988) Transesophageal two-dimensional echocardiography and color Doppler flow velocity mapping in the evaluation of cardiac valve prostheses. Circulation 78:848–855
10. Mohr-Kahaly S, Erbel R, Drexler M, Wittlich N, Steller D, Szydlowski D, Meyer J (1989) Vergleich der diagnostischen Wertigkeit von transthorakaler und transösophagealer Echokardiographie für die Funktionsbeurteilung von Herzklappenprothesen. In Grube E (Hrsg) Farbdoppler und Kontrastechokardiographie. Georg Thieme Verlag Stuttgart. 259–265
11. Kyo S, Takamoto S, Matsumura M, Asano A, Yokote Y, Motoyama T, Omoto R (1987) Immediate and early postoperative transesophageal two-dimensional Doppler echocardiography. Circulation 76 (Suppl V):113–121
12. Jones M, McMillan ST, Eibdo EE, Woo YR, Yoganathan AP (1986) Evaluation of prosthetic heart valves by Doppler flow imaging. Echocardiography 3:513–525

13. Mohr-Kahaly S, Erbel R, Kupferwasser I, Wittlich N, Henrichs J, Meyer J (1988) Regurgitation of prosthetic heart valves analyzed by transesophageal 2d color Doppler (Abstract). Eur Heart 9 (Suppl I):274
14. Switzer DF, Yoganathan AP, Nanda NC, Woo YR, Ridgway AJ (1987) Calibration of color Doppler flow mapping during extreme hemodynamic conditions in vitro: a foundation for a reliable quantitative grading system for aortic incompetence. Circulation 75:837−846
15. Lange HW, Olson J, Kane M, Daniel JA, Goldenberg IF (1988) Transesophageal color Doppler evaluation of transvalvular regurgitation of the normally functioning St. Jude bileaflet mechanical prosthesis in aortic and mitral position. Abstracts of the proceedings of transesophageal echocardiography, Mainz

**Transesophageal Echocardiography
in Critically Ill Patients, Monitoring
by Transesophageal Echocardiography**

Diagnostic Value of Transesophageal Echocardiography in Critically Ill Patients

P. HANRATH, A. KREIS, B. SCHNEIDER, B. LANGENSTEIN, and W. KRÜGER

The idea of scanning the heart from the esophagus is not new [7, 13, 16, 19, 22, 38]. The underlying concept is that superior image quality should be obtained by scanning the target organ with the transducer very close to it. This can be done using high-frequency transducers which give a much better resolution from this position than with the common transthoracic echocardiographic approch, avoiding interference from air-filled pulmonary structures and bones [14, 33, 34]. The decisive breakthrough towards wide application of transesophageal echocardiography (TEE) was the incorporation of a miniaturized phased-array transducer into a flexible endoscope in the early 1980s [18, 28, 30, 42]. Recently, through the additional use of color-coded Doppler echocardiography TEE has gained, increasing importance, not only as an intraoperative monitoring system [5, 6, 20, 23, 24, 27, 31,39] but also as an alternative method in the intensive care unit.

In the following the value of this technique as a routine diagnostic method in the intensive care unit is demonstrated showing its diagnostic capabilities and the immediate therapeutic conclusions that can be arrived at using TEE.

Diseases of the Thoracic Aorta

It was the work of the group in Mainz which showed the unique capabilities of TEE in detecting acute aortic dissection in comparison with conventional imaging techniques [4, 14, 29]. In contrast to conventional echocardiography, which shows aortic wall dissection only under ideal scanning conditions in the ascending aorta, with TEE almost the whole thoracic aorta can be visualized without problems. TEE is capable of showing the morphology and extent of the dissection and the entrance and exit of the false lumen, and can be used to evaluate the results of treatment without exposing a dangerously ill patient to the risk of transportation to other imaging facilities.

Only the superior ascending aorta and parts of the aortic arch with the brachiocephalic arteries cannot always be visualized because of the interposition of the right main bronchus between the transducer and the target organ, this being most frequent in type II dissection. This method can also be used to demonstrate or rule out complicating aortic insufficiency and pericardial effusion.

Using TEE, recurrent peripheral arterial embolization was shown to be due to free-floating thrombotic material in the descending aorta, probably

Transesophageal Echocardiography
Edited by R. Erbel et al.
© Springer-Verlag Berlin Heidelberg 1989

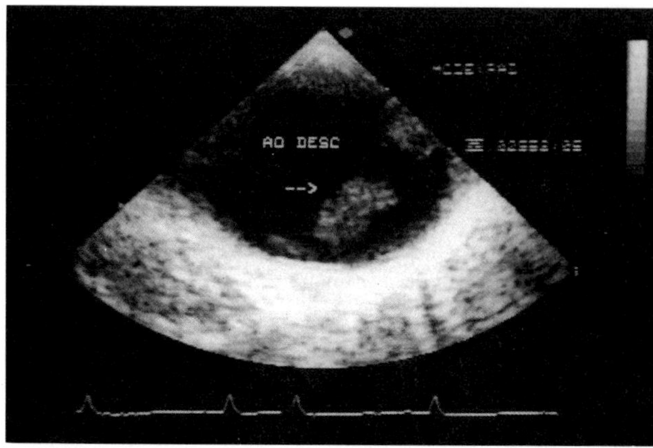

Fig. 1. Cross-sectional view of the aorta descendens (*Ao DESC*) with free-floating thrombotic material (*arrow*)

originating from advanced-stage arteriosclerosis in the aorta [21] (Fig. 1). Using the same investigation procedure, the left atrial appendage and the left ventricular cavity were ruled out as sources of cardiac embolization.

Diseases of Native Valves

Today there is no doubt that echocardiography is the diagnostic procedure of choice to prove the existence of bacterial endocarditis [2, 3]. Even if the age and underlying morphology of the process cannot be assessed by ultrasound, endocarditis can be confirmed by a combination of external echocardiography and the clinical findings in two-thirds of all cases. With the additional use of TEE the sensitivity may be increased up to 90%. The echocardiographic information combined with the clinical pattern leads in most cases to a certain diagnosis followed by successful therapeutic intervention [3]. Worldwide experience with TEE in the past few years has shown that when acute endocarditis is suspected on the basis of clinical symptoms, negative results of transthoracic echocardiography need to be confirmed or the disease ruled out by TEE.

An extremely life-threatening and diagnostically difficult situation is the development of valvular ring abscesses. In this special form of acute endocarditis, TEE is at present the method of choice [8, 9, 12]. Figure 2 shows a case of abscess formation in the posterolateral wall of the aorta which was confirmed during operation.

It is not rare for aortic valve endocarditis with flail ruptured valves or attached vegetations prolapsing into the left ventricular outflow tract in diastole to be found using TEE. These structures may be difficult to differentiate from congenital subaortic fibrous membranes. With TEE these structures can be identified and their morphology characterized, resulting in clear differentiation of the two disease forms [32, 43].

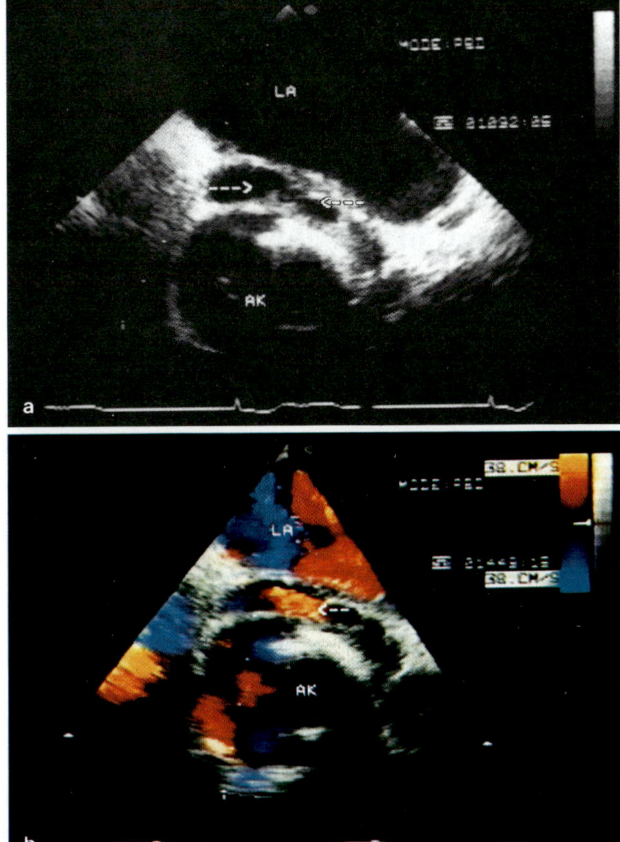

Fig. 2. a Abscess formation (*arrow*) in the posterolateral wall of the aorta ascendens. **b** Connection of the abscess hole (*arrow*) with the lumen of the aorta, demonstrated by color-coded Doppler flow. *AK*, aortic valve; *LA*, left atrium

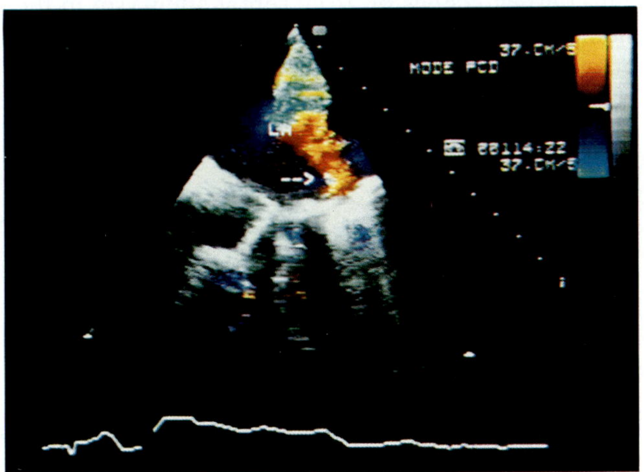

Fig. 3. Artificial valve in the mitral position with paravalvular leakage (*arrow*) shown by two-dimensional color Doppler analysis from the esophagus. *LA*, left atrium

Acute mitral insufficiency may lead to life-threatening left ventricular heart failure. One of the many causes of acute mitral insufficiency is rupture of the chordae tendineae supporting a leaflet [35]. With color two-dimensional TEE, ruptured chordae of the mitral leaflets and the resulting regurgitation during ventricular systole can be easily shown.

Dysfunction of Prosthetic Valves

Acute left ventricular dysfunction due to a stenotic or insufficient prosthetic mitral valve is often a cause for emergency treatment being given in the cardiac care unit. TEE is very useful in scanning prosthetic valves, especially ones in the mitral position, because there are no interfering structures between the atrial side of the prosthesis and the transducer [11, 25, 36, 37].

An other life-threatening complication easily detected using TEE is thrombus formation within the left atrium or the left atrial appendage due to stenosis of an artificial valve. The transesophageal approach combined with color-coded Doppler analysis also allows valvular and paravalvular leakages to be differentiated easily and safely (Fig. 3) [11].

Cardiac Sources of Embolization

The most frequent source of cardiac embolization is a thrombus in the left atrial appendage, which cannot be visualized using the transthoracic approach. With TEE this structure is easily visualized [1]. Because of the great depth using the apical or parasternal approaches and the resulting decreased resolution, small thrombi within the anterosuperior and lateral left atrium are difficult to identify using transthoracic echocardiography. So-called spontaneous contrast echoes or atrial septal aneurysm in the left atrium [15, 17], which cannot be shown using the transthoracic approach, are significant indicators of a higher risk of embolization, so evidence of these must be taken into account in determining the therapeutic strategy [10].

Morphology and Function of the Ventricles During Acute Myocardial Infarction

Infarction of the right ventricle together with left ventricular inferior wall infarction − so-called right ventricular infarct − is clinically and electrocardiographically difficult to diagnose and needs a different therapeutic approach. With the help of TEE it is possible to show wall motion abnormalities and impairment of right ventricle function in more detail (Fig. 4). A dangerous,

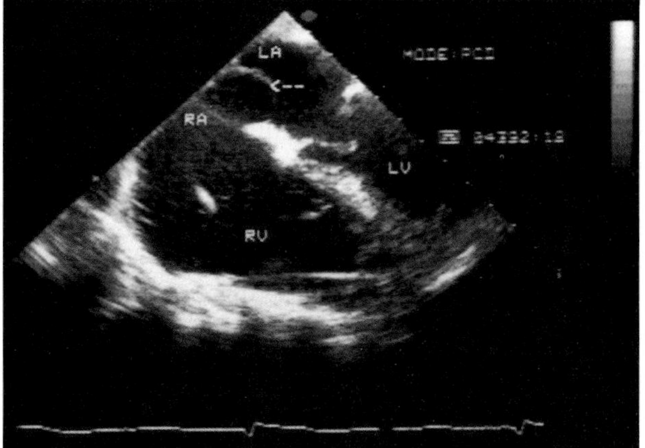

Fig. 4. Akinesis of the lateral wall of the right ventricle (*RV*) in inferior wall infarction, resulting in right ventricle (*RV*) and right atrial (*RA*) dilatation with paradoxical motion of the interatrial septum (*arrow*). *LA*, left atrium; *LV*, left ventricle

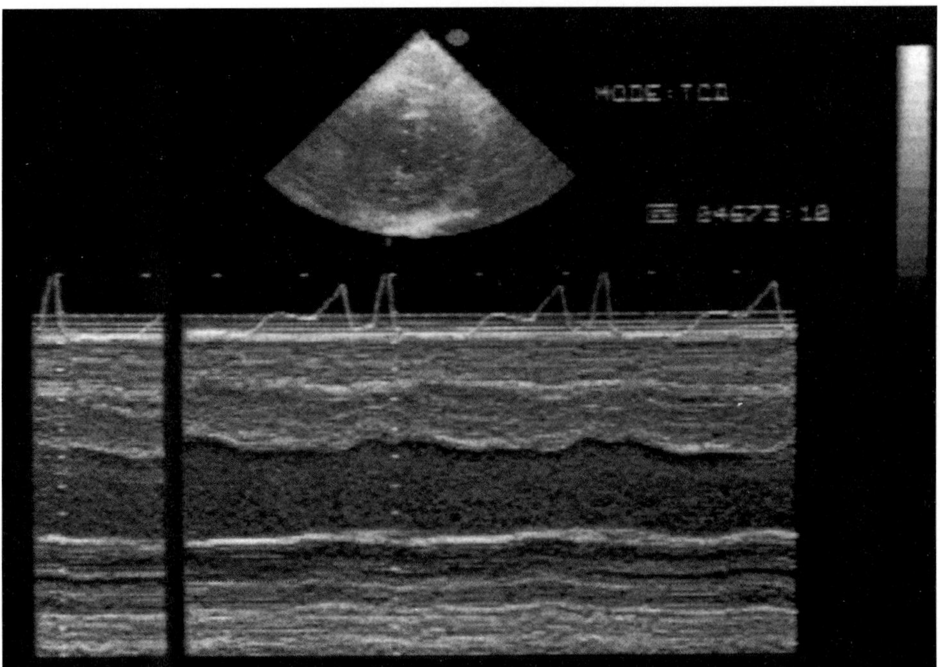

Fig. 5. Transesophageal M-mode recording in a patient with myocardial infarction with akinesis of the anteroseptal wall and hypokinesis of the inferior wall (*IW*) intraoperatively (*top* of the M-mode and two-dimensional recordings)

usually fatal, complication of myocardial infarction is acute cardiac rupture. If the rupture is limited to the intraventricular septum with consecutive shunt or if a pseudoaneurysm develops the patient's survival depends on quick diagnosis and immediate therapy. These findings are easily detected with TEE.

Postoperative Follow Up

Postoperative follow up of patients after implantation of prosthetic valves or coronary artery bypass grafting (CABG) is usually based mainly on the clinical and radiologic findings, as well as on left atrial pressure measurements or blood gas analysis. In the diagnostic and therapeutic management of postoperatively difficult patients, TEE has proven in our hands to be a very useful tool. Intra- and postoperative myocardial infarction can occur during CABG procedures and are often a considerable diagnostic and therapeutic problem [41]. The use of TEE in these cases allows a rough evaluation of the infarcted area and the functional state of the resting myocardium, which may have implications for the future drug treatment of the patient [25, 26].

Figure 5 shows a large expanded anteroseptal akinesis in a 45-year-old patient after CABG and intraoperative infarction, which was judged as mild based on ECG and enzymatic criteria. The TEE findings provided a plausible

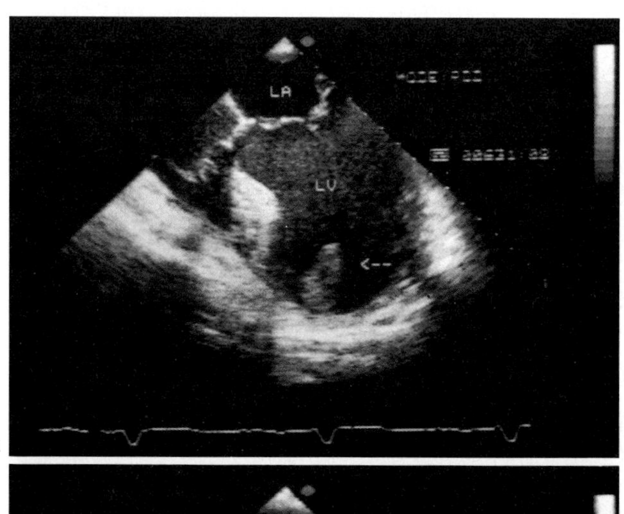

a

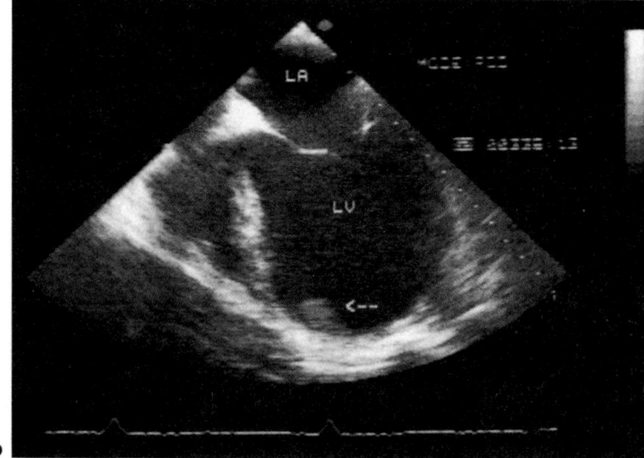

b

Fig. 6 a, b. Thrombus formation (*arrow*) in the apex of the left ventricle (*LV*) before *a* and *b* after heparinization. *LA*, left atrium

explanation for the poor postoperative recovery and the high dosage of catecholamines the patient needed.

Intra- and postoperative cerebral strokes are potentially dangerous events after cardiac surgery. If the embolus is of cardiac origin, it can be of air or thrombus. Figure 6 shows a lance-shaped thrombus emerging into the left ventricle (Fig. 6a) of a 42-year-old patient who had had a severe intraoperative cerebral embolization. After high-dose heparin therapy over several weeks the thrombus was abolished almost totally (Fig. 6b).

Conclusions

The increasing clinical use of TEE as a cardiac imaging technique in the past few years has clearly shown that TEE is not only of importance as an alternative to the well-known transthoracic approach as a routine procedure but is especially useful in the intensive care unit where, because of the difficulty of transthoracic access, it is of greater clinical relevance.

Recording of the pulmonary wedge pressure by Swan-Ganz catheterization combined with morphologic information derived from TEE allows quick diagnostic and therapeutic decisions to be made on a causal basis in individual patients.

References

1. Aschenberg W, Schlüter M, Kremer P, Schröder E, Siglow V, Bleifeld W (1986) Transesophageal two-dimensional echocardiography for the detection of left atrial appendage thrombus. J Am Coll Cardiol 7:163−166
2. Becher H, Polster J, Langenstein BA, Hanrath P, Bleifeld W (1983) Stellenwert der Echokardiographie in der präoperativen Diagnostik der akuten bakteriellen Endokarditis. Dtsch Med Wochenschr 108:363
3. Becher H, Hanrath P, Bleifled W, Bleese N (1984) Correlation of echocardiography and surgical findings in acute bacterial endocarditis. Eur Heart J 5 (suppl C):67
4. Börner N, Erbel R, Braun B, Henkel B, Meyer J, Rumpelt J (1984) Diagnosis of aortic dissection by transesophageal echocardiography. Am J Cardiol 54:1157
5. Bruijn P de, Clements FM, Kisslo JA (1987) Intraoperative transesophageal color flow mapping: initial experience. Anesth Analg 66:386
6. Cahalan MK, Litt L, Botvinik EH, Schiller NB (1987) Advances in noninvasive cardiovascular imaging: implications for the anesthesiologist. Anesthesiology 66:356
7. Daigle RE, Miller CW, Histand MB et al (1975) Non-traumatic aortic blood flow sensing by use of an ultrasonic esophageal probe. J Appl Physiol 38:1153
8. Daniel WG, Schröder E, Nonnast-Daniel B, Lichtlen PR (1987) Conventional and transesophageal echocardiography in the diagnosis of infective endocarditis. Eur Heart J 8 (suppl J):287
9. Daniel WG, Schröder E, Mügge A, Lichtlen PR (1988) Transesophageal echocardiography in infective endocarditis. Am J Cardiac Imaging 2:78
10. Daniel WG, Nellessen U, Schröder E, Nonast-Daniel B, Bednarski P, Nikutta P, Lichtlen PLR (1988) Left atrial spontaneous echo contrast in mitral valve disease: an indicator for an increased thromboembolic risk. J Am Coll Cardiol 11:1204

11. Daniel WG, Hanrath P, Mügge A, Langenstein B, Engel H, Grote I (1988) Assessment of mitral prosthetic valve dysfunction by transesophageal color coded dopplerechocardiography (abstract). Circulation 78 (suppl part II):II−607

12. Drexler M, Erbel R, Rohmann S, Mohr-Kahaly S, Meyer J (1987) Diagnostic value of two-dimensional transesophageal versus transthoracic echocardiography in patients with infective endocarditis. Eur Heart J 8 (suppl J):303

13. Eggleton RC (1973) Ultrasonic visualization of the dynamic geometry of the heart. Proceedings 2nd world congress on ultrasonics in medicine. Excerpta Medica, Amsterdam, p 10 (International congress series 277)

14. Erbel R, Mohr-Kahaly S, Drexler M, Pfeiffer C, Börner N, Schuster S (1987) Diagnostischer Stellenwert der transoesophagealen Echokardiographie. Dtsch Med Wochenschr 112:23

15. Erbel R, Stern H, Ehrenthal W, Schreiner G, Treese N, Kramer G, Thelen M, Schweizer P, Meyer J (1986) Detection of spontaneous echocardiographic contrast within the left atrium by transesophageal echocardiography: spontaneous echocardiographic contrast. Clin Cardiol 6:245

16. Frazin L, Talano JV, Stephanides (1976) Esophageal echocardiography. Circulation 54:102

17. Gallet B, Malergue MC, Adams C, Saudemont JP, Collot AM, Druon MC, Hiltgen M (1985) Atrial septal aneurysm − a potential cause of systemic embolism. An echocardiographic study. Br Heart J 53:292

18. Gussenhoven WJ, Roeland JRTC, Ligtvoet CM, McGhie J, van Herwerden LA, Cahalan M (1986) Transesophageal two-dimensional echocardiography: its role in solving clinical problems. J Am Coll Cardiol 8:975

19. Gussenhoven EJ, van Herwerden LA, Roeland JRTC, Ligtvoet KM, Bos E, Witsenburg M (1987) Intraoperative two-dimensional echocardiography in congenital heart disease. J Am Coll Cardiol 9:656

20. Hanrath P, Kremer P, Langenstein BA, Matsumoto M, Bleifeld W (1981) Transoesophageale Echokardiographie. Ein neues Verfahren zur dynamischen Ventrikelfunktionsanalyse. Dtsch Med Wochenschr 106:523

21. Hanrath P, Schneider B, Langenstein B, Poppele G, Krüger W (1989) Diagnostische Wertigkeit der transoesophagealen Echokardiographie in der internistischen Intensivmedizin. Dtsch Med Wochenschr, 114:515−523

22. Hisanaga K, Hisanaga A, Hibi N (1980) High speed rotating scanner for transesophageal crossectional echocardiography. Am J Cardial 46:10

23. Kaplan JA (1984) Transesophageal echocardiography. Mt Sinai J Med 51:5

24. Koenig K, Kasper W, Hofmann T, Meinertz T, Just H (1987) Transesophageal echocardiography for diagnosis of rupture of the ventricular septum of left ventricular papillary muscle during acute myocardial infarction. Am J Cardiol 59:330

25. Koolen II, Visser CA, Wever E, von Wezel H, Meyne NG, Dünning AJ (1987) Transesophageal echocardiographic evaluation of biventricular dimension and function during PEEP-pressure ventilation after coronary bypass grafting. Am J Cardiol 59:1047

26. Kremer P, Cahalan M, Hanrath P (1985) Die intraoperative Erkennung von Myokardischämien mittels transoesophagealer 2-D-Echokardiographie. In: Erbel R, Meyer J, Brennecke R, (eds) Fortschritte der Echokardiographie. Springer, Berlin Heidelberg New York, p 218

27. Krüger W, Plettenberg A, Poppele G, Langenstein BA, Hanrath P (1987) Funktionsbeurteilung von Mitralklappenprothesen durch transoesophageale Farbdopplerechokardiographie. Z Kardiol 76 Supp II:51

28. Langenstein BA, Poppele G, Hanrath P (1986) Nachweis einer Malfunktion von Mitral-Bioklappen durch transoesophageal 2-D-Echokardiographie. Z Kardiol 75 (suppl 4)

29. Matsumoto M, Oka Y, Strom J (1980) Application of transesophageal echocardiography. Am J Cardiol 46:95

30. Matsumoto M, Hanrath P, Kremer P, Tamms C, Langenstein BA, Schlüter M, Bleifeld W (1982) Evaluation of left ventricular performance during bicycle exercise by transesophageal M-mode echocardiography in normal subjects. Br Heart J 48:61

31. Mohr-Kahaly S, Erbel R, Börner N, Drexler M, Wittlich N, Iversen S, Oelert H, Meyer J (1986) Kombination von Farb-Doppler- und transoesophagealer Echokardiographie in der Notfalldiagnostik bei Aortendissektion vom Typ I. Z Kardiol 75:616
32. Poppele G, Krüger W, Langenstein B, Hanrath P (1988) Membranöse subvalvuläre Aortenstenose. Dtsch Med Wochenschr 113:1224
33. Roewer N, Beck H, Kochs E, Kremer P, Schröder E, Schöntag H, Jungbluth KH, Schulte am Esch J (1985) Nachweis venöser Embolien während intraoperativer Überwachung mittels transoesophagealer zweidimensionaler Echokardiographie. Anasth Intensiver Notfallmed 20:200
34. Schlüter M, Langenstein BA, Polster J, Kremer P, Souget I, Engel S, Hanrath P (1982) Transesophageal cross-sectional echocardiography with a phased array transducer system. Technique and initial clinical results. Br Heart J 48:67
35. Schlüter M, Thier W, Kremer P, Siglow V, Hanrath P (1984) Klinischer Einsatz der transoesophagealen Echokardiographie. Dtsch Med Wochenschr 18:722
36. Schlüter M, Hanrath P (1984) The clinical application of transesophageal echocardiography. Echocardiography 1:427
37. Schlüter M, Kremer P, Hanrath P (1984) Transesophageal 2-D-echocardiographic feature of flail mitral leaflet due to ruptured chordae tendineae. Am Heart J 3:609
38. Schlüter M, Langenstein BA, Hanrath P, Kremer P, Bleifeld W (1982) Assessment of transesophageal pulsed Doppler echocardiography in the detection of mitral regurgitation. Circulation 66:784
39. Schuster S, Weilemann LS, Schinzel H, Schreiner G, Henkel B, Erbel R, Meyer J (1985) Transoesophageale Echokardiographie zur Analyse des Effektes der Beatmung mit positiv endexspiratorischem Druck. In: Erbel R, Meyer J, Brennecke R (eds) Fortschritte der Echokardiographie Springer, Berlin Heidelberg New York, p 238
40. Side CD, Gosling RG (1971) Non-surgical assessment of cardiac function. Nature 232:335
41. Smith JS, Michael K, Benefiel DJ, Bird BF, Lurz FW, Shapiro WA, Rizen MF, Bouchard A, Schiller NB (1985) Intraoperative detection of myocardial ischemia in high risk patients: electrocardiography versus two-dimensional echocardiography. Circulation 72:1015
42. Souquet J, Hanrath P, Zitelli L, Kremer P, Langenstein BA, Schlüter M (1982) Transesophageal phased array for imaging the heart. IEEE Trans Biomed Eng 29:707
43. Sutherland GR, Poppele G, Langenstein B, Taams M, Roelandt J, Hanrath P (1988) Transesophageal echo, an improved diagnostic technique for sub arotic membranes. Circulation 78:(suppl part II) II−441

Complications of Acute Myocardial Infarction and the Role of Transesophageal Echocardiography

J. K. OH

Introduction

Acute myocardial infarction disturbs the functional and structural integrity of the heart. The type and severity of the disturbance influence the treatment modalities and the prognosis of the patients with acute myocardial infarction.

Echocardiography has become a major diagnostic tool in the detection of complications of myocardial infarction. M-mode and two-dimensional echocardiography enables us to assess regional as well as global ventricular function and to detect mechanical complications such as ventricular aneurysm, pseudoaneurysm, ventricular septal defect, papillary muscle rupture, mural thrombus, and pericardial effusion [1]. Furthermore, Doppler and color flow imaging help us to assess hemodynamic and blood flow abnormalities resulting from a complication so that the presence of a defect and its severity are more confidently evaluated [2]. The advantage of echocardiography over other noninvasive as well as invasive imaging modalities in patients with a suspected complication of acute myocardial infarction is that the study can be performed and interpreted readily at the patient's bedside. Hence, immediate feedback is given to the primary physician without transporting patients frequently in a critical condition. The utility of echocardiography by the transthoracic approach is, however, limited in this setting because of suboptimal quality or the lack of a satisfactory imaging window. The majority of these patients in the coronary care unit are connected to a cardiac rhythm monitor, a Swan-Ganz balloon catheter, a temporary pacemaker, intraaortic balloon pump, and/or a mechanical ventilator. Transesophageal echocardiography offers an alternative imaging window to the heart when the transthoracic approach is not entirely satisfactory [3, 4]. Without any intervening structures between the esophagus and the heart, transesophageal echocardiography provides superb images and fine details of the normal and abnormal cardiac anatomy.

Feasibility and Safety

Since many of these patients are mechanically ventilated and confined to a certain position (usually supine), the procedure for introduction of a transesophageal probe is frequently modified from that for awake patients. They

Transesophageal Echocardiography
Edited by R. Erbel et al.
© Springer-Verlag Berlin Heidelberg 1989

are more heavily sedated and it is occasionally necessary to use a laryngoscope to aid intubation in the supine position (as opposed to the left lateral decubitus position in the awake patients). They receive lidocaine sprays to the posterior pharynx and 0.2 mg glycopyrrolate for secretion control. Unless sedated beforehand, it is preferable to give adequate sedation. It has been noted that the heart rate increases mildly during intubation if the patient is not sedated satisfactorily. No significant change in blood pressure, mixed venous oxygen saturation, or pulmonary artery pressure occurs. Therefore, transesophageal echocardiography should be feasible in all patients except when prohibited by esophageal pathology, and is well tolerated by patients with acute myocardial infarction [5].

Mitral Regurgitation from Papillary Muscle Dysfunction or Rupture

Mitral regurgitation is the most frequent indication for transesophageal echocardiography in patients with acute myocardial infarction and unstable hemodynamics. It is well known that even the most severe mitral regurgitation may not produce a significant murmur. The left atrium, located immediately anterior to the esophagus, is always clearly visualized by transesophageal echocardiography from the basal short-axis and the four-chamber view. Tomographic sections of the left atrial cavity can be obtained at multiple levels by adjusting the position of the transesophageal transducer. Due to the superb visualization, color flow imaging detects not only the area and the extent but also the origin of any mitral regurgitation jet. The mitral valve apparatus is best seen from the four-chamber view, and its structural abnormalities (prolapse, flail, papillary muscle dysfunction, or rupture) can be readily evaluated.

Ventricular Septal Defect

The treatment of choice for infarcted ventricular septal defect is surgical repair immedialy after diagnosis. The ventricular septum is best visualized from the four-chamber and the transgastric views. However, it should be noted that the apical septum may not be visualized by the transesophageal approach. Due to the oblique tomographic transesophageal image, a ventricular septal defect located at the distal end of the septum may not be a true apical septal defect, but rather a midventricular septal defect. The location of ventricular septal defects should be described in relation to other adjacent cardiac structures such as the papillary muscle. Color flow imaging supplements two-dimensional echocardiographic diagnosis of a ventricular septal defect by demonstrating any left to right shunt through the defect. In our experience, the cardiac surgeons have been satisfied with the clarity and the confidence of transesophageal echocardiographic diagnosis of infarcted ventricular septal defects, so that no further diagnostic procedure, with the exception of coronary angiography, is required prior to surgical repair.

Ventricular Aneurysm

The entire apex of the heart may not be visualized by the current transesophageal echocardiography with the capability of only a cross-sectional view. This will change when longitudinal section is available. Therefore, caution should be exercised in detecting an apical aneurysm or apical thrombus. Except for the apex, both right and left ventricular segments are clearly seen from the four-chamber and the transgastric view, so that free wall rupture or pseudoaneurysm is easily diagnosed and distinguished from true aneurysm.

Right Ventricular Infarction

We found the transgastric view to be useful in detecting right ventricular dilatation and wall motion abnormalities. In comparison to right ventricular contusion where the predominant wall motion abnormality occurs anteriorly, a hemodynamically significant right ventricular infarct (in association with inferior wall infarction) occurs in the posterior wall, which makes the transesophageal approach an ideal means to detect it.

Conclusion

The management of a mechanical complication of acute myocardial infarction is frequently a shared responsibility among the primary physician, cardiologist, cardiac surgeon, and other medical disciplines. The urgency with which a hemodynamically compromising complication must be surgically repaired dictates a prompt diagnosis. In order for echocardiography to be a complete diagnostic imaging tool rather than one used to recommend a further study (such as left ventriculography) to confirm the findings, it should have a satisfactory image to convince both the echocardiographer performing the study and others of its diagnosis. I believe that transesophageal echocardiography can meet that challenge.

References

1. Freeman WK, Miller FA, Oh JK, Seward JB, Tajik AJ (1987) Postinfarct ventricular septal rupture: diagnosis and management facilitated by two-dimensional and Doppler echocardiography. Echocardiography 4:75−81
2. Reeder GS, Seward JB, Tajik AJ et al. (1982). The role of two-dimensional echocardiography in coronary artery disease. Mayo Clin Proc 57:247
3. Schluter M, Hinrichs A, Thier W, Kremer P, Schroder S et al. (1984) Transesophageal two-dimensional echocardiography: comparison of ultrasonic and anatomic sections. Am J Cardiol 53:1173−1178
4. Seward JB , Khandheria BK, Oh JK, Abel MD et al. (1988) Transesophageal echocardiography: technique, anatomic correlations, implementation, and clinical applications. Mayo Clin Proc 63:649−680
5. Oh JK, Seward JB, Khandheria BK, Freeman WK, Tajik AJ (1988) Transesophageal echocardiography in the intensive care unit. Circulation 11:78

Monitoring During PEEP Ventilation in Patients with Severe Left Ventricular Failure Using Transesophageal Echocardiography

S. Schuster, R. Erbel, L. S. Weilemann, W. Lu, and S. Wellek

Mechanical ventilation with positive end-expiratory pressure (PEEP) considerably reduces cardiac output [1–6]. This has been attributed to reduction of venous return and transmural right and left ventricular (LV) pressure [1, 2, 7, 8], but unchanged or even increased transmural right or LV pressure has also been found [8–11]. A reduction in myocardial contractility and ventricular interdependence has been discussed [9, 12, 13].

The aim of the present study was to investigate the effect of PEEP ventilation on cardiac function using transesophageal echocardiography in patients with severe LV failure. Limitations of transthoracic echocardiography related to pulmonary emphysema, obesity, thoracic deformaties, and mechanical ventilation have been overcome by transesophageal echocardiography. Transesophageal echocardiography has been found to be highly accurate for both diagnostic purposes and monitoring of cardiac and valve function [14–17], as well as for anesthesia [18, 19] because of its excellent resolution.

Patients and Methods

The investigation was carried out in 11 patients with severe LV failure requiring ventilation after resuscitation (Table 1). Clinical and hemodynamic subsets were assigned according to the classification of Forrester [40] before starting specific therapy. Ventilation was maintained using a Servo 900 B respirator (Siemens, Erlangen) which provided constant flow and inspired volume, inspiration-expiration ratio, and arterial oxygen tension. Sedation and analgesia were maintained using diazepam and opiates. Hemodynamic and two-dimensional transesophageal echocardiographic measurements were performed on the second day after hemodynamic and metabolic stabilization. Management with inotropic drugs, vasodilators and diuretics followed accepted practices [40]. All parameters were recorded simultaneously after 2 min ventilation at PEEP levels of 0, 4, 8, 12, and 16 cm H_2O.

Transesophageal Echocardiography

Echocardiographic measurements were obtained with a 3.5-MHz real-time 84° sector scanner (Diasonic Cardiovue). The scanner, placed laterally at the end of a modified gastroscope, was easily inserted with the patient in the supine

Transesophageal Echocardiography
Edited by R. Erbel et al.
© Springer-Verlag Berlin Heidelberg 1989

Table 1. Clinical data

Patient	Age (years)	Sex (m/f)	Diagnosis	Hemodynamic subsets (PAEDP/CI)	Hemodynamic therapy	Outcome
1	76	m	Chronic left heart failure resuscitation	IV (26/2.2)	Dopa. = 1200 µg/min, NPN = 40 µg/min, Dobu. = 600 µg/min	Died
2	53	m	Cardiogenic shock, posterior myocardial infarction	IV (30/1.8)	Dopa. = 200 µg/min, Nitro = 3 mg/h, Dobu. = 500 µg/min	Survived
3	78	m	Chronic left heart failure	III (16/2.1)	Dobu. = 600 µg/min, NPN = 60µg/min	Died
4	66	m	Cardiogenic shock, anterior myocardial infarction	IV (25/1.6)	Dopa. = 600 µg/min, NPN = 40 µg/min, Dobu. = 1800 µg/min	Survived
5	71	m	Anterior myocardial infarction	II (22/3.3)	Nitro. = 3 mg/h, NPN = 45 µg/min	Died
6	58	m	Endocarditis, left heart insufficiency	II (23/2.9)	NPN = 50 µg/min, Eurosemide = 60 mg/day	Died
7	62	f	Cardiogenic shock, anterior myocardial infarction	IV (26/2.1)	Dopa. = 600 µg/min, Nitro. = 6 mg/h, Dobu. = 800 µg/min, NPN = 60 µg/min	Died
8	58	m	Left heart insufficiency	II (27.2.6)	Dopa. = 200 µg/min, Nitro. = 4 mg/h	Died
9	55	m	Trichloroethylene intoxication	III (15/1.8)	NPN = 50 µg/min	Died
10	44	m	Posterior myocardial infarction	II (24/2.3)	Dobu. = 700 µg/min, Nitro. = 5 mg/h	Survived
11	53	m	Posterior myocardial infarction	II (26/2.6)	Nitro. = 6 mg/h	Survived

NPN, Nitroprusside; Nitro, Nitroglycerin; Dopa, Dopamine; Dobu, Dobutamine;
PAEDP (mm Hg), Pulmonary artery end-diastolic pressure; CI(l/min m^2), cardiac index

position. The probe was placed in the standard positions for evaluation of the left and right atria and ventricles in the four chamber view, and for monitoring LV cross sections in the transgastric view. Videotape recordings were made of cross-sectional measurements of the right atrium during gradual increase of the PEEP level and of the LV at the level of the cordae tendineae of the mitral valve during stepwise reduction of the PEEP to the initial level. In each case, the position of the transducer was adjusted to maximize the dimension of the atrium or ventricle. When PEEP altered the position of the heart relative to the transducer, the position and direction of the transducer were adjusted so that the maximal chamber dimension could be obtained. The endocardial contours were examined in slow motion and stop frame video projection and analyzed by two observers independently. End-diastolic and end-systolic cross-sectional areas were calculated semiautomatically as the mean of three determinations using a desk computer (Kontron 200). Fractional shortening of the LV was calculated. In one patient, cross sections of the left atrium and left and right ventricles along the long axis were recorded during an increase of PEEP from 0 to 16 cmH_2O and during decrease of PEEP from 16 to 0 cm cmH_2O.

Hemodynamics

Mean right atrial pressure (RAP) and pulmonary arterial systolic and diastolic pressure (PAP) were measured using a Swan-Ganz thermodilution catheter. The pressures were measured using an external pressure transducer. The zero reference was placed at midchest level and pressure values were measured at end-expiration. Cardiac output was determined in triplicate by a thermodilution technique using the Edwards cardiac computer 9520 A. With each injection of 5 ml cold sodium chloride 0.9% solution being started at the end of expiration. The cardiac index (CI) and stroke index (SI) were calculated. Heart rate was derived from ECG, and blood pressure was measured with a cuff. Transesophageal pressure was recorded using an external transducer connected with a closed-end angiographic catheter (Cordis femoral aortic flush F8×65 cm) placed behind the left atrium. During measurement, the catheter was perfused with 4 ml saline solution / 60 min [41].

Statistical Analysis

The null hypothesis (no influence of PEEP level) was testes against the alternative of a monotonic trend for each of the 13 hemodynamic variables (Table 2), using the nonparametric test of Page [20] with adjustment for bias. This was calculated by summation of the intrablock variation and determination of Spearman's rank correlation for the dependent variable and PEEP level. Statistical significance of the observed $p$values was checked against a multiple significance level of $\alpha = 0.01$. Whether a given $p$value was significant was determined on the basis of Holm's [21] sequential rejection procedure. Values are given as mean ± standard deviation.

Table 2. Hemodynamic data (mean $\pm$ SD) at different levels of psoitive end expiratory pressure

	PEEP (cm H$_2$O)					
	0	4	8	12	16	p value
CI	3.5 $\pm$ 0.7	3.4 $\pm$ 0.8	3.1 $\pm$ 0.7	3.0 $\pm$ 0.8	2.8 $\pm$ 0.7	< 0.001
SI	43.8 $\pm$ 12	40.7 $\pm$ 10	37.4 $\pm$ 10	35.0 $\pm$ 11	32.9 $\pm$ 11	< 0.0001
PA$_s$	30 $\pm$ 6	32 $\pm$ 8	33 $\pm$ 12	34.8 $\pm$ 10	35.4 $\pm$ 10	< 0.01
PA$_d$	15 $\pm$ 5	15.4 $\pm$ 4	18 $\pm$ 4	18.3 $\pm$ 4	19.6 $\pm$ 4	n.s.
P$_{RA}$	6.2 $\pm$ 3	6.8 $\pm$ 3	8.3 $\pm$ 3	10.5 $\pm$ 3	11.3 $\pm$ 4	< 0.0001
P$_{esoph}$	3.3 $\pm$ 2.0	4.7 $\pm$ 2.5	5.7 $\pm$ 2.5	7.3 $\pm$ 3.4	9.0 $\pm$ 3.5	< 0.001
T$_{RA}$	4 $\pm$ 0.8	3.7 $\pm$ 0.5	3.3 $\pm$ 0.6	3.7 $\pm$ 1.8	3 $\pm$ 0.8	n.s.
BP$_s$	133 $\pm$ 21	129 $\pm$ 21	129 $\pm$ 21	121 $\pm$ 20	119 $\pm$ 19	< 0.001
BP$_d$	79 $\pm$ 15	78 $\pm$ 16	76 $\pm$ 13	77 $\pm$ 16	76 $\pm$ 16	< 0.01
HR	83 $\pm$ 20	87 $\pm$ 20	86 $\pm$ 21	88 $\pm$ 21	89 $\pm$ 21	n.s.
A$_{LVES}$	18.5 $\pm$ 5.6	17.7 $\pm$ 6.2	16.4 $\pm$ 5.6	15.8 $\pm$ 5.9	15.1 $\pm$ 5.9	< 0.0001
A$_{LVED}$	25.5 $\pm$ 7.2	22.9 $\pm$ 6.5	21.0 $\pm$ 5.9	20.1 $\pm$ 6.0	19.3 $\pm$ 5.8	< 0.0001
A$_{RAES}$	12.4 $\pm$ 4.9	11.9 $\pm$ 5.2	10.4 $\pm$ 4.1	8.9 $\pm$ 3.7	8.4 $\pm$ 3.6	< 0.0001
A$_{RAED}$	18.6 $\pm$ 5.1	16.1 $\pm$ 4.3	14.6 $\pm$ 3.6	12.7 $\pm$ 3.8	11.5 $\pm$ 3.4	< 0.0001
F	26.4 $\pm$ 8.7	24 $\pm$ 12.6	23 $\pm$ 13.5	23 $\pm$ 14.5	24 $\pm$ 16.8	n.s.

CI, cardiac index; SI, stroke index; PA$_{s/d}$, pulmonary artery pressure systole/diastole; P$_{RA}$, right atrial pressure, T$_{RA}$, transmural right atrial pressure; BP, blood pressure; HR, heart rate; A$_{LVES/LVED}$, left ventricular area end-systole/end-diastole (cm^2); A$_{RAES/RAED}$, right atrial area end-systole/end-diastole (cm^2); F, fractional shortening of LV area (%); P$_{esoph}$, esophageal pressure; n.s., not significant

Results

Hemodynamic and echocardiographic results are shown in Table 2. Figure 1a–c show in the original echocardiograms and 1d, e in schematic drawings the cross-sectional areas and diameters of the left atrium and ventricle and the right ventricle along its long axis. Examination of the heart after application of 16 cmH$_2$O PEEP showed an acute decrease of the right ventricular area, the septal-lateral diameter, and a displacement of the ventricular septum to the right. The LV area decreased only slightly without marked change in septal-lateral diameter. On discontinuation of 16 cmH$_2$O PEEP, massive volume loading of the right ventricle occurred, accompanied by a displacement of the septum to the left and a distinct change of the LV geometry. Analysis of all heart activity after application and removal of 16 cmH$_2$O PEEP demonstrated an acute change in size of the right and left ventricles within one to five heart beats (Fig. 2). There was a marked increase in volume of the left atrium under 16 cmH$_2$O PEEP, accompanied by a prompt initial decrease of the left and right ventricular volume.

Systolic and diastolic area of the right atrium decreased considerably with rising PEEP levels. Right atrial pressure increased significantly, but transmural filling pressure did not change. A high negative correlation between right atrial pressure and cross-sectional area was found during stepwise increase of PEEP. The correlation coefficients ranged between -0.75 and -0.99. End-diastolic and end-systolic area of the LV decreased progressively with increasing PEEP levels; thus, areas were considerably smaller at the highest PEEP levels in all patients. Fractional shortening was not related to PEEP level. Mean cardiac index decreased significantly $P < 0.001$). As regards individual cases, the cardiac index was at a maximum at a PEEP level of 4 cmH$_2$O in three patients, at 8 cmH$_2$O in one patient and at 12 cmH$_2$O in one patient. The pulmonary artery end-diastolic pressures in these patients were 10, 11, 17, 18, and 27 mmHg, respectively. Only in one patient did the cardiac index fall below the critical value at a PEEP level of 8 cmH$_2$O (Fig. 3). The decrease in cardiac index was caused by a decrease in stroke index. Blood pressure decreased and pulmonary artery pressure and heart rate increased significantly (Table 2).

Discussion

Echocardiography is a practical and semi-invasive technique for evaluation of heart morphology and performance. The diagnostic value of the standard precordial technique is limited by thoracic deformation, obesity, or emphysema in 20%–30% of the patients, particularly during mechanical ventilation. By contrast, the transesophageal echocardiography transducer can be placed behind the heart and enables continuous evaluation of all four heart chambers without hindrance from lung tissue even during mechanical ventilation. The

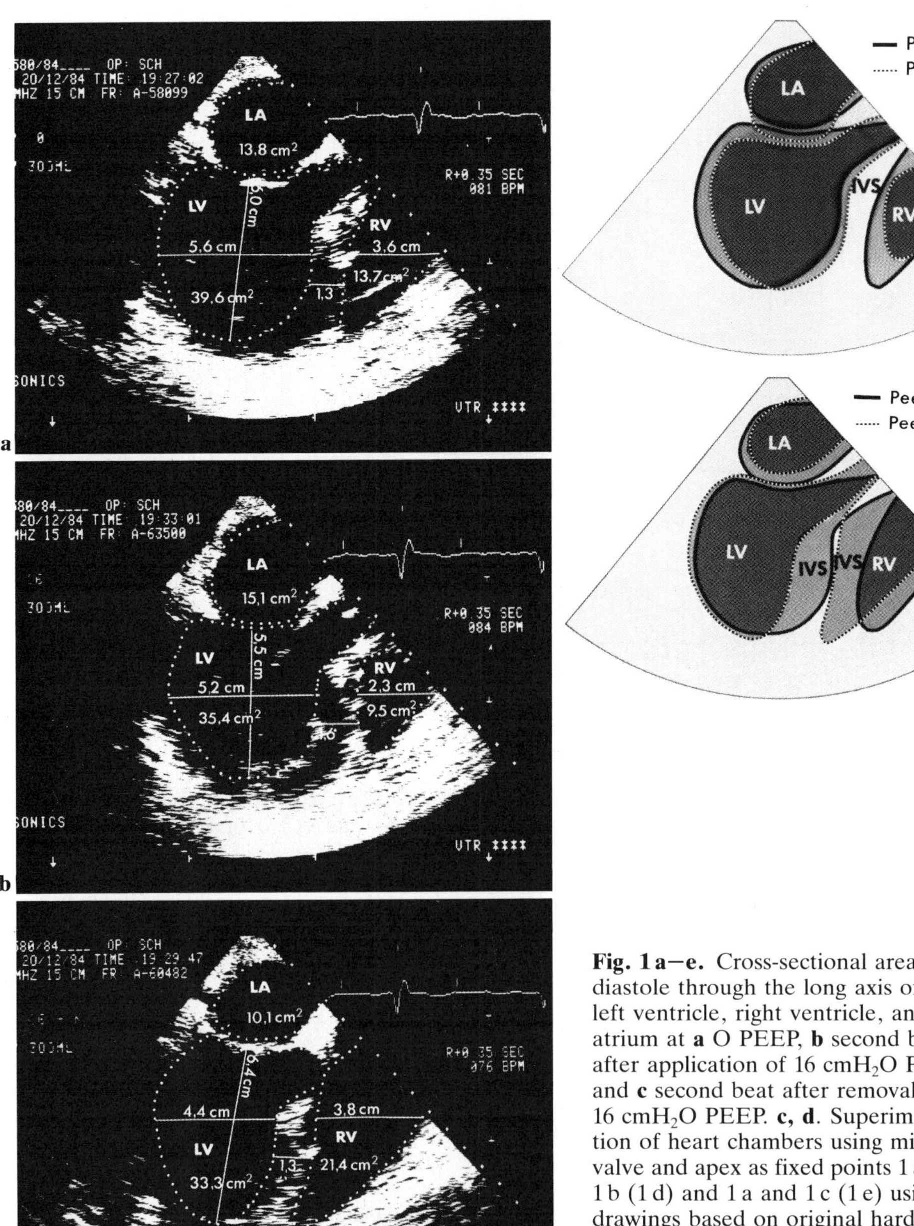

Fig. 1a–e. Cross-sectional area at diastole through the long axis of the left ventricle, right ventricle, and left atrium at **a** O PEEP, **b** second beat after application of 16 cmH$_2$O PEEP, and **c** second beat after removal of 16 cmH$_2$O PEEP. **c, d**. Superimposition of heart chambers using mitral valve and apex as fixed points 1a and 1b (1d) and 1a and 1c (1e) using drawings based on original hard copies: **d** from **a** and **b**; **e** from **a** and **c**. *LA*, left atrium; *LV*, left ventricular; *RV*, right ventricle; *IVS*, interventricular septum

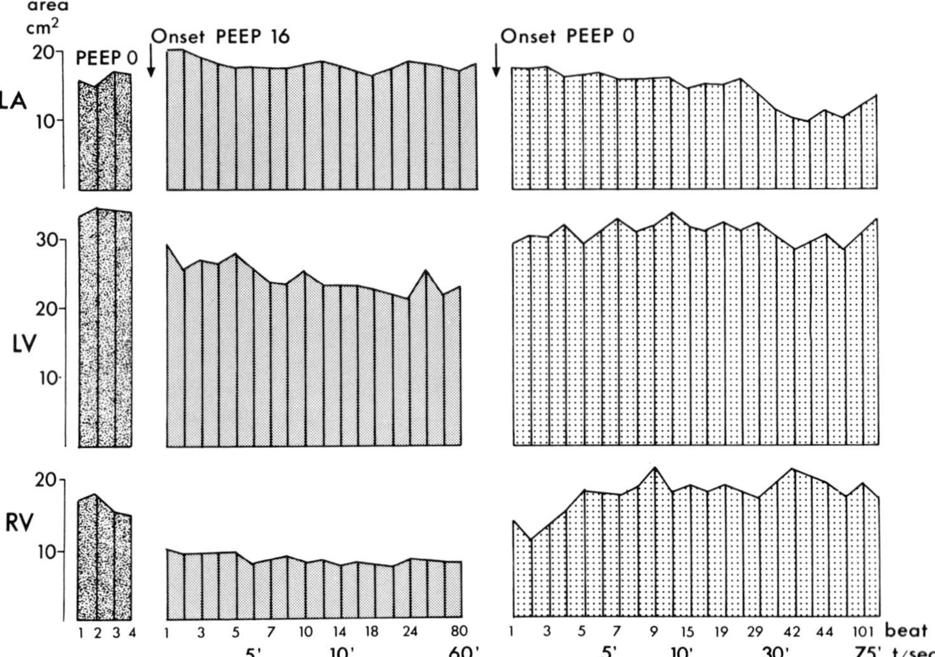

Fig. 2. Cross-sectional areas of left atrium (*LA*), left ventricle (*LV*), and right ventricle (*RV*) for each heart beat during consecutive periods with O PEEP, 16 cmH$_2$O PEEP for 60 and after removal of 16 cmH$_2$O PEEP for 75 s. Analysis of all heart activity demonstrated the acute change in size of the right and left ventricles within one to five heart beats after the first respiratory cycle with PEEP. The ratio RV/LV area decreased from 48.6% under zero end-expiratory pressure to 36.5% under 16 cmH$_2$O PEEP (average of the first four cardiac cycles) and increased to 57.9% upon discontinuation of 16 cmH$_2$O PEEP (average of the first four cardiac cycles). After 1 min, the initial value had almost been reached (50.9%)

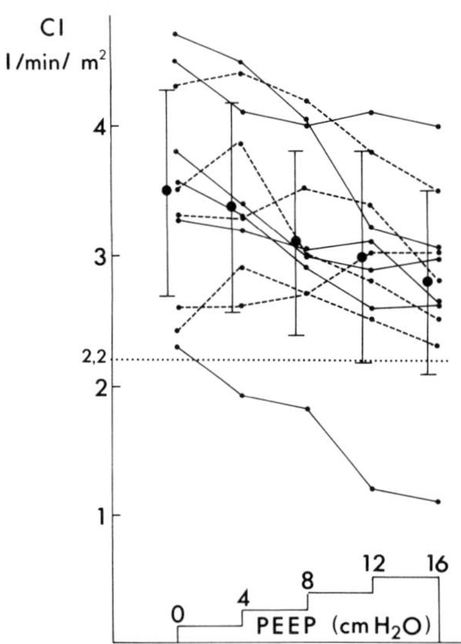

Fig. 3. Individual changes of cardiac index during stepwise increase to 16 cmH$_2$O PEEP. In five patients, the cardiac index (*CI*) increased under 4–12 cmH$_2$O PEEP (*broken line*). One patient developed a low output syndrome with a fall in CI to below 2.2 l/min m^2 under 8 cmH$_2$O PEEP. The CI under 16 cmH$_2$O PEEP was significantly lower than under zero end-expiratory pressure ($p < 0.001$). The *filled circles* and *bars* represent the mean and standard deviation

validity and reproducibility of transesophageal echocardiography in evaluating left heart performance has been demonstrated during open heart surgery and dynamic exercise [22, 23].

The good correlation between left and right atrial dimension (LAD and RAD) as measured by M-mode transesophageal echocardiography and angiographic volumes during spontaneous ventilation, and between LV dimensions as measured by transesophageal echocardiography by the standard precordial method, indicated the feasibility of transesophageal echocardiography for evaluation of right atrial and LV dimensional changes also during PEEP [24, 25]. Therefore, we assumed that during PEEP the values for right atrial and LV dimensions obtained by transesophageal echocardiography were reliable after proper manipulation of the transducer.

In our study, the cardiac index decreased significantly during ventilation with PEEP. Other authors have also reported a reduction in the cardiac index during PEEP [26−31]. It decreased significantly with increased PEEP steps, but even when the PEEP level was raised to 16 cmH$_2$O, only one patient showed a critical fall in cardiac index. The relation was not linear. In half the patients, the influence on cardiac index was dependent on the PEEP level, the cardiac index increasing in the range 4−12 cmH$_2$O and decreasing at higher levels. No relationship between the increase in cardiac index under PEEP and the pulmonary artery end-diastolic pressure) under zero endexpiratory pressure was observed. This may be related to the fact that our measurements were taken after stabilization of LV function by vasodilators, diuretics, or inotropic agents. In contrast, Nishimura et al. [32] demonstrated a relationship by examination of six myocardial infarction patients with serious left heart failure (Killipp classes III and IV). In four patients with a high pulmonary capillary pressure and a low stroke work index, the cardic index increased at 5 cmH$_2$O PEEP, whereas in two patients with a low pulmonary capillary pressure and high initial stroke work index, the cardiac index decreased.

In this group of patient with severe LV failure, a decrease in fractional shortening, which is a sign of reduced LV performance, was not found. Other authors have also demonstrated unchanged contractility under PEEP ventilation [10, 34]. In animal experiments, Qvist et al. [7] only found a shift along the same ventricular function curve at different PEEP levels and Fewell et al. [33] were unable to show a change in the pressure/volume relationship, ejection fraction, or maximum (DP/dt) at 12 cmH$_2$O PEEP. Dainant et al. [10] found no reduction of DP/dt/dp, a parameter of contractility, in ten adult respiratory distress syndrome (ARDS) patients.

The adverse effects of PEEP ventilation on hemodynamics as a function of end-expiratory pressure were reported in the early literature [2, 26]. The primary cause of these effects is the increase in intrathoracic pressure.

Animal experiments showed that a decrease in transmural filling pressure was the reason for the decrease in stroke and cardiac index [7]. Fewell et al. [34] observed a prompt decrease in cardiac index after application of PEEP within one or two respiratory cycles; this was followed by a decrease in aortic blood flow relative to blood flow in the pulmonary artery. Since a decrease in end-diastolic right and left ventricular volume occurred, they attributed these effects to a primary decrease in preload. The experimental results are in accordance with those of our study, where a decrease in end-diastolic and end-systolic size of the left and right ventricles was shown by transesophageal echocardiography. Similar results were previously reported in patients with ARDS [35–37]. In addition to the effects shown by these studies, a decrease in right atrial size proportional to the rise in PEEP level occurs together with an increase in right atrial pressure. An unchanged transmural filling pressure was demonstrated. This phenomenon must be related to the effects of external pressure on the right atrium, which results in a reduction in filling volume and an increase in intravascular pressure because of the incompressibility of liquids. The high negative correlation between right atrial pressure and cross-sectional area during stepwise increase of PEEP supports this explanation. This balance of forces is maintained as long as right ventricular function does not fail and the caval vessels do not collapse. A change in transmural filling pressure would not be expected under these conditions, and therefore transmural filling pressure cannot be a reliable measure for assessing ventricular end-diastolic volume under PEEP conditions.

The continuous transesophageal echocardiographic recordings impressively demonstrate the acute impairment in filling with PEEP and an acute volume overloading of the heart after removal of PEEP. With echocardiography, only can the size of the chamber be analyzed, but also the geometry and, particularly, the behavior of the intraventricular septum. During transthoracic echocardiographic examination of ARDS patients under high PEEP treatment, Jardin et al. [38] found a left shift of the ventricular septum as a consequence of pressure loading on the right ventricle together with a decrease in the cardiac index due to reduced filling of the LV. However, a plausible explanation was not found, since the transmural right ventricular end-diastolic pressure decreased up to 30 cmH_2O PEEP and the end-systolic pressure at 30 cmH_2O was only 3 mm Hg above the initial value. In contrast, the present investigation has shown movement of the ventricular septum at 16 cmH_2O PEEP in the reverse direction, that is, toward the right ventricle. A shift of the ventricular septum to the right under ventilation with PEEP must be due to the greatly impaired filling of the right atrium and right ventricle when there is excess external pressure. The increase in the septal curvature radius, used by Jardin et al. [38] as an index of a leftward shift, appears to result from an increase in septum thickness and a reduction in size of both ventricles as our measurements showed. However, the reason why the left atrial area increased during the acute phase after 16 cmH_2O PEEP and the LV decreased remains unclear and it seems that other factors affecting LV size must be involved. It is possible that there is a change in ventricular geometry, as has been shown in recent animal experiments [39], or reduced LV compliance.

Conclusion

PEEP leads to a decrease in the cardiac index and a right shift of the ventricular septum caused by a primary reduction of the right atrial and ventricular filling volumes by external compression. The transmural filling pressure remains unchanged. PEEP does not reduce LV contractility. Patients with severe LV failure can be ventilated with $8-10$ cmH$_2$O PEEP after hemodynamic stabilization with drugs. Careful hemodynamic control at PEEP levels above 10 cmH$_2$O is therefore always necessary, since neither blood pressure nor central venous pressure can be used as indices of shock. Transesophageal echocardiography gives precise information on ventricular function even during PEEP ventilation, thus facilitating suitable treatment.

References

1. Ashbaugh DG, Petty TL (1973) Positive end-expiratory pressure. J Thorac Cardiovasc Surg 65:165−170
2. Cournand A, Motley HL, Werko L, Richards DW (1948) Physiological studies of the effects of the intermittent positive pressure breathing on cardiac output in man. Am J Physiol 152:162−173
3. Kirby RR, Downs JB, Civetta JM et al. (1975) High level positive end-expiratory pressure (PEEP) in acute respiratory insufficiency. Chest 67:156−163
4. Kumar A, Falke KJ, Geffin B et al. (1970) Continuous positive-pressure ventilation in acute respiratory failure. N Engl J Med 283:1430−1436
5. Tucker HJ, Murray JF (1972) Effects of end-expiratory pressure on organ blood flow in normal and diseased dogs. J App. Physiol 34:573−577
6. Walkinshaw M, Shoemaker WC (1980) Use of volume loading to obtain preferred levels of PEEP: preliminary study. Crit Care Med 8:81−86
7. Qvist J, Pontoppidan H, Wilson RS, Lowenstein E, Laver MB (1975) Hemodynamic responses to mechanical ventilation with PEEP. The effect of hypervolemia. Anaesthesiology 42:45−55
8. Simonneau G, Lemaire F, Harf A, Teisseire C, Teisseire B (1982) A comparative study of the cardiorespiratory effects of continuous positive airway pressure breathing and continuous positive pressure ventilation in acute respiratory failure. Intensive Care Med 8:61−67
9. Cassidy SS, Robertson CH, Pierce AK, Johnson RL (1978) Cardiovascular effects of positive end-expiratory pressure in dogs. J Appl Physiol 44:743−750
10. Dhainaut JF, Bricard C, Monsallier FJ et al. (1982) Left ventricular contractility using isovolumic phase indices during PEEP in ARDS patients. Crit Care Med 10: 631−635
11. Scharf SM, Caldini P, Ingram HR (1977) Cardiovascular effects of increasing airway pressure in the dog. Am J Physiol 232:H35−H43
12. Manny JM, Patten MT, Liebman PR, Hechtmann HB (1978) The association of lung distenion, PEEP and biventricular failure. Ann Surg 187:151−157
13. Laver MB, Strauss HW, Pohost GM (1979) Right and left ventricular geometry: adjustments during acute respiratory failure. Crit Care Med 7:509−519
14. Matsumoto M, Oka Y, Strom J et al. (1980) Application of transesophageal echocardiography to continuous intraoperative monitoring of left ventricular performance. Am J Cardiol 46:05
15. Schlüter M, Hanrath P (1984) The clinical application of transesophageal echocardiography. Echocardiography 1:427

16. Beaupré PN, Kremer P, Cahalan MK, Lurz FW, Schiller B, Hamilton WK (1984) Intraoperative detection of changes in left ventricular sequential wall mition by transesophageal two-dimentional echocardiography. Am Heart J 107:1021
17. Smith JS, Benefiel DJ, Lurz W et al. (1984) Detection of intraoperative myocardial ischemia: ECG vs. 2-D transesophageal echocardiography (abstr). Anesthesiology 61:A 158
18. Cronelly R, Kremer PF, Baupré PN, Cahalan MK, Salvatierra O, Feduska N (1983) Hemodynamic response to anesthesia in patients with end-state renal disease. Anesthesiology 59:A 47
19. Beaupré P, Cahalan M, Kremer P, et al. (1983) Contractility depression during anesthesia: compaison of haolthane, enflurane and isoflurane by transesophageal echocardiography (abstr). Circulation [Suppl] 11:332
20. Page EB (1963) Ordered hypotheses for multiple treatments: a significance test for linear ranks. J Am Statist Assoc 58:216−230
21. Holm S (1979) A simple sequentially rejective multiple test procedure. Scand J Statist 6:65−70
22. Matsumoto M, Osa Y, Strom J et al. (1980) Application of transesophageal echocardiography to continuous intraoperative monitoring of left ventricular performance. Am J Cardiol 46:95−105
23. Matsumoto M, Hanrath P, Kremer P et al. (1982) Evaluation of left ventricular performance during supine exercise by transesophageal M-mode echocardiography in normal subjects. Br Heart J 48:61−66
24. Toma Y, Matsuda Y, Matsuzaki M et al. (1983) Determination of atrial size by esophageal echocardiography. Am J Cardiol 52:878−880
25. Terai C, Uenishi M, Sugimoto H, Shimazu T, Yoshioharu T, Sugimoto T (1985) Transesophageal echocardiographic dimensional analysis of four cardiac chambers during positive end-expiratory pressure. Anaesthesiology 63:640−646
26. Barach AL, Echman M, Ginsberg E (1946) Positive pressure respiration studies on general aspects and types of pressure breathing. J Aviat Med 17:290
27. Lutch JS, Murray JF (1972) Continuous positive-pressure ventilation: effects on systemic oxygen transport and tissue oxygenation. Ann Int Med 76:193−202
28. Powers SR, Mannal R, Neclerio M et al. (1973) Physiologic consequences of positive end-expiratory pressure (PEEP) ventilation. Ann Surg 178:265−272
29. Braunwald E, Binion JT, Morgan WL et al. (1957) Alterations in central blood volume and cardiac output induced by positive pressure breathing and counteracted by metaraminol (Aramine). Circ Res 5:670−675
30. Morgan BC, Crawford EW, Guntheroth WG (1969) The hemodynamic effects of changes in blood volume during intermittent positive-pressure ventilation. Anaesthesiology 30:297−305
31. Sykes MK, Adams AP, Finley WEI et al. (1970) The effect of variations in end-expiratory inflation pressure on cardiorespiratory function in normo-, hypo- and hyper-volemic dogs. Br J Anaesth 42:669−677
32. Niskimura N, Obayashi K, Takano T (1980) Hemodynamic effect of positive end-expiratory pressure (PEEP) in severe heart failure due to acute myocardial infarction (AMI). Crit Care Med 8:229
33. Fewell JE, Abendschein DR, Carlson CJ, Rapaport E, Murray JF (1981) Continuous positive pressure ventilation does not alter ventricular pressure volume relationship. Am J Physiol 240:H821−H826
34. Fewell JF, Abendschein DR, Carlson CJ, Murray JF, Rapaport E (1980) Continuous positive pressure ventilation decreases right and left ventricular end-diastolic volumes in dog. Cir Res 46:125−132
35. Dhainaut JF, Devaux JY, Schlemmer B et al. (1983) Effects of PEEP on right ventricular function in ARDS patients (abstr). Intensive Care Med 9:149
36. Viquerat CE, Righetti A, Suter PM (1983) Biventricular volumes and function in patients with adult respiratory distress syndrome ventilated with PEEP. Chest 3:509−514
37. Koolen JJ, Visser CA, Wever E, van Wezel H, Meyne NG, Dunning AJ (1987) Transesophageal two-dimensional echocardiographic evaluation of biventricualr dimension

and function during positive end-expiratory ventilation after coronary artery bypass grafting. Am J Cardiol 59:1047−1051
38. Jardin F, Farcot J, Bosiante L, Curien N, Margiaraz A, Bourdarias JP (1981) Influences of positive end-expiratory pressure on left ventricular performance. N Engl J Med 304:387−392
39. Robotham JL, Bell RC, Badke FR, Kindred MK (1985) Left ventricular geometry during positive end-expiratory pressure in dogs. Crit Care Med 13:617−624
40. Forrester JS, Diamond G, Chatterjee K, Swan JC (1976) Medical therapy of acute myocardial infarction by application of hemodynamic subsets. N Engl J Med 295:1404−1412
41. Skarvan K, Hasse J, Wolf G (1981A) Myocardial transmural pressure in ventilated patients. Intensive Care Med 7:277−283

Transesophageal Echocardiographic Monitoring During Positive Inotropic Drug Intervention and Balloon Pumping

M. Drexler, E. Mayer, H. Oelert, R. Erbel, and J. Meyer

Introduction

Positive inotropic drugs and intraaortic balloon pump (IABP) counterpulsation may become necessary in patients with postoperative low cardiac output syndrome following coronary artery bypass surgery. In these patients, the maximum information about the functional state of the heart is required. Hemodynamic parameters like cardiac output and pulmonary arterial pressure demonstrate the consequences, but not the myocardial function itself.

With echocardiography, the myocardial contractility can be assessed by demonstration of changes of the regional and global left ventricular wall motion. Because of its well-known advantages, transesophageal echocardiography (TEE) is superior to the transthoracic approach in the detection of wall motion abnormalities in postoperatively ventilated patients.

Methods

For the TEE examination we used a 12-mm echoscope with a 3.5-MHz transducer at the distal end connected to a phased array sector scanner (Diasonics V6400 or Toshiba SSH-65A).

The study was performed in ten patients (six men and four women, age range 52–72 years). They all underwent coronary artery bypass surgery and required intraaortic balloon pumping as well as high dosages of positive inotropic drugs because of low cardiac output syndrome. Seven patients had three-vessel disease, and in three patients two vessels were involved. Three patients had anterior (2) or inferior (1) wall aneurysm.

The left ventricle was analyzed echocardiographically in the short-axis view at the level of the papillary muscles. We measured the end-diastolic and end-systolic areas of the left ventricular short axis using different ratios of IABP counterpulsation. The optimal ratio was thought to be achieved when at least a 10% decrease of both the end-diastolic and end-systolic left ventricular areas (LV_{ed}, LV_{es}) could be demonstrated on the transesophageal echocardiogram compared to the left ventricular areas without IABP assistance. The cardiac output was measured simultaneously.

Transesophageal Echocardiography
Edited by R. Erbel et al.
© Springer-Verlag Berlin Heidelberg 1989

Results

In four patients a significant decrease of the end-diastolic and end-systolic left ventricular short axis areas could be demonstrated at an IABP ratio of 1:1 by TEE, and in one patient at a ratio of 1:2. Only in one of those patients there was an increase of cardiac output of about 10% (Table 1). In two patients we saw neither on the transesophageal echocardiogram nor by the hemodynamic parameters any effect of the balloon pumping. In these cases early weaning from the IABP was performed.

In two similar cases with no effect of the intraaortic counterpulsation an additional intravenous bolus of 50 or 60 mg Enoximone, a new positive inotropic agent, led to a marked increase of the cardiac index (1.2 to 1.9 l/min m^2 and 2.1 to 3.7 l/min m^2) and a decrease of the systemic vascular resistance (2170 to 1650 dyn and 1460 to 762 dyn). In these patients, an increase of the

Table 1. Transesophageal echocardiography (TEE) and cardiac output (CO) monitoring in eight patients with low cardiac output syndrome and different ratios of intraaortic balloon pump counterpulsation (IABP)

Patient		IABP			Therapeutic consequences
		1:1	1:2	1:3	
A.H.	TEE systole	+ +	+	−	IABP 1:1
	diastole	+ + + + +	−	+	
	CO	+	−	−	
B.K.	TEE systole	+ + +	−	−	IABP 1:1
	diastole	+ +	+	−	
	CO	+	−	−	
S.W.	TEE systole	+ +	+ +	+ +	IABP 1:1
	diastole	+ + +	+	−	
	CO	+	+ +	−	
G.G.	TEE systole	+ + + + +	+ +	+ + +	IABP 1:1
	diastole	+	+ +	+ + + +	
	CO	+ +	−	+	
U.B.	TEE systole	+	+ + + + +	−	IABP 1:2
	diastole	+ +	+ + + + +	+	
	CO	−	+	−	
K.A.	TEE systole	−	−	−	Early weaning from IABP
	diastole	−	−	−	and IABP explantation
	CO	+	−	−	
K.K.	TEE systole	−	−	+	Early weaning from IABP
	diastole	+	+	−	and IABP explantation
	CO	+	−	+	
H.L.	TEE systole	LV hypertrophy, increased			IABP and epinephrine in-
	diastole	contractility			fusion stopped; verapamil
	CO	−	−	−	infusion

+: for TEE, 5% decrease in left ventricular area compared to status without IABP assistance; for CO, 5% increase in CO
−: no change

ejection fraction area ($LV_{ed} - LV_{es}/LV_{ed}$) of about 10% was demonstrated by TEE. These effects could be sustained by continuous infusion of Enoximone.

Another patient with coronary artery disease, failed coronary angioplasty of the left anterior descending artery, and consecutive anterior wall ischemia had low cardiac output syndrome after emergency coronary bypass grafting, in spite of the intraaortic balloon pumping and high dosages of epinephrine. Two hours after surgery TEE showed an extensively hypertrophied left ventricle with increased contractility. Because of the TEE findings the IABP and epinephrine infusion were stopped and verapamil was given intravenously, resulting in an increase of cardiac output and a stabilization of the circulation.

Conclusion

TEE is an effective diagnostic method in the management of patients after cardiac surgery with ventricular dysfunction requiring IABP circulation support. It is useful for the direct analysis of the left ventricular function and regional wall motion. It is helpful in making the decisions about the optimal IABP triggering mode and the time setting for weaning from the IABP, and also in the management and control of specific drug therapy.

Transesophageal Doppler Echo Monitoring of Cardiac Function During Assist Circulation

S. KYO, M. MATSUMURA, S. TAKAMOTO, K. NEYA, and R. OMOTO

Introduction

Weaning a patient from mechanical assist circulation (MAC) at the optimal time is a determining factor for his survival. However, information available to determine the optimal timing is usually limited in an intensive care unit (ICU), because the patient is supported by a heavy circulation assist system, which prevents him or her being transfered to the cardiac examination laboratories. Transthoracic echocardiography may be effective in evaluating perioperative cardiac function in some cases, but in an ICU the echo penetration is usually poor because the patients are on ventilators and receiving some positive end-expiratory pressure assistance. Transesophageal echocardiography (TEE) can usually give a reasonably good echo window even in such a circumstance in ICU, because with this technique there is no obstruction by the lung, sternum, or ribs and so distinct and stable images can be obtained in the deeper area of the thoracic cavity [1, 7]. The purpose of this study was to evaluate the clinical feasibility and effectiveness of TEE, including color flow mapping Doppler [9], in management of patients during MAC.

Materials and Methods

In the past 5 years we have evaluated 33 patients who were supported by MAC after cardiac surgery by postoperative TEE. Twenty-one were men and 12 were women; ranged from 41 to 76 years, with an average of 61 years. Twenty-eight patients were on intra-aortic balloon pumping (IABP) support, four were on left ventricular assist device (VAD) support combined with IABP, and one patient was on right VAD support. Of the 33 patients examined, 22 had ischemic heart disease (IHD), including 11 with acute myocardial infarction, ten had valular heart disease (VDH), and one had left atrial myxoma (Table 1). Thirteen of 22 IHD patients and three of ten VHD patients were already in shock when transferred to us with IABP support before undergoing cardiac surgery (Table 2). IABP support was indicated in 12 because cardiopulmonary bypass could not be discontinued. Among five patients who were supported by VAD, two were operated on in two of our affiliated hospitals for left atrial myxoma (case 3) and ischemic heart disease (case 4), and because cardiopulmonary bypass could not be discontinued even

Transesophageal Echocardiography
Edited by R. Erbel et al.
© Springer-Verlag Berlin Heidelberg 1989

Table 1. Type of Disease

1.	Ischemic heart disease	22
	Angina pectoris	4
	Unstable angina	6
	LV aneurysm	1
	Acute MI	11
	Unstable angina	2
	PTCA accident	2
	VS rupture	6
	Cardiac rupture	1
2.	Valvular heart disease	10
	Aortic valve	2
	Mitral valve	2[a]
	Aortic + mitral valve	2[a]
	Mitral + tricuspid valve	2[a]
	Aortic + mitral + tricuspid valve	2
3.	Miscellaneous	1
	LA myxoma	1

[a] Severe pulmonary hypertension present in one patient. MI, myocardial infarction; PTCA, percutaneous transluminal coronary angioplasty; VS, ventricular septum; LV, left ventricle; LA, left atrium

with the support of IABP, the Saitama Medical School VAD team was requested to assist them (Table 3).

At the initial postoperative TEE examination after the necessity of MAC support had been recognized, we examined the results of surgery to determine whether the surgical correction was complete, or whether further surgical repair was required for uncorrected minor lesions. Ventricular function

Table 2. TEE findings during mechanical assist circulation

IABP assist	28 cases
Good Recovery of LV Function	25 cases
Mild AR (grade 1)	4 cases
Perioperative MI	2 cases
Moderate MR (grade 2−3)	2 cases
Severe TR (grade 3)	1 case
VAD Assist	5 cases
Good recovery of LV Function	2 cases
(LVAD discontinued at 4th POD & 9th POD)	
Good recovery of RV function	1 case
(RVAD discontinued at 4th POD)	
Moderate right to left shunt through PFO	1 case

LVAD, left ventricular assist device; RVAD, right ventricular assist device; IABP, intra-aortic balloon pumping; LV, left ventricle; RV, right ventricle; AR, aortic regurgitation; MI, myocardial infarction; MR, mitral regurgitation; TR, tricuspid regurgitation; POD, postoperative day; PFO, patent foramen ovale

Table 3. Results of VAD support

Case	Age	Sex	Disease	VAD	Duration(h)	Discontinued	Result
1	58	M	VSR	LVAD	250	No	Death
2	76	F	VSR	LVAD	278	No	Death
3	41	F	Myxoma	LVAD	219	Yes	Survival
4	56	M	IHD	LVAD	107	Yes	Death
5	57	M	VHD+PH	RVAD	98	Yes	Survival

LVAD, left ventricular assist device; RVAD, right ventricular assist device; VSR, ventricular septal rupture; IHD, ischemic heart disease; VHD, valvular heart disease; PH, pulmonary hypertension

was evaluated intermittently by measuring the size of the ventricles and wall motion analysis.

The systems used for MAC were the Kontron IABP systems (Model-10, K-2000) and the Japanese National Cardiovascular Center Type VAD system (Model VCT-100, Toyobo, Osaka, Japan). The system used for TEE evaluation was Aloka Models SSD-880, SSD-860, and SSD-870.

Results

IABP Support

IABP was successfully introduced in 28 patients, but could not be introduced in three patients due to aortic dissection (two patients) and thoracic aneurysm at the diaphragm level which was not be detected preoperatively (one patient). The aortic lesions in these three could be detected only by TEE evaluation, which was performed because of the difficulty of inserting the IABP balloon catheter. In 25 patients, IABP support was successfully discontinued with good functional recovery, which could be confirmed not only by hemodynamic data but also by TEE wall motion analysis. In three patients, IABP support could not be withdrawn because of failure of left ventricular function recovery. In four patients, grade 1 mild aortic regurgitation which did not have any adverse effects on the hemodynamics was observed with TEE during IABP support. In two patients, segmental posterior wall motion abnormality due to perioperative myocardial infarction was observed by TEE after elective aortocoronary bypass surgery. In two patients, one after left ventricular aneurysmectomy and the other after repair of left ventricular free wall rupture, moderate to severe mitral regurgitation was observed. Although these patients were successfully disconnected from IABP support in the early postoperative stage, they died due to development of cardiac failure within 1 year. In one patient who underwent aortic and mitral valve replacements and tricuspid valvuloplasty, the postoperative TEE examination demonstrated severe residual tricuspid regurgitation which prevented withdrawal of IABP support.

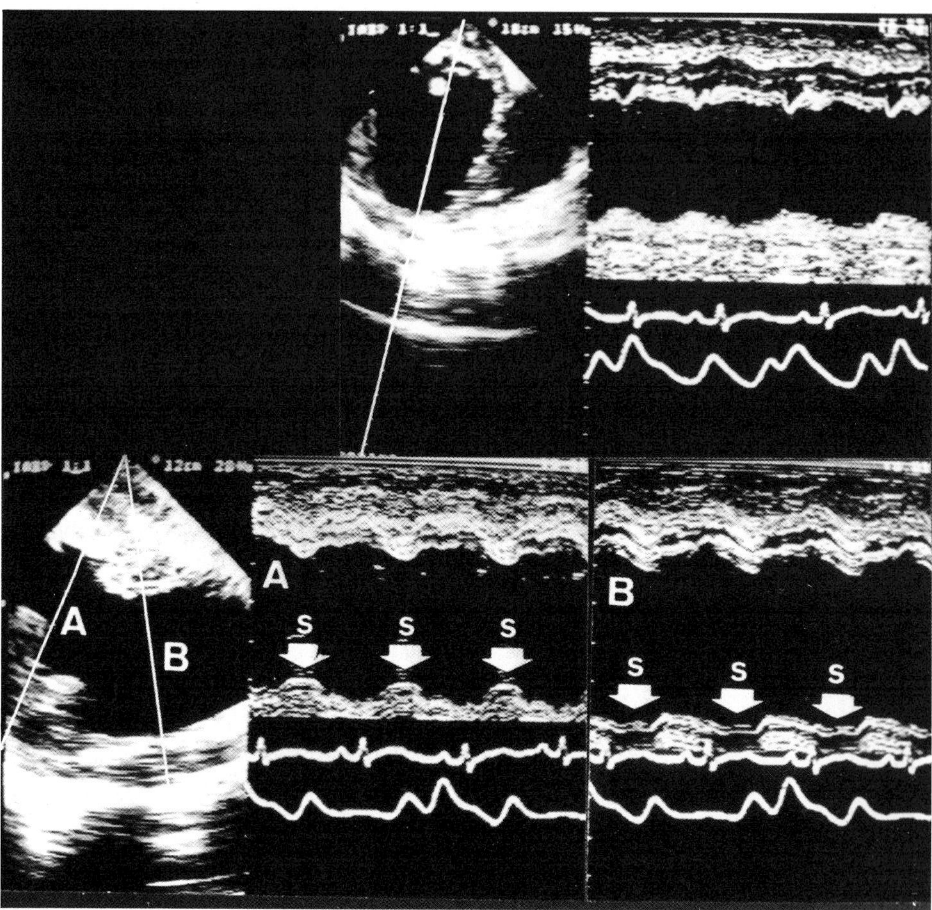

Fig. 1. Evaluation of left ventricular function by bi-plane TEE during IABP support 4 days after surgical repair of left ventricular free wall rupture in a 69-year-old woman. The gastric short-axis view shows a large dyskinetic area in the anterior wall. However, the long-axis view at the same level demonstrates good recovery of the wall motion in the base area (*A*), although a segmental aneurysmal formation was observed in the apical area (*B*). *S*, Systole

Wall motion analysis by TEE with a single-plane transducer to evaluate ventricular function three-dimensionally has not been easy because of the lack of a left ventricular long-axis view. Therefore, we have recently developed a bi-plane TEE transducer. With a bi-plane echo-image, we can easily obtain a three-dimensional concept of ventricular wall motion, which enables abnormalities in left ventricular segmental wall motion to be detected more easily and precisely. Figure 1 shows an example of left ventricular wall motion analysis by bi-plane TEE. The traditional transverse view only indicates dyskinesis in the LV anterior wall. However, a longitudinal view at the same level showed clearly an apical aneurysm in the anterior wall of the left ventricle. IABP support was successfully withdrawn from this patient and good functional recovery of the non-infarcted area was confirmed.

VAD Support

Five patients were supported by VAD for 98 to 278 hours after surgery, and in three VAD support was successfully withdrawn on the 5th postoperative day (POD) (cases 4, 5) or 9th POD (case 3) with good recovery of ventricular function. In one case of ventricular septal rupture (case 1), a moderate right to left shunt (maximum shunt ratio 29%) through the patent foramen ovale (PFO) was observed which had a detrimental effect on the arterial blood oxygen saturation. Due to severe hypoxemia, multiple organ failure developed in this patient, who died on the 10th POD. Figure 2 demonstrates a successful recovery of left ventricular function following left VAD support (case 3). This patient was operated on in one of our affiliated hospitals for myxoma in the left atrium. The patient developed acute left ventricular dysfunction despite the short aortic cross-clamping time and the cardiopulmonary bypass could be discontinued even with IABP support. It was thought that the patient was suffering from acute myocardial damage secondary to a tumor thrombus in the coronary artery during surgery. Postoperatively, the patient was supported

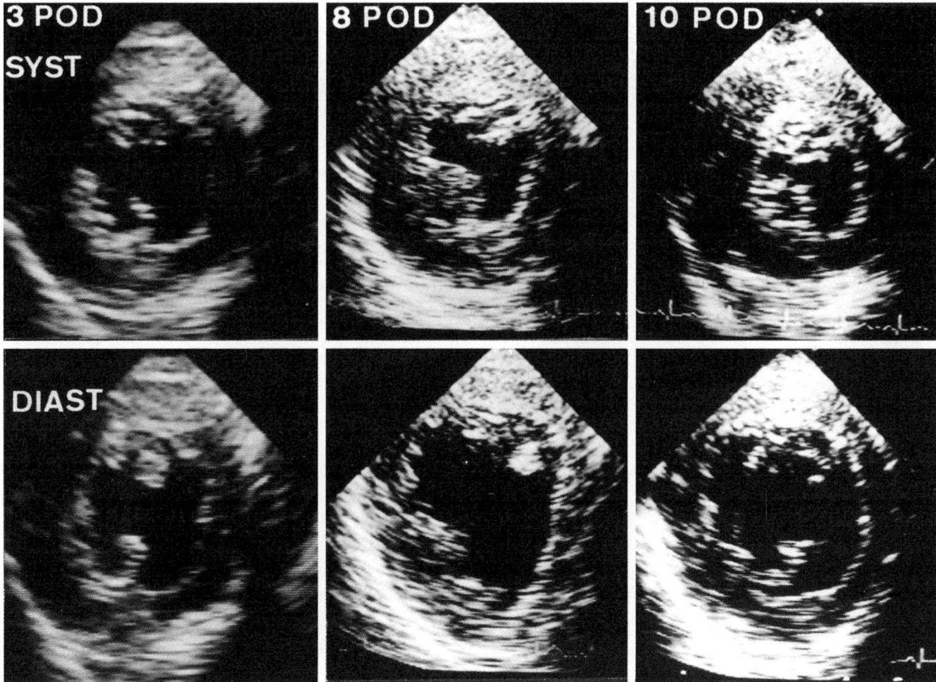

Fig. 2. Evaluation of left ventricular function by TEE in a case of left atrial myxoma (case 3) during left VAD support. On the 3rd POD the LVEF was still less than 20%, but on the 8th POD marked improvement of left ventricular function was noticed, with a LVEF of 60%. VAD was successfully dicontinued on the 9th POD and further improvement of left ventricular function to an LVEF of about 70% was confirmed on the 10th POD. *SYST*, Systole; *DIAST*, diastole

by left VAD and left ventricular function was intermittently monitored by TEE. Until the 3rd POD, the left ventricular ejection fraction (LVEF) was still less than 20%, but from the 5th POD on left ventricular function gradually started to improve; on the 8th POD marked LV function improvement was noticed, with a LVEF of 60%. On the 9th POD VAD support was sucessfully withdrawn and on the 10th POD further improvement of left ventricular function to a LVEF of about 70% was confirmed by TEE.

Evaluation of Left Main Coronary Artery and Its Flow

In five of six pts with ventricular septal rupture and one with left ventricular free wall rupture following acute myocardial infarction, surgery was performed without coronary angiography. Good patency of the left main coronary artery and the proximal left anterior descending coronary artery (LAD) was confirmed by TEE examination in these six patients. Coronary blood flow

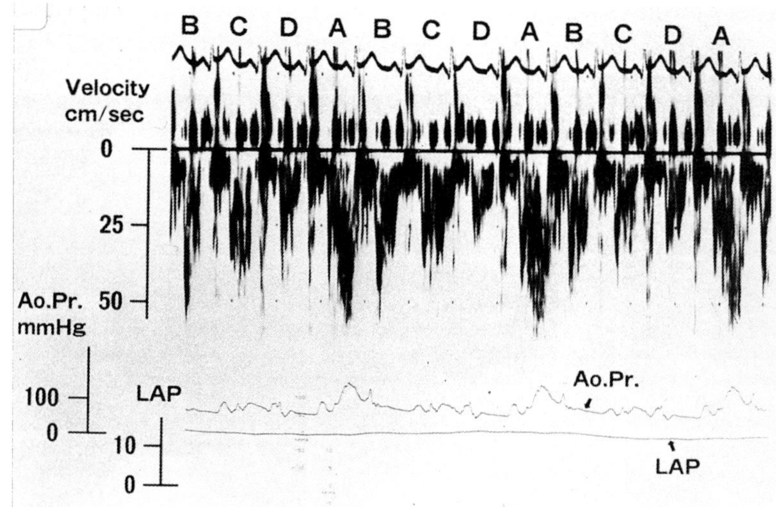

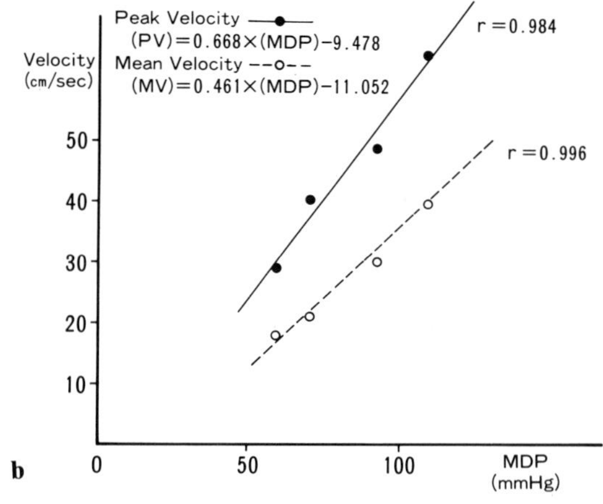

Fig. 3. a Fast Fourier transform spectral analysis of proximal LAD flow and aortic (*Ao.Pr*) and left atrial pressures (*LAP*) during MAC with LVAD (4:1) and IABP (2:1). The peak velocity of LAD flow was 64.6 cm/s with combined IABP and LVAD support (*A*), 48.8 cm/s with LVAD support only (*B*), 40.4 cm:s with IABP support only (*C*), and 29.2 cm/s without MAC support (*D*). **b** Relationship between mean diastolic pressure (*MDP*) and peak velocity (*PV*) and mean velocity (*MV*) of proximal LAD flow during combined VAD and IABP support. (From [8])

was measured during IABP support in seven patients with an assist ratio of 2:1. The peak velocity of diastolic coronary flow in the proximal LAD was increased by approcimately 34% through diastolic augmentation during IABP support. In the case of combined IABP and VAD support (case 3), more marked effects of MAC on coronary blood flow were noticed (Fig. 3), Figure 3a shows the change of flow velocity in the proximal LAD with changes of assistance between IABP and VAD. The peak velocity of the LAD flow was 64.6 cm/s with combined IABP and left VAD support, 48.8 cm/s with left VAD support only, 40.4 cm/s with IABP support only, and 29.2 cm/s without any support. Thus, the peak and mean velocity of LAD flow demonstrated very good linear correlations with mean aortic diastolic pressure (MDP) (Fig. 3b).

Discussion

The information available to confirm the surgical results [4] and safe introduction of MAC during surgery, to confirm the maintenance of adequate circulation to promote recovery from low output syndrome, and to determine the optimal time to discontinue MAC is usually limited in the ICU. This information is very pertinent and useful in critically ill patients. Transthoracic echocardiography can only give limited information due to poor echo penetration with for example, mechanical ventilation. In this study, we found that for TEE there is usually a reasonably good echo window even in these cases in the ICU, and it provides useful information to help in the maintenance of critically ill patients with multiple organ failure [5]. Magovern [6] reported that right to left shunt through PFO has a detrimental effect on the arterial blood oxygen saturation, but before introduction of intraoperative color flow mapping it was not easy to detect PFO during surgery [3]. During emergency surgery following acute myocardial infarction without cardiac catheterization, it is valuable to at least exclude the existence of left main coronary artery disease. Direct measurement of coronary blood flow by TEE is also valuable to detect effective diastolic augmentation during MAC, which cannot be done with any other medical diagnostic tool [4, 8]. Further important information that can be obtained by TEE concerns evaluation of LV function. TEE examination can be performed daily during MAC without any difficulty, and at a reasonable cost. The major limitation of traditional TEE, which could provide only M-mode and transverse sectional views for evaluating ventricular function [1, 2, 7, 9], was mostly resolved by the development of the new bi-plane TEE transducer. The bi-plane TEE probe is particularly important in the evaluation of segmental wall motion abnormalities following acute and/or chronic myocardial infarction. In Japan, the use of radioactive substances in the ICU has been totally prohibited. Therefore, TEE examination is the only currently available diagnostic tool for immediate evaluation of overall cardiac function during MAC. It can provide important information for patient management including the safe introduction of MAC, appropriate maintenance of MAC, and determination of optimal timing for discontinuation of MAC.

References

1. Hisanga K, Hisanga A, Nagata K, Ichie Y (1980) Tranesophageal cross-sectional echocardiography. Am Heart J 100:605—609
2. Kremer P, Schwartz L, Cahalan MK, Gutman J, Schiller NB (1982) Intraoperative monitoring of left ventricular performance by transesophageal M-mode and 2-D echocardiography (abstract). Am J Cardiol 49:956
3. Kyo S, Handa N, Takamoto S, Adachi H, Ueda K, Yokote Y, Omoto R (1988). The reversed shunt flow through the patent foramen ovale in left ventricular assist circulation: evaluation by transesophageal color Doppler echo. Jpn J Artif Organs 17:888—891
4. Kyo S, Takamoto S, Matsumura M, Yokote Y, Omoto R (1986). Visualization of coronary blood flow by transesophageal Doppler color flow mapping. J. Cardiogr 16:831—840
5. Kyo S, Takamoto S, Matsumura M, Asano H, Yokote Y, Motoyama T, Omoto R (1987). Immediate and early postoperative evaluation of results of cardiac surgery by transesophageal two-dimensional Doppler echocardiography. Circulation 76 (Suppl V): 113
6. Magovern JA, Pae WE Jr, Pichenbacher WE, Pierce WS (1986). The importance of a foramen ovale in left ventricular assist pumping. Trans Am Soc Artif Intern Organs 32:449—453
7. Matsumoto M, Oka Y, Strom J, Frishman W, Kadish A, Becker RM, Frater RWM, Sonnenblick EH (1980). Application of transesophageal echocardiography to continuous intraoperative monitoring of left ventricular performance. Am J Cardiol 46:95
8. Neya K, Takamoto S, Harada M, Nakano R, Kyo S, Yokote Y, Omoto R (1989). Effect of left ventricular assist device and intra-aortic balloon pumping on the coronary flow. Jpn J Artif Organs (in press) 18(2):503—506
9. Omoto R, Yokote Y, Takamoto S, Kyo S, Ueda K, Asano H, Namekawa K, Kasai C, Kondo Y, Koyano A (1984). The development of real-time two-dimensional Doppler echocardiography and its clinical significance in acquired valvular disease with special reference to the evaluation of valvular regurgitation. Jpn Heart J 25:325—340
10. Takamoto S, Kyo S, Adachi H, Matsumura M, Yokote Y, Omoto R (1985). Intraoperative color flow mapping by real-time two-dimensional Doppler echocardiography for evaluation of valvular and congenital heart disease and vascular disease. J Thorac Cardiovasc Surg 90:802—812

Transesophageal Two-Dimensional and Doppler Echocardiography During Percutaneous Transluminal Coronary Angioplasty

J. J. Koolen, C. A. Visser, G. K. David, G. Hoedemaker, H. J. van Wezel, and A. J. Dunning

Introduction

More than fifty years ago, Tennant and Wiggers [1] were the first to demonstrate that "the ventricular zone affected by ligation of a large coronary branch not only appears cyanotic and dilated, but that it seems to alter in its mode of contraction". Since then, the function of ischemic and nonischemic myocardium has been studied extensively in animal models by a variety of techniques [2−6], including M-mode and two-dimensional echocardiography. Similar data in humans on the effect of transient ischemia on left ventricular function have been limited to observations during spontaneous or provoked attacks of angina pectoris. Using two-dimensional echocardiography, Gerson et al. [7] demonstrated in a patient with Prinzmetal's angina, akinesia of the previously normally contracting left ventricular posterior wall during a provoked attack of pain.

The advent of percutanous transluminal coronary angioplasty provides the opportunity to assess the time course of changes in myocardial wall motion during transient, total interruption of coronary flow in humans, and its relation to clinical and electrocardiographic signs of ischemia. Two-dimensional echocardiograhic studies performed during coronary angioplasty have recently demonstrated that systolic dysfunction starts early after occlusion [8−10]. In addition, ischemia may occur without pain and/or electrocardiographic abnormalities.

As transesophageal echocardiography usually provides high-quality images, is highly reproducible and does not interfere with the procedure [11], the present study was undertaken to determine the effects of ischemia, in a quantitative fashion, on both global and regional left ventricular function and left ventricular filling.

Methods

Eleven patients were selected for this study. All were men, the mean age being 52 ± 8 years. All had normal global left ventricular function on transthoracic echocardiography without regional wall motion abnormalities. Seven patients had one-vessel disease, in five proximally located in the left anterior

Transesophageal Echocardiography
Edited by R. Erbel et al.
© Springer-Verlag Berlin Heidelberg 1989

descending artery (LAD) and in two in the right coronary artery (RCA). Four patients had a significant obstruction in two coronary arteries; in five patients there were lesions in the LAD and RCA, and in one patient in the LAD and circumflex artery.

Transesophageal Echocardiography

After induction of general anesthesia a transesophageal echocardiographic transducer (5.0 MHz) was introduced into the esophagus and connected to a Hewlett-Packard ultrasonic system, which has two-dimensional and Doppler color flow imaging capabilities. Since depression of myocardial function may occur directly after intubation echocardiographic baseline data were obtained at least 20 min after intubation [12]. Twenty-six ischemic periods were monitored; the balloon inflation time ranged from 45 to 60 s. Just before every ischemic period the transducer was positioned at the level of the papillary muscles; this position was noted relative to the incisors to ensure reproducibility. Cross sections obtained at this level were used for quantitative analysis later on, see below. Continuous recordings were obtained just before and during approximately 25-s balloon inflation. Then the transducer was pulled backwards to record transmitral flow at the level of the mitral valve annulus in a four-chamber view (Fig. 1).

Quantitative Analysis

Analysis of the cross sections obtained at the level of the papillary muscles as well as the transmitral flow recordings was performed with a commercially available computer-aided, contouring system (Digisonics). The peak of the R wave of the simultaneously displayed electrocardiogram was used to select end-diastolic stopframes. End-systolic stopframes were defined as the minimal cross-sectional area of the left ventricle. The outlines of the papillary muscles were excluded from the contour. End-diastolic and end-systolic area were calculated as well as the percent area reduction (PAR) [13]. Cross sections were then subdivided into eight equal areas and the regional area shrinkage or ejection fraction (RAEF; Fig. 2) was calculated using a floating axis system [14]. Percentage area reduction and regional area ejection fraction measurements were calculated for three beats and averaged. Finally, the early to atrial peak flow velocity ratio (E/A) of the transmitral flow was calculated as well as the time velocity integral (TVI) in at least five beats.

Statistical Analysis

All data are given as mean $\pm$ 1 standard deviation. The Student's t test was used for testing the significance of differences.

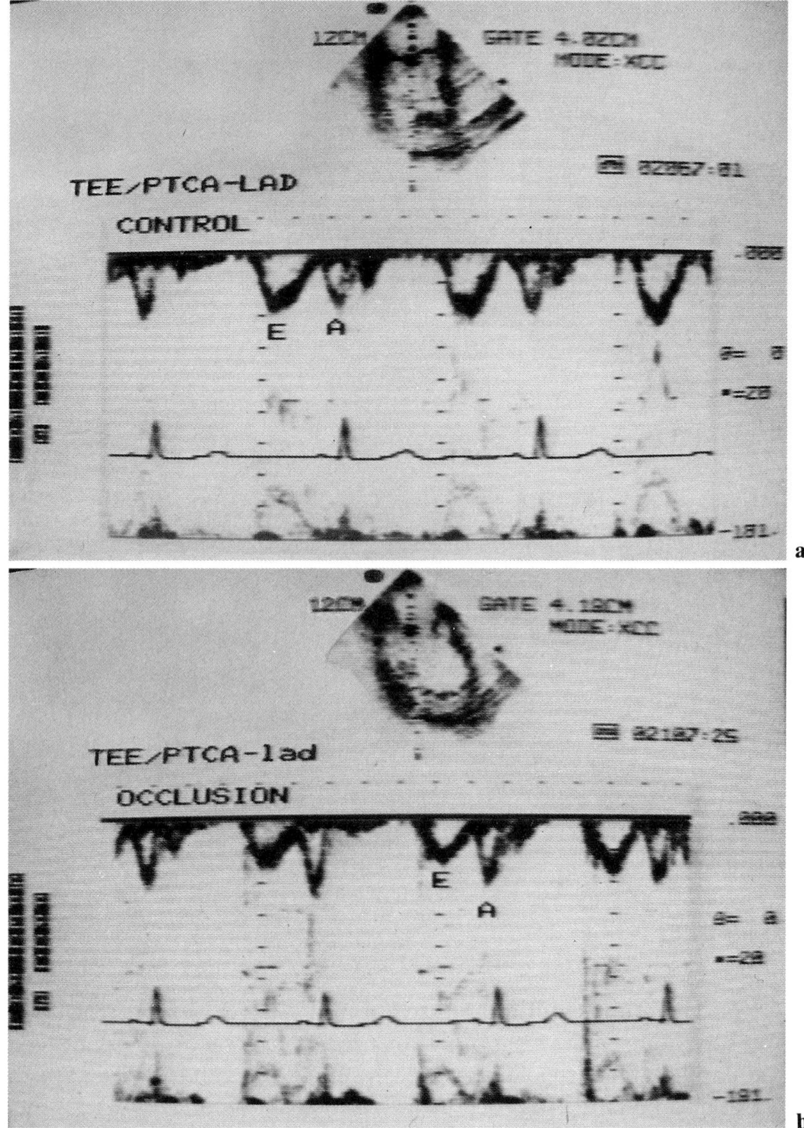

Fig. 1a, b. Transesophageal pulsed Doppler recording of transmitral flow obtained at the level of the mitral valve annulus before occlusion of the left anterior descending artery (**a**). During occlusion (**b**) there is rearrangement of left ventricular inflow with E/A less than 1

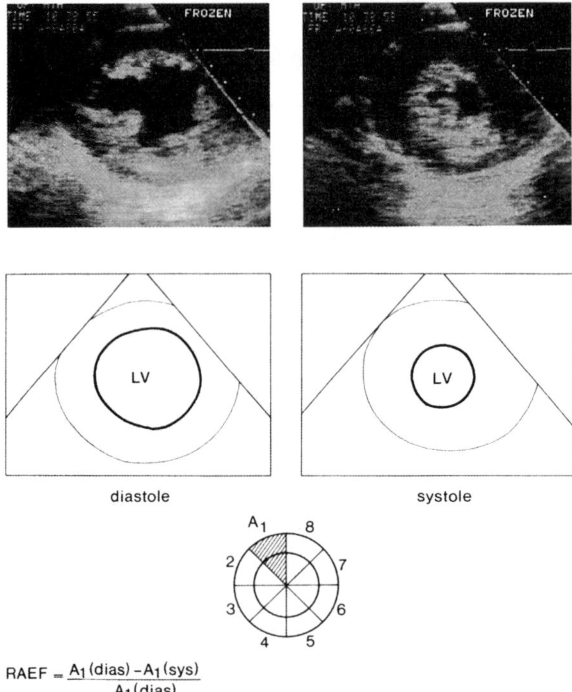

Fig. 2. End-diastolic and end-systolic stopframes including endocardial outlines of images obtained at the level of the papillary muscles. The schematic diagram demonstrates the eight areas (A) evaluated at this level. The regional area ejection fraction (RAEF) was calculated using a floating-axis analysis system and defined as [(diastolic area − systolic area)/(diastolic area)] × 100%

Results

In the 11 patients studied, 36 balloon inflations were performed. During 26 of these ischemic periods both transmitral flow recordings and cross sections at the papillary muscles level were obtained. Eleven of these 26 ischemic periods were obtained during occlusion of the RCA and the remaining 15 during occlusion of the LAD.

Global and Regional Left Ventricular Function

Figure 3 clearly demonstrates what happens following LAD occlusion. The end-systolic frame in A was obtained before occlusion and left ventricular configuration in this four-chamber view is normal. This is contrast to the still-frame in B, which was obtained approximately 20 following proximal LAD occlusion and which demonstrates overt end-systolic bulging. Quantitative analysis of all ischemic periods demonstrated that global left ventricular func-

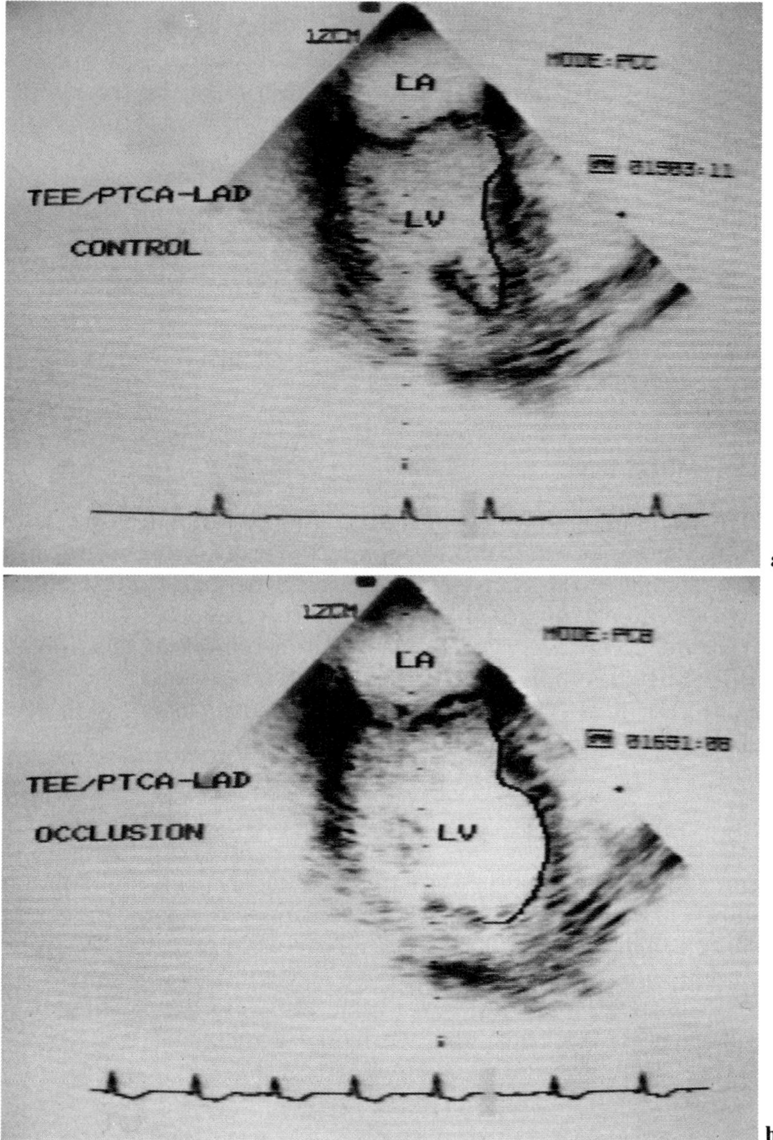

Fig. 3a, b. End-systolic transesophageal echocardiogram obtained **a** before and **b** during occlusion of the left anterior descending artery. Note the overt bulging of the septum during occlusion. *LA*, left atrium; *LV*, left ventricle

tion, as assessed by PAR, decreased from $59 \pm 6\%$ to $46 \pm 8\%$ ($p < 0.01$) (Table 1). Regional myocardial function was assessed by RAEF (Fig. 1), and the lowest value obtained in the ischemic zone was used for this purpose. During RCA occlusion this usually was area 1, and during LAD occlusion area 6 or 7. RAEF decreased from $55 \pm 8\%$ to $43 \pm 18\%$ ($p < 0.01$).

Table 1. Changes of left ventricular dynamics during percutaneous transluminal coronary angioplasty

	Control	Ischemia
PAR (%)	59 ± 6	46 ± 8
RAEF (5%)	55 ± 8	43 ± 18
E/A	1.23 ± 0.27	0.87 ± 0.26
TVI (cm)	11.8 ± 1.8	10.6 ± 1.5

Differences between control and ischemia were all significant at $p < 0.01$.
PAR, percentage area reduction; RAEF, regional area ejection fraction; E/A, early to atrial peak flow velocity ratio; TVI, time velocity integral of transmitral flow.

Transmitral flow

Figure 2 demonstrates a transmitral flow recording on the left, as obtained by pulsed Doppler echocardiography at the level of the mitral valve annulus in a four-chamber view, before occlusion of the LAD. Note that the early peak flow velocity is higher than the peak flow velocity due to atrial contraction. Following LAD occlusion there is rearrangement of this flow pattern resulting in E/A being less than 1. E/A for all occlusions was 1.23 ± 0.27 and dropped to 0.87 ± 0.26 ($p < 0.01$). The TVI also decreased significantly, from 11.8 ± 1.8 cm to 10.6 ± 1.5 cm ($p < 0.01$).

LAD Versus RCA Occlusion

Percentage increases or decreases of the variables evaluated in this study are shown in Table 2. All variables were affected significantly more by LAD occlusion than by RCA occlusion. RAEF decreased by 96% following LAD occlusion and by 60% following RCA occlusion. The percentage changes of PAR and E/A following LAD occlusion were approximately twice as high as following RCA occlusion. TVI decrease following LAD occlusion was 16%, versus 2% following occlusion of the RCA.

Table 2. Percentage increase/decrease of all variables during occlusion of left anterior descending (LAD) and right coronary artery (RCA)

	LAD	RCA
PAR	23	11
RAEF	96	60
E/A	37	28
TVI	16	2

Differences between LAD and RCA were all significant at $p < 0.01$.

Discussion

Percutaneaous transluminal coronary angioplasty is not only a therapeutic tool but can also be used as a source of information hitherto unavailable. Transthoracic two-dimensional echocardiography performed during coronary angio-plasty has recently demonstrated that, in line with the classic study of Tennant and Wiggers [1] who used an optical myograph, transient regional asynergy rapidly occurs following occlusion of a coronary artery [8–10].

In addition, the paradoxic systolic motion of the affected myocardium once described by them has also been documented in man, in particular following LAD occlusion. The majority of these studies, however, were not quantitatively analyzed, most likely due to image quality.

As ischemia affects both left ventricular ejection and filling, Doppler-derived transmitral flow velocities may provide information on diastolic performance of the left ventricle. Animal studies have shown that following the onset of ischemia a transient shift is seen of diastolic filling from early to late diastole [15–17]. A drop of the E/A ratio to below 1 occurred 20 $\pm$ 10 beats after occlusion. Comparable changes have been described recently in humans undergoing coronary angioplasty. Raisano et al. [17] noted the beginning of a decrease in the E/A ratio in a group of eight patients with isolated LAD stenosis as early as 8 $\pm$ 5 s after occlusion. Bowman et al. [18] also studied patients undergoing LAD angioplasty and found the onset of diastolic dysfunction as early as 15–20 after balloon inflation. It is conceivable, however, that the transthoracic approach during this type of intervention, with patients hyperventilating during pain, may have affected the position of the transducer and thus the sample volume postion and the quality of the cross section obtained. With anesthetized patients and using the transesophageal approach, images of both transmitral flow and left ventricular cross section are usually highly reproducible and of sufficient quality to analyze in a quantitative fashion. The present study was not undertaken to assess the time of onset of diastolic/systolic dysfunction but rather to quantify it. Systolic function parameters were evaluated as soon as the worst degree of asynergy had occured; this was invariably within 20 s following occlusion. All our patients developed regional myocardial dysfunction, the degree and extent of which was most prominent in patients undergoing coronary angioplasty of the LAD. RAEF dropped in these patients from 57 $\pm$ 6% to 3 $\pm$ 10%, and ranged during occlusion from -15% to 22%, indicating a paradoxic motion pattern. This type of asynergy was never encountered in patients undergoing coronary angioplasty of the RCA; in these patients RAEF during occlusion ranged from 15% to 25%, indicating hypokinesis. This apparent preference is also found in acute myocardial infarction and cannot be explained by myocardial involvement alone [19, 20].

Other factors such as different myocardial thickness and myocardial support by both the pericardium and surrounding structures might play a role [21]. In addition, the anterior shift of the heart during systole may result in cancellation of a paradoxic motion of the posterior wall and in aggravation of anteriorly localized asynergy.

Global left ventricular function was assessed by means of the PAR at the level of the papillary muscles. This cross section was chosen as this area of the left ventricle is supplied by the three major coronary arteries. One must bear in mind, however, that this approach is a simplification, as changes in the long axis of the ventricle are neglected. PAR was more affected by LAD occlusion than by RCA occlusion. This can be explained by differences in both degree and extent of asynergy. The extent of asynergic area, as assessed in a previous study by a "myocardial risk area" [10], was indeed significantly larger during LAD occlusion. This is in line with studies on the size of individual coronary vascular beds in humans [22] and may also explain the differences found in left ventricular inflow.

We conclude that coronary angioplasty combined with transesophageal echocardiography provides an unique opportunity to study the effects of temporary ischemia in humans. Systolic and diastolic dysfunction are invariably linked and more profound following LAD occlusion.

References

1. Tennant R, Wiggers J (1935) The effect of coronary occlusion on myocardial contraction. Am J Physiol 112:351−361
2. Prinzmetal M, Schwartz LL, Corday E, Spritzler R, Bergman HC, Krueger HE (1949) Studies on the coronary circulation. I. Loss of myocardial contractility after coronary artery occlusion. Ann Intern Med 31:429−449
3. Hood WG, Corelli VH, Abelmann WH, Normal JC (1969) Persistance of contractile behaviour in acutely ischmic myocardium. Cardiovasc Res 3:249−260
4. Theroux P, Franklin D, Ross J, Kemper WS (1974) Regional myocardial function during acute coronary artery occlusion and its modifications by pharmacologic agents in the dog. Circ Res 35:896−908
5. Kerber RE, Marcus ML, Abboud FM (1977) Echocardiography in experimentally induced myocardial ischemia. Am J Med 63:21−28
6. Pandian NG, Kieso RA, Kerber RE (1982) Two-dimensional echocardiography in experimental coronary stenosis. II. Relationships between systolic wall thinning and regional myocardial perfusion in severe coronary stenosis. Circulation 66:603−611
7. Gerson MC, Nobele RJ, Wann LS, Faris JN, Morris SN (1979) Noninvasive documentation of Prinzmetal angina. Am J Cardiol 43:323−334
8. Hauser AM, Gangadharan V, Ramos RG, Gordon S, Timmis GC Sequence of mechanical, electrocardiographic and clinical effects of repeated coronary artery occlusion in human beings: echocardiographic observations during coronary angioplasty. J Am Coll Cardiol 5:193−197
9. Wohlgelernter D, Cleman M, Ainsley Highman H, Fetterman RC, Duncan JS, Zaret BL, Jaffe CC (1986) Regional myocardial dysfunction during coronary angioplasty: evaluation by two-dimensional echocardiography and 12-lead electrocardiography. J Am Coll Cardiol 7:1245−1254
10. Visser CA, David GK, Kan G, Meltzer RS, Koolen JJ, Dunning AJ (1986) Two-dimensional echocardiography during percutaneous transluminal coronary angioplasty. Am Heart J 111:1035−1041
11. Visser CA, Koolen JJ, van Wezel HB, Dunning AJ (1988) Transesophageal echocardiography: technique and clinical applications. J Cardiothor Anesth 2:74−91
12. Giles R, Berger H, Barash P (1982) Continuous monitoring of left ventricular performance with the computerized nuclear probe during laryngoscopy and intubation before coronary artery bypass surgery. Am J Cardol 50:735−741

13. Koolen JJ, Visser CA, Wever E, van Wezel HB, Meyne NG, Dunning AJ (1987) Transesophageal two-dimensional echocardiographic evaluation of biventricular dimension and function during positive end-expiratory pressure ventilation after coronary bypass grafting. Am J Cardiol 59:1047–1051
14. Koolen JJ, Visser CA, van Wezel HB, Meyne NG, Dunning AJ (1987) Influence of coronary bypass surgery on regional left ventricular wall motion: an intraoperative transesophageal two dimensional echocardiographic study. J Cardiothor Anesth 1:276–283
15. Visser CA, Janse MJ, Koolen JJ, Dunning AJ (1986) Comparison of left ventricular systolic and diastolic dysfunction sequence following transient ischemia. Circulation (Suppl 2) 74:II–403
16. Armstrong WF, Ryan T, Feigenbaum H (1987) Doppler evaluation of left ventricular inflow during transient myocardial ischemia. 9:213A
17. Raisaro A, Bargiggia G, Deservi S, Bramucci E, Recusani F, Valdes-Crusz LM (1987) Doppler evaluation of left ventricular diastolic filling function during angioplasty. J Am Coll Cardiol 9:213A
18. Bowman LK, Cleman MW, Cabin HS, Zaret BL, Jeffe C (1987) Evaluation of left ventricular diastolic filling during coronary angioplasty using Doppler echocardiography. J Am Coll Cardiol 9:213A
19. Visser CA, Lie KI, Kan G, Meltzer RS, Durrer D (1981) Detection and quantification of acute, isolated myocardial infarction by two dimensional echocardiography. Am J Cardiol 47:1020–1026
20. Gibson RS, Bishop HL, Stamm RB, Crampton RS, Beller GA, Martin RP (1982) Value of early two dimensional echocardiography in patients with acute myocardial infarction. Am J Cardiol 49:1116–1122
21. Bulkley BH (1981) Size and sequelae of myocardial infarction. N Engl J Med 305:337–338
22. Kalbfleish H, Horst W (1977) Quantitative study on the size of coronary artery supply area postmortem. Am Heart J 94:1983–1992

Transsesophageal Echocardiographic Monitoring of Aortic Valvuloplasty

K. J. Henrichs, N. Wittlich, S. Sack, R. Erbel, and J. Meyer

Introduction

Balloon valvuloplasty is considered a palliative treatment for patients with severe aortic stenosis and in whom the risk of surgery would be unacceptably high (Cribier et al. 1986; Serruys et al. 1988; Pop et al. 1988). Apart from there being a high rate of restenosis, the procedure itself may be accompanied by cardiac and noncardiac complications (Serruys et al. 1988; McKay et al. 1987). Cardiac complications such as ventricular perforation, aortic insufficiency, and progressive heart failure have been described (McKay et al. 1987; Serruys et al. 1988). In a minority of patients, worsening of left ventricular contraction was observed after aortic balloon valvuloplasty in comparison with prevalvuloplasty conditions.

The present study was performed to assess the acute effects of balloon dilatation of the aortic valve on left ventricular performance using transesophageal echocardiographic monitoring in a group of adult patients with severe aortic valve stenosis.

Methods

Study Population

The study group comprised 20 patients (7 men, 13 women) with a mean age of 74 years (range 55–92 years). All patients were symptomatic, with a history of either syncope, angina or dyspnea at exertion, or congestive heart failure. Echocardiographic and hemodynamic evaluation revealed critical aortic stenosis in all patients. Eight patients were offered valve replacement but refused such a procedure. Seven patients who were offered a choice of either valvuloplasty or surgical valve replacement preferred the valvuloplasty procedure. All patients gave informed consent for balloon aortic valvuloplasty after being informed of the risks and potential complications of the procedure.

Aortic Valvuloplasty Procedure

All patients underwent left heart catheterization from a percutaneous femoral approach. The left ventricular cavity was approached using either a pigtail

Transesophageal Echocardiography
Edited by R. Erbel et al.
© Springer-Verlag Berlin Heidelberg 1989

catheter (USCI) or Sones catheter with a straight-tipped guide wire to cross the aortic valve.

The valvuloplasty procedure was begun by exchanging the left chamber catheter for a 300-cm guidewire. Balloon dilatation was performed by advancing a 15-mm valvuloplasty balloon catheter (Mansfield, BSIC, Hilden, FRG) over the guidewire and positioning the balloon in the plane of the aortic valve. Balloon inflations were performed by hand injection of a saline-contrast medium mixture. The duration of balloon inflation varied between 10 and 30 s. Repeated inflations were performed using larger balloon catheters (up to 23 mm), depending on the outcome of repeated evaluations of the aortic valve area.

Transesophageal Echocardiography

Transesophageal echocardiographic studies were performed using a Toshiba SSH-65A phased array sector scanner and a fiber echoscope (ESB-37SR, Toshiba, Delft, Netherlands) with a 3.75-MHz transducer.

Each patient's history was evaluated to exclude any esophageal disease, which was considered a contraindication for the procedure. Before insertion of the probe, local anesthetic spray (Lidocain, Astra Chemicals) was applied to the pharyngeal region and 0.3 mg buprenorphine (Temgesic®, Boehringer Mannheim) was administered intravenously. The echoscope was advanced blindly. For the esophageal studies, informed consent from the patients was also obtained. After advancing the scope to a distance of 35–40 cm from the patient's incisors into the stomach, and at anteflexion of the distal portion of the scope, cross-sectional images of the left ventricle (short-axis views) at the midpapillary muscle level were obtained; care was taken that the ventricular cavity appeared to have a circular rather than an elliptical shape. After drawing back the scope until the tip was at a distance of 25–30 cm from the patient's incisors, the left ventricle was imaged in the long-axis view and the transducer was focused on the mitral valve. Doppler flow patterns across the mitral valve were obtained. During each balloon inflation, the echoscope was kept in one or other position for continuous monitoring. Periods of interest (preinflation, during inflation, postinflation) were recorded on videotape for later detailed analysis. ECG, left ventricular pressure, and aortic pressure were continuously recorded during the procedure.

Quantitative Assessment of Left Ventricular Function

Epicardial and endocardial borders were traced, and with the aid of a graphics tablet and a semiautomatic computer system (Kontron 200, Munich, FRG), end-diastolic and end-systolic areas of the short-axis view of the left ventricle were calculated. End-diastole was defined at the peak of the R wave in the electrocardiogram, which was recorded simultaneously. End-systole was defined as the smallest ventricular silhouette. From these variables, left ventricular area ejection fraction and endocardial circumferential shortening were calculated. Short-axis views of the left ventricle at the midpapillary muscle level were considered indicative of left ventricular volume, because previous papers confirm that minor axis shortening is closely related to stroke volume (Rankin et al.1976; De Bruijn and Clements (1987).

Turbulent regurgitant jets across the mitral valve were traced and the area of the regurgitant jet was used as a semiquantitative measure of mitral regurgitation. Left ventricular short-axis dimensions and mitral regurgitation were evaluated throughout the cardiac cycle before, during, and after balloon inflation.

Documentation

The end-diastolic and end-systolic left ventricular areas and the area ejection fractions were obtained before and during balloon inflation and 90—120 s after deflation of the valvuloplasty balloon. Individual values and means ± standard error are presented in Figs. 1—3.

Results

The mean peak-to-peak pressure gradient across the aortic valve was found to be 86 ± 6 mmHg, and the mean aortic valve area was $0.59 ± 0.03$ cm^2 in our patient group. After the procedure, the aortic valve area was found to be $1.02 ± 0.09$ cm^2 with a mean peak-to-peak gradient of 44 ± 5 mmHg. End-diastolic left ventricular cavity area increased considerably during balloon inflation, but returned to nearly preinflation levels within 2 min after balloon deflation, as shown in Fig. 1; accordingly, left ventricular area ejection fraction decreased during the balloon inflation period, but left ventricular func-

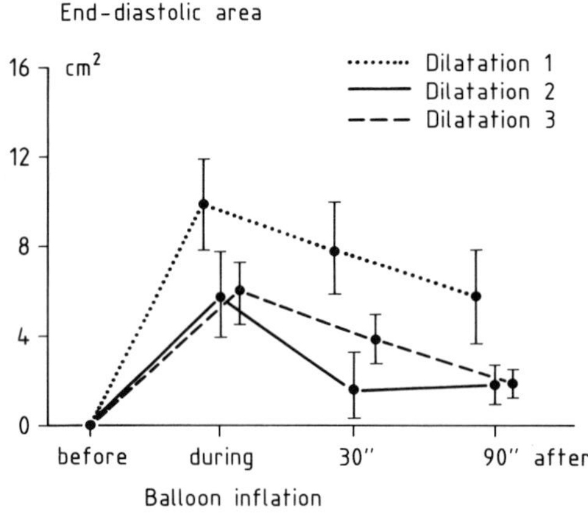

Fig. 1. End-diastolic left ventricular cavity area as measured from the short-axis view shows an increase during balloon inflation during valvuloplasty of the aortic valve; after balloon deflation, end-diastolic left ventricular cavity area gradually returned to near baseline levels

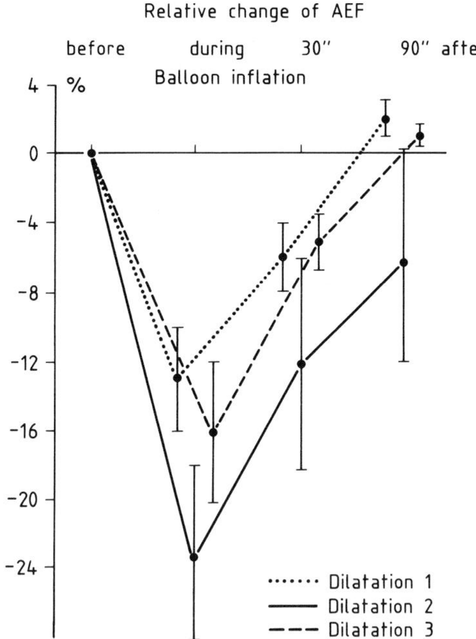

Fig. 2. Left ventricular area ejection fraction decreased as a result of increased afterload and returned to preinflation levels within 2 min of balloon deflation during aortic valvuloplasty

tion returned to nearly preinflation levels after balloon deflation (Fig. 2). Recovery of left ventricular function was not impaired with successive balloon inflations.

Evaluation of color Doppler flow across the mitral valve showed an increase of mitral regurgitation during balloon inflation in the majority of cases,

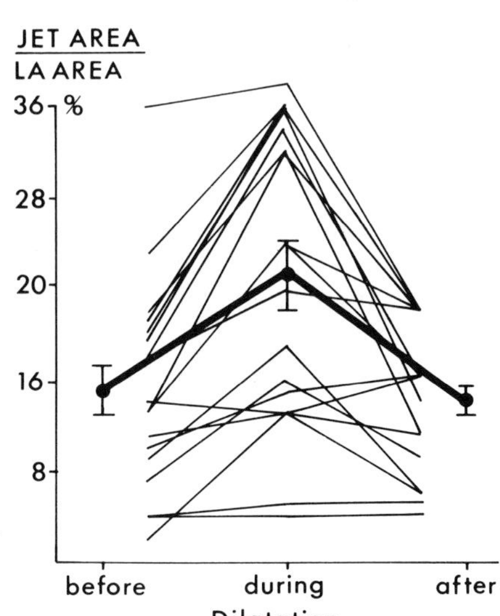

Fig. 3. Mitral regurgitation, as assessed by color Doppler imaging, increased during aortic valvuloplasty as a result of increased afterload, but returned to baseline levels after balloon deflation. *LA*, left atrium

with a return to preinflation levels within 2 min after balloon deflation (Fig. 3). In one patient, a considerable decrease of mitral regurgitation was found after valvuloplasty when compared with prevalvuloplasty values.

Discussion

Percutaneous aortic valvuloplasty appears to be a feasible treatment in a selected group of patients with critical aortic stenosis, but it remains palliative because of its limited immediate and long-term efficacy (Serruys et al. 1988). A variety of procedure-related complications such as heart failure have also been observed (Isner et al. 1987; McKay et al. 1987; Pop et al. 1988). Heart failure was related to ischemic events caused by compromised coronary perfusion which resulted from reduced perfusion pressure during prolonged balloon inflation; also, left ventricular perforation has been observed during aortic valvuloplasty.

Transesophageal echocardiography has been proven to be a valuable method for continuous and on-line observation of regional and global left ventricular function during cardiological interventions. Complications such as ventricular perforation with subsequent pericardial effusion or tamponade can be readily detected by this approach. Furthermore, transesophageal echocardiography allows direct visualization of the valvuloplasty balloon, which can be used for optimal transvalvular balloon placement (Cyran et al. 1988). Imaging of aortic valve leaflets and planimetry of the aortic valve area appear to be useful for immediate evaluation of the valvuloplasty effect, obviating the need for repeat angiography.

Our data show that in all cases balloon inflation results in an abrupt and considerable increase of left ventricular afterload with increases in end-diastolic and end-systolic left ventricular volumes. Reduction of contraction was marked during the balloon inflation period. An increase in left ventricular afterload causes an increase in left ventricular wall stress, and this − together with a reduction in coronary perfusion pressure − could result in ischemic alterations during prolonged periods of balloon inflation. In our series where balloon inflation time did not exceed 30 s, ischemic alterations of left ventricular function were not observed. Left ventricular contraction variables returned to preinflation levels within 2 min of balloon deflation. Interestingly, with the increase of left ventricular afterload during balloon inflation, mitral regurgitation was shown to be considerably increased, but it returned to preinflation levels in most cases with the reduction of left ventricular afterload after balloon deflation.

References

Cribier A, Saouch N, Berland J, Savin T, Rocha P, Letac B (1986), Percutaneous transluminal valvuloplasty of aquired aortic stenosis in elderly patients: an alternative to valve replacement? Lancet 1:63−67

Cyran SE, Kimball TR, Schwartz DC et al. (1988). Evaluation of balloon aortic valvuloplasty with transesophageal echocardiography. Am Heart J 115:460−462

De Bruijn NP, Clements FM (1987). Transesophageal echocardiography. Nijhoff, Boston

Isner JM, Salem DN, Desmayers MR et al. (1987). Treatment of calcific aortic stenosis by balloon valvuloplasty. Am J Cardio 59:313−317

McKay RG, Safian RD, Lock JE et al. (1987). Assessment of left ventricular and aortic valve function after aortic balloon valvuloplasty in adult patients with critical aortic stenosis. Circulation 75:192−203

Pop T, Erbel R, Henrichs KJ, Todt M, Bednarczyk I, Meyer J (1988). Perkutane Valvuloplastie der stenosierten Aortenklappe: Ergebnisse, haemodynamische Auswirkungen, Komplikationen. Z Kardiol 77:337−345

Rankin JS, McHale PA, Arentzen CE et al. (1976). Three dimensional dynamic geometry of the left ventricle in the conscious dog. Circ Res 39:304−313

Serruys PW, Kijten HE, Beatt KJ et al. (1988). Percutaneous balloon valvuloplasty for calcific aortic stenosis. A treatment "sine cure"? Eur Heart J 9:782−794

Transesophageal Echocardiographic Observations During Percutaneous Balloon Mitral Valvuloplasty

C. A. VISSER, W. JAARSMA, F. D. H. HAAGEN, and S. M. P. G. ERNST

Introduction

Percutaneous balloon dilatation of the mitral valve has been shown to be a promising new approach to the management of patients with rheumatic mitral stenosis [1–5]. Although the mitral valve orifice determines the hemodynamic condition of these patients, the outcome of this procedure appears to be highly associated with the two-dimensional echocardiographic features of the mitral valve apparatus [6]. The immediate results of valvuloplasty can indeed be predicted by assessment of leaflet thickness and mobility, subvalvular thickening, and extent of calcifications [7], and hence may be used to select suitable candidates for this procedure. In addition, Doppler echocardiographic evaluation after valvuloplasty can readily be performed and it has been shown that mitral valve area may increase to values similar to those obtained after surgical commissurotomy [8].

Limited data are to hand concerning the application of transthoracic echocardiography during mitral valvuloplasty. Pandian et al. [9] recently reported successful delivery of the valvular dilatation catheter across the atrial septum and through the valve orifice using subcostal echocardiography. As transesophageal echocardiography provides highquality images of the interatrial septum, left atrial appendage, and mitral valve morphology [10], and does not interfere with the valvuloplasty procedure, we undertook the present study to determine the value of this imaging modality in this setting.

Patients and Methods

The original population consisted of 18 patients, the mean age being 46 ± 11 years. There were 16 women and 2 men. All had a severe symptomatic rheumatic mitral stenosis as shown by both hemodynamics and Doppler echocardiography. The electrocardiogram showed a sinus rhythm in 15 patients and atrial fibrillation in three patients. Right and left heart catheterization including selective coronary angiography and left ventriculography was performed in all patients before the mitral valvulplasty procedure.

Transesophageal Echocardiography
Edited by R. Erbel et al.
© Springer-Verlag Berlin Heidelberg 1989

Echocardiography

Transthoracic echocardiography was performed for patient selection; patients with heavily calcified, immobile leaflets with subvalvular involvement were excluded. In addition, the presence of a thrombus in the left atrium or appendage demonstrated by transesophageal echocardiography was also an exclusion criterion. The final population comprised 15 patients, of whom only one had mild calcifications. Approximately 24 h before and after mitral valvuloplasty the size of the mitral valve orifice was calculated by continuous wave Doppler, as described previously [11]. During the mitral valvuloplasty procedure, a commercially available transesophageal transducer (Hewlett-Packard) was introduced after induction of general anesthesia. This device provides both two-dimensional and color-coded Doppler flow imaging capabilities. Presence and degree of mitral regurgitation was visually assessed, before and after valvuloplasty. In addition, the "maximal leaflet separation" of the mitral valve leaflets during diastole was calculated. During the procedure continuous two-dimensional echocardiographic monitoring was used to facilitate positioning of the sheath and balloon. After termination of the procedure the degree of interatrial shunting was visually estimated, depending on the extent into the right atrium.

Mitral Valvuloplasty

From the left femoral vein a Swan-Ganz catheter was positioned in the pulmonary artery. A pig tail angiographic catheter was positioned in the aorta from the left femoral artery. Transseptal left heart catheterization was performed from the right common femoral vein with a 8F Mullens transseptal sheath and dilator and a modified Brockenbrough needle. Systemic anticoagulation was obtained by 10000 U heparin. After the transseptal procedure, a long 16F Schneider sheath containing a septal dilator was positioned in the mitral orifice over a "back-up" wire. Through this sheath a two-foil Schneider

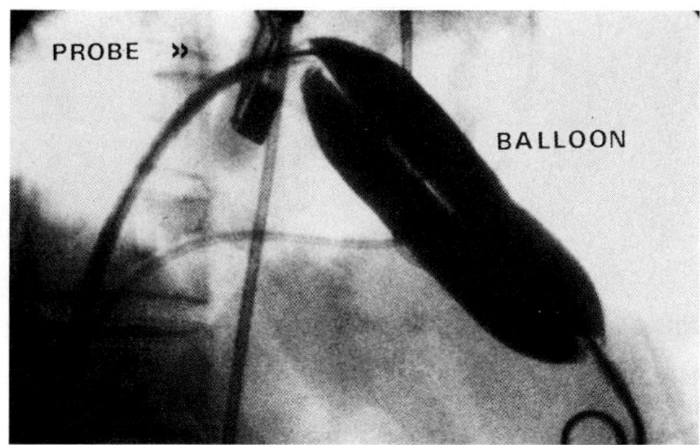

Fig. 1. Inflated two-foil balloon in the mitral valve orifice. Note the position of the echocardiographic probe in relation to the balloon. See also Fig. 3

balloon catheter was introduced into the mitral orifice during continuous fluroscopic and echocardiographic monitoring. Then, balloon inflations of 3 atmospheres over approximately 30 s were repeated until indentation of the balloon due to the stenotic mitral valve was no longer present (Fig. 1).

Results

Visualization of the interatrial septum, in particular of the oval fossa, was possible in all but one patient. The top of the transseptal device could readily be localized as well as the triangular configuration of the septum as soon a some pressure was applied on the needle (Fig. 2). Once the needle had successfully crossed the atrial septum this typical configuration disappeared and some bright echoes usually originated within the left atrium from the puncture site. In only two patients was transesophageal echocardiography important for the positioning of the septostomy device. In these two patients resistance was encountered due to a suboptimal position beyond the oval fossa in the muscular part of the interatrial septum.

Balloon Positioning Through Mitral Valve

After crossing the interatrial septum the sheath was positioned through the mitral valve orifice after using a combination of fluroscopic and echocardiographic imaging. Then, the two-foil balloon catheter was introduced and positioned with the proximal end approximately 2 cm above the mitral valve

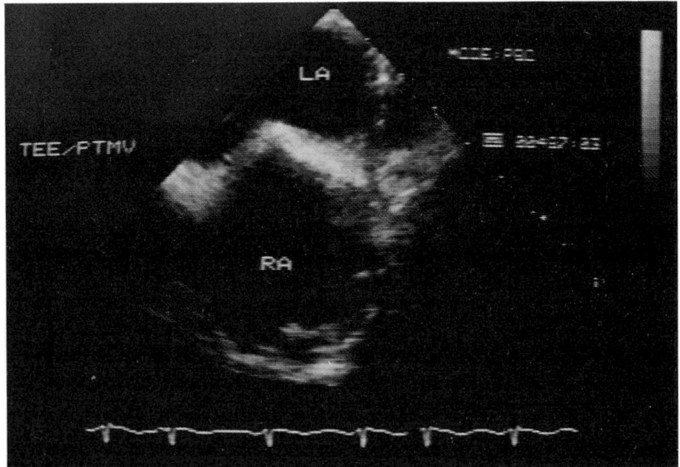

Fig. 2. "Biatrial view" with the right atrium (*RA*), left atrium (*LA*) and interatrial septum that did not show the usual horizontal orientation but the typical triangular configuration due to the transseptal device (*arrow heads*)

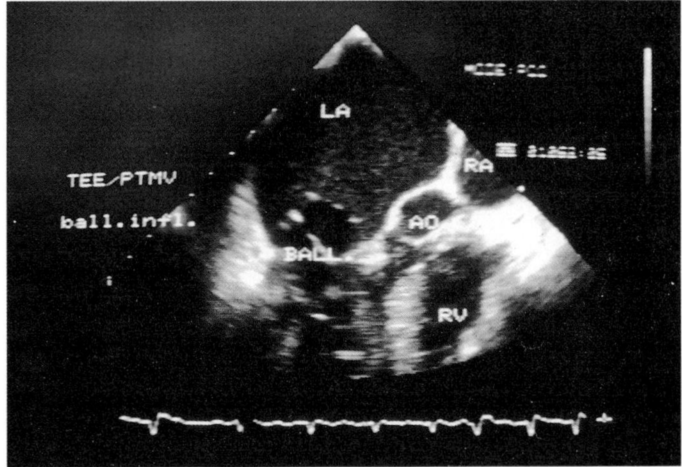

Fig. 3. Transesophageal echocardiogram demonstrating the inflated balloon as "negative contrast" positioned within the mitral valve orifice. Note the 8-like configuration of the balloon due to identation of the stenotic valve, and the distance between the annulus and the proximal end of the balloon. The left atrium (*LA*) is filled with "spontaneous contrast" due to stagnant blood. *AO*, aorta; *RA*, right atrium; *RV*, right ventricle

annulus (Fig. 3). When the distance between the annulus and the proximal part of the balloon was more, the balloon, once fully inflated, was usually pushed backwards into the left atrium.

Maximal Leaflets Separation and Mitral Valve Orifice

During the valvuloplasty procedure maximal leaflet separation was obtained just before and at the end of the dilatation procedure. Before valvuloplasty this separation was 0.6 ± 0.3 cm and after valvuloplasty, 1.4 ± 0.7 cm ($p<0.01$) (Fig. 4). The mitral valve orifice within 24 h before valvuloplasty measured 0.9 ± 0.2 cm^2 and within 24 h after valvuloplasty, 1.9 ± 0.5 cm^2 ($p < 0.01$). The correlation between these two variables, however, was poor, both before and after valvulplasty, with *r* values of 0.3 and 0.1, respectively.

Mitral Regurgitation and Interatrial Shunting

During the procedure, presence and degree of mitral regurgitation was visually estimated before and after valvuloplasty. Before there was no regurgitation present in 15 patients; the remaining two patients had a mild regurgitation. After the procedure 13 patients had a mild regurgitation, one patient a moderate regurgitation, and the other a severe regurgitation.

In all but one patient a jet, originating from the oval fossa, was present. The maximal jet length within the right atrium measured 1.7 ± 1.0 cm.

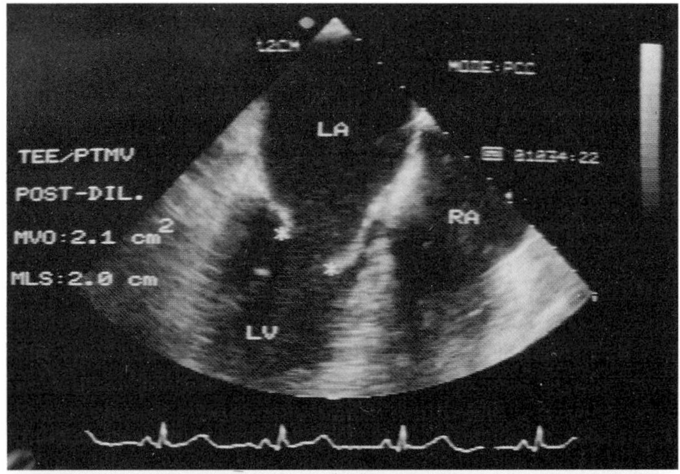
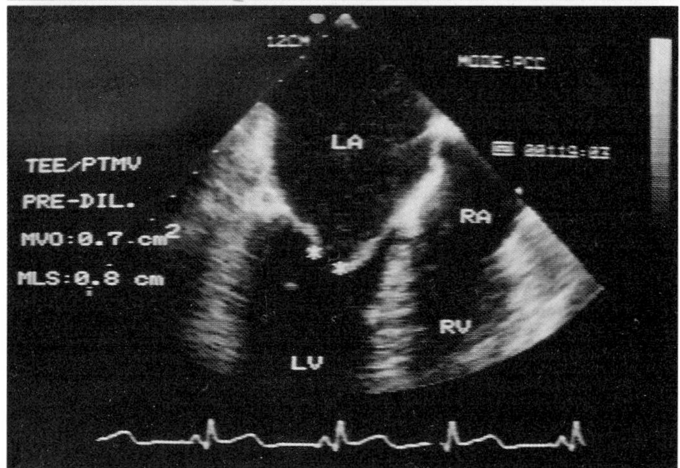

Fig. 4. Four-chamber transesophageal echocardiograms obtained during the mitral valvulo-plasty procedure. The maximal leaflet separation (*MLS*) before dilatation was 0.8 cm and after dilatation, 2.0 cm. The mitral valve orifice, as examined by Doppler echocardiography the day before valvuloplasty, measured 0.7 cm^2 (**a**) and 1 day after the procedure, 2.1 cm^2 (**b**). *LA*, left atrium; *LV*, left ventricle; *RA*, right atrium; *RV* right ventricle

Discussion

Transesophageal echocardiography is now widely used in both clinical and outpatient settings [10]. Limited data are available, however, about the utility of this imaging modality in the setting of cardiac intervention, such as val-vuloplasty and coronary angioplasty.

Although the adventages, being i.e., the high quality of the images and the capability for continuous monitoring without interference with the proce-dure, are obvious, transesophageal echocardiography can only be used in this particular setting in anesthetized patients. Apart from echocardiographic guidance, general anesthesia in this setting is now highly appreciated in both situations.

The atrial septum and the stenotic mitral valve both constitute potential sites of resistance to advancement of the valvular dilatation catheter. In only two patients was echocardiographic monitoring necessary to guide the catheter across the oval fossa. The short distance and sharp bend from the fossa ovalis to the mitral valve orifice, however, usually provides difficulties when only fluroscopy is used. Guidance at this stage by transesophageal echocardiography facilitated greatly the delivery of the dilatation catheter through the initial mitral valve orifice, and hence reduced the X ray radiation time. In addition, by assessing the distance between the proximal end of the mildly inflated balloon and the mitral valve annulus, unsuccessful inflations can be avoided.

Furthermore, the degree of mitral regurgitation as well as the interatrial shunting can be readily assessed at the end of the procedure, making cineangiography of the left ventricle and left atrium not necessary. Finally, in one patient of left ventricle was perforated by the dilatation device; in both patients right atrial collapse could be readily seen before hemodynamic deterioration had occurred. Until a continuous wave modality is available in transesophageal transducers, evaluation of mitral valvuloplasty during the procedure should be performed by two-dimensional imaging and color Doppler flow. The maximal leaflet separation, however, appeared to be highly specific but insensitive for assessment of the mitral orifice increase. Although we had no control group, we think that the use of transesophageal echocardiography greatly reduced X ray exposure. The advantages of this echocardiographic support should be weighed against the need for general anesthesia in this setting.

References

1. Lock JE, Khalilullah M, Shrivasta S, Bahl V, Keane JF (1985) Percutaneous catheter commissurotomy in rheumatic mitral stenosis. N Engl J Med 313:1515−1518
2. McKay RG, Lock JE, Keane JF, Safian RD, Aroesty JM, Grossmann W (1986) Percutaneous mitral valvotomy in an adult patient with calcific rheumatic mitral stenosis. J Am Coll Cardiol 7:1410−1415
3. Al-Zaibag M, Ribeiro PA, Al-Kasab S, Al-Fagih MR (1986) Percutaneous double balloon mitral valvotomy for rheumatic mitral valve stenosis. Lancet 1:757−761
4. Babic UU, Pejcic P, Djurisic Z, Vucinic M, Grujicic S (1986) Percutaneous transarterial balloon valvuloplasty for mitral valve stenosis. Am J Cardioal 57:1101−1104
5. Inoue K, Owaki T, Nakamura T, Kitamura F, Miyamoto N (1984) Clinical application of transvenous mitral commissurotomy by a new ballon catheter. J Thorac Cardiovasc Surg 87:299−402
6. Wilkins GT, Weyman AE, Abascal VM, Block PC, Palacios I (1988) Percutaneous balloon dilatation of the mitral valve: an analysis of echocardiographic variables related to outcome and the mechanism of dilatation. Br Heart J 60:299−308
7. Reid CL, Mc Kay C, Chandraratna AN, Kawamishi DT, Rahimtoola SH (1987) Prediction of immediate results of double balloon catheter balloon valvuloplasty by echocardiographic analysis of mitral valve morphology. Circulation [Suppl 2] 74:II−209

8. Hegar JJ, Wann LS, Weyman AE, Dillon JC, Feigenbaum H (1979) Long-term changes in mitral valve area after successful mitral commissurotomy. Circulation 59:443−448
9. Pandian NG, Isuer JM, Hougen TJ, Desnoyers MR, McInerney K, Salem DV (1987) Percutaneous balloon valvuloplasty of mitral stenosis aided by cardiac ultrasound. Am J Cardiol 59:380−382
10. Visser CA, Koolen JJ, van Wezel HB, Dunning AJ (1988) Transesophageal echocardiography: technique and clinical applications. J. Cardiothor Anesth 2:74−91
11. Hattle L, Angelsen B, Tromsdal A (1979) Non-invasive assessment of atrioventricular pressure half-time by Doppler ultrasound. Circulation 60:1096−1105

Transesophageal Echocardiography in the Operating Room

Automated Contour Detection on Short-Axis Transesophageal Echocardiograms*

H. G. Bosch, J. H. C. Reiber, G. van Burken, J. J. Gerbrands, and J. R. T. C. Roelandt

Introduction

Manual contour tracing in echocardiograms suffers from large inter- and intraobserver variation and is a tedious, time-consuming procedure. As a result, quantitative assessment of left ventricular (LV) wall motion is not routinely performed in echocardiographic studies. Various groups have attempted to detect the endocardial contours automatically in echocardiograms (Adam et al. 1987; Chu et al. 1987; Ezekiel et al. 1987; Grube et al. 1985; Kuwahara et al. 1980; Skorton et al. 1986), but these efforts have not yet resulted in routinely applicable approaches. Automated contour detection on echocardiograms is rather difficult because of the relatively poor image quality, the possible occurrence of dropouts, the high noise level, and disturbances in the images by valves, papillary muscles, etc.

The goal of our project has been the development of an off-line echocardiographic workstation for automated LV contour detection, and the subsequent quantitation of clinically relevant parameters such as regional LV wall motion and regional ejection fraction.

Our first approach has been directed towards the processing of esophageal echocardiograms because of the great clinical interest in quantification of these images and their relatively high image quality. The basic principles of our approach and the result from a preliminary validation study will be described in this paper.

Two models for analysis of LV wall motion in short-axis echocardiograms have been implemented: a regional area ejection fraction model (Koolen et al. 1987) and a centerline model (Bolson et al. 1980).

Methods

Configuration of the Analysis System

The edge detection and analysis algorithms have been developed on an IBM-AT-compatible personal computer equipped with a simple frame grabber

* This research was supported by a research grant from the Netherlands Heart Foundation (NMS 86.080)

Transesophageal Echocardiography
Edited by R. Erbel et al.
© Springer-Verlag Berlin Heidelberg 1989

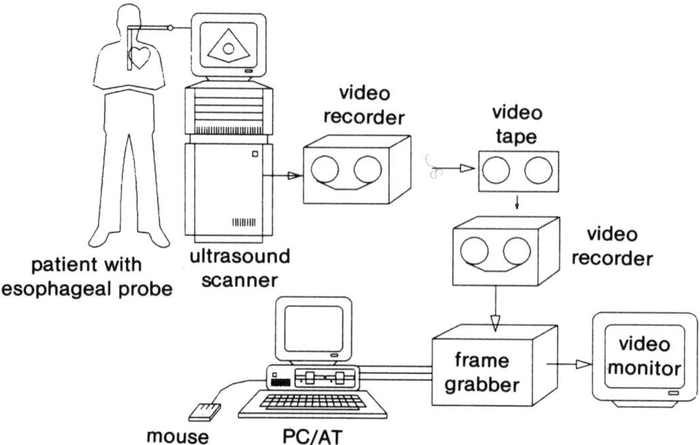

Fig. 1. System configuration

(Fig. 1). The short-axis esophageal echocardiographic images were recorded on video tape at the clinical site. The end-diastolic (ED) and end-systolic (ES) images were selected visually from tape and digitized with the frame grabber. The images and the detected contours were displayed on a separate color monitor. User interaction was performed with a mouse. No proprietary hardware was used.

Automated Endocardial Contour Detection

The method that we have implemented for the automated endocardial contour detection is based on minimum-cost contour detection using a novel iterative approach. Minimum-cost contour detection has been used earlier with success in our laboratory on coronary and left ventricular angiograms and on technetium-99m and thallium-201 scintigrams (Gerbrands et al. 1981; Van Leeuwen and Reiber 1986; Reiber et al. 1985; Reiber 1985). This technique is not very sensitive to image noise and small disturbances, and it may be tailored to specific characteristics of the image. This suggest that it will also be suitable for echocardiographic images.

The minimum-cost method requires the definition of a model for the contour to be detected. Due to certain restrictions, the detected contour cannot differ very much in shape from the model. For short-axis echocardiograms, a simple circular model may be proposed: a circle with a fixed radius around a manually indicated centerpoint of the left ventricle. However, some parts of the endocardial contour, especially at the papillary muscles,have a shape that differs significantly from the circular mode land therefor would give rise to problems in the automated edge detection procedure. To overcome this problem, we have developed an iterative approach: the minimum-cost contour detection procedure is applied twice. After the first iteration the simple circular model is replaced by the first approximation of the endocardial contour, which ist then used as a model in the second iteration, and a better approximation of the true endocardial contour is found. In this way, complex nonconvex contours can be found with a very simple model. It has been our experience that two iterations suffice in most cases; additional iterations did not improve the contours substantially. The automated contour detection algorithm has been described in detail in a previous publication (Bosch et al. 1989).

LV Wall Motion Analysis

As mentioned earlier, two models for analyzing the endocardial contours in short-axis echocardiograms have been implemented: a regional area ejection fraction (RAEF) model and a centerline model.

RAEF Model. For both the ES and ED contours, the luminal area is divided into a number ob wedge-shaped segments. Regional area ejection fractions are defined by the relative area differences of corresponding segments within the ES and ED boundaries (Koolen et al. 1987) (Fig. 2 b):

$$\text{RAEF }(n) = \frac{\text{RAED}(n) - \text{RAES}(n)}{\text{RAED}(n)} \times 100\%$$

where n is segment number, RAEF is regional area ejection fraction, RAED is regional area within ED boundary, and RAES is regional area within ES boundary.

Centerline Model. A centerline is computed between the ES and ED contours and wall motion is quantified by determining for 100 points along this centerline the signed local distances between the two contours in directions perpendicular to the local direction of this centerline. These distances are normalized by the length of the ED contour. The centerline is computed following the procedure described by Sheehan (Bolson et al. 1980), with some adaptations to allow for the analysis of closed contours (Fig. 2 b).

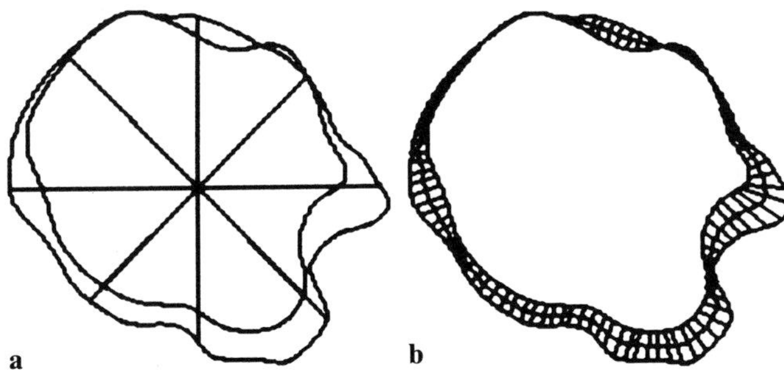

a   **b**

Fig. 2 a, b. LV wall motion models. (**a**) Regional area ejection fraction model with wedge-shaped segments; (**b**) centerline model

Validation of the Technique

An intermediate evaluation of the implemented contour detection procedure
has been carried out, which has focused primarily on the stability of the contour detection method as a function of the variation in the manually defined
LV centerpoints. From ten routinely acquired studies stored on video tape
(short-axis view at papillary muscle level), the ES and ED images were
selected and digitized. These 20 images were analyzed automatically as described above. The analysis was carried out independently by two operators,
one of whom analyzed the images twice with a time interval of two days. The
only operator interaction allowed was the manual definition of the LV centerpoint, i.e., corrections to the otherwise automatically detected contours were
not allowed. Inter- and intraoperator variabilities in the automatic contour
detection technique were described quantitatively by determining the 100
signed local distances between pairs of corresponding contours and by calculating the mean distance and the standard deviation per contour pair. Results for the ten ES and ten ED images were summarized into a mean value
(accuracy) and a pooled standard deviation (precision), for both the intra-
and interoperator variabilities.

Results

As an example, in Fig. 3 two different images are shown with the automatically detected contours. At present, the processing time for the contour detection (two iterations) is approximately 6 s on a 20-MHz Compaq 386 equipped
with an Imaging Technologies FG-100 frame grabber.

The results of the evaluation study are presented in Table 1. None of the
differences between the ED and ES data, or between the inter- and intraoperator variabilities, were found to be statistically significant. Overall, the
accuracy and precision of the automated contour detection technique are very
high, which means that the algorithm is only minimally sensitive to small variations in the manually defined centerpoint positions.

Table 1. Inter- and intraoperator variation in the detection of the
endocardial contours

	ES		ED	
	Accuracy	precision	Accuracy	precision
Intraoperator variation (mm)	− 0.066	0.89	0.11	1.28
Interoperator variation (mm)	− 0.27	1.42	0.21	0.82

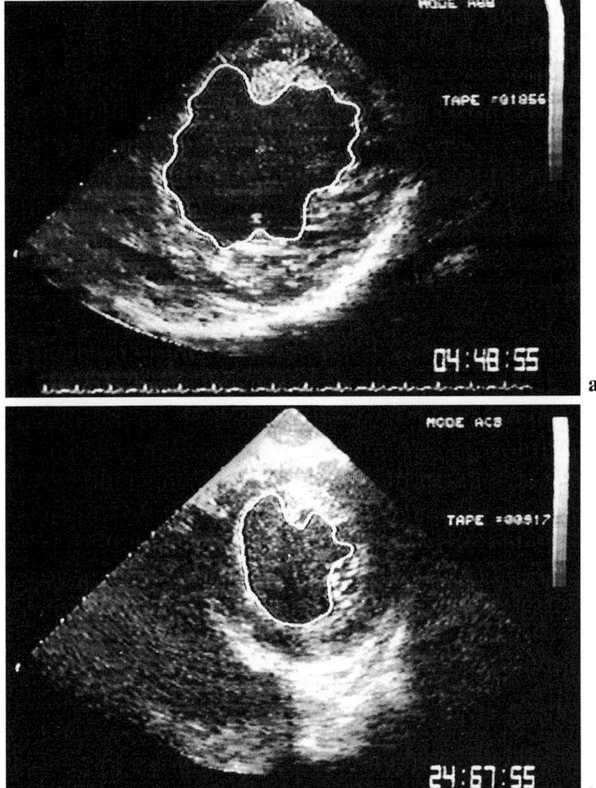

Fig. 3a, b. Selected images with automatically detected contours

Visual interpretation of the detected contours showed that the variations were not distributed evenly over the contours. They occurred only in relatively small image regions, under the following circumstances:

- Large dropouts in endocardial contour
- Epicardial contour much more prominent than endocardial contour
- Complex merging of papillary muscle with endocardial contour

Apparent deviations in the detected contours, according to our own observations, were found in seven out of 20 images; these occurred in the regions mentioned above.

Current Developments

Currently, developments are taking place in three directions. First, we are trying to locate two concentric contours (i.e., endocardium and epicardium) simultaneously in the image. This will not only provide us with both endo- and epicardial contours (allowing wall thickening measurement), but will also eliminate the most important drawback of the algorithm at present: sometimes parts of the epicardium are interpreted erroneously as endocardial contour sections. Secondly, we are extending the method to precordial images. To do this, the improvement mentioned above is essential because of the nature of the precordial images. Thirdly, the method will be extended towards frame-to-frame analysis (tracking the contour(s) during the whole cardiac cycle). This will allow analysis of asynchrony and will probably provide more reliable contour detection, since information from several consecutive images may be combined.

Conclusions

Overall, the accuracy ($\leq$ 0.2 mm) and precision ($\leq$ 1.42 mm) of automatic contour detection are very high. Apparently, the algorithm is not very sensitive to small variations in the manually defined LV centerpoint.) The variabilities in the ES and ED data, as well as in the inter- and intraoperator results, were not statistically significant. The automated contour detection method is both stable and accurate in most cases, but requires some further improvements for the problematic image regions mentioned above.

Acknowledgements. The authors wish to thank Mrs. B. Smit-van der Deure for her secretarial assistance with the preparation of this manuscript.

References

Adam D, Hareuveni O, Sideman S (1987) Semiautomated border tracking of cine echocardiographic ventricular images. IEEE Med Imaging 3:266–271

Bolson EL, Kliman S, Sheehan F, Dodge HT (1980) Left ventricular segmental wall motion – a new method using local direction information. Comp Cardiol: 245–248

Bosch JG, Reiber JHC, Burken G van, Gerbrands JJ, Gussenhoven WJ, Bom N, Roelandt JRTC (1989) Automated endocardial contour detection in short-axis 2-D echocardiograms: methodology and assessment of variability. Comp Cardiol: (in press)

Chu CH, Delp EJ, Buda AJ (1987) Detecting left ventricular endocardial and epicardial boundaries by two-dimensional echocardiography. Comp Cardiol: 393–396

Ezekiel A, Areeda JS, Garcia EV, Corday SR (1987) Intelligent left ventricular contour detection results from two-dimensional echocardiograms. Comp Cardiol: 603–606

Gerbrands JJ, Hoek C, Reiber JHC, Lie SP, Simoons ML (1982) Automated left ventricular boundary detection from technetium-99 m gated blood pool scintigrams with fixed or moving regions of interest. In: Jaffee CC (ed) 2nd International conference on visual psychophysics and medical imaging, Brussels (B), Cat No 81 Ch 1676–6, pp 155–159

Grube E, Mathers F, Backs B, Luederitz B (1985) Automatische und halbautomatische Konturfindung des linken Ventrikels im zweidimensionalen Echokardiogramm. Invitro Untersuchungen an formalinfixierten Schweineherzen. Z Kardiol 74:15–22

Koolen JJ, Visser CA, Wezel HB van, Meyne NG, Dunning AJ (1987) Influence of coronary bypass surgery on regional left ventricular wall motion: an intraoperative transesophageal two-dimensional echocardiographic study. In: Left ventricular monitoring by transesophageal echocardiography. Thesis, University of Amsterdam, pp 35–54

Kuwahara M, Eiho S, Kitagawa H, Ishimi K (1980) Automatic analysis of two-dimensional echocardiograms. In: Lindberg DAB, Kaihara S (eds) Medinfo 80, Proc 3rd world conference on medical informatics, North-Holland, Amsterdam, pp 210–213

Reiber JHC (1985) Quantitative analysis of left ventricular function from equilibrium gated blood pool scintigrams: an overview of computer methods. Eur J Nucl Med 10:97–110

Reiber JHC, Serruys PW, Kooijman CJ, Wijns W, Slager CJ, Gerbrands JJ, Schuurbiers JCH, Boer A den, Hugenholtz PG (1985) Assessment of short-, medium-, and long-term variations in arterial dimensions from computer-assisted quantitation of coronary cineangiograms. Circulation 71:280–288

Skorton DJ, Collins SM, Kerber RE (1986) Digital image processing and analysis in echocardiography. In: Collins SM, Skorton DJ (eds) Cardiac imaging and image processing. McGraw-Hill, New York, pp 172–205

Van Leeuwen PJ, Reiber JHC (1986) Automated detection of left ventricular boundaries from 35 mm contrast cine-angiograms. In: Young IT, Biemond J, Duin RPW, Gerbrands JJ (eds) Signal processing III: theories and applications. Eusipco-86. North-Holland, Amsterdam pp 1409–1412

Continuous and Noninvasive Monitoring of Cardiac Output by Transesophageal Doppler Ultrasound

M. HAUDE, Th. GERBER, R. BRENNECKE, R. ERBEL, and J. MEYER

Introduction

The determination of cardiac output (CO) and related measures is of great relevance especially under intensive care conditions. Various approaches to determining cardiac output have been developed but lack of performance prevented a wide acceptance in clinical medicine. The present method of choice for measuring cardiac output is the thermodilution method which involves transvenous insertion of pulmonary artery catheters [15, 7]. A major disadvantage of this method apart from its invasiveness [5] is the requirement for interactive central venous fluid injections to measure cardiac output, which makes continuous measurement impossible from the practical point of view. Furthermore, the presence of valve insufficiencies may result in underestimation of cardiac output [13].

Thus, an optimal method for monitoring cardiac output, especially when applied to critically ill patients, should allow *continuous* and *noninvasive* determination of cardiac output with little need of personal interaction.

Determination of Cardiac Output by Doppler Ultrasound

Since the technique of either pulsed-wave (pw) or continuous wave (cw) Doppler ultrasound, especially when combined with two-dimensional echocardiography, was introduced to clinical cardiology, different attempts have been made to determine cardiac output on this basis [2, 8].

Methodological Aspects

Doppler ultrasound allows the assessent of blood flow velocity (v) using the formula [11]:

$$V = \frac{\Delta F \cdot c}{2 \cdot F_0 \cdot \cos\alpha}$$

where ΔF = change in frequency of ultrasound, c = velocity of ultrasound in human tissue, F_0 = initial frequency of ultrasound, and α = angle between Doppler ultrasound and flow direction.

Transesophageal Echocardiography
Edited by R. Erbel et al.
© Springer-Verlag Berlin Heidelberg 1989

Based on this relation, cardiac output can be calculated using the following formula [11]:

$$CO = ET \cdot HR \cdot v \cdot 0.25 \cdot \pi \cdot D^2,$$

where ET = systolic ejection time, HR = heart rate, v = blood flow velocity determined by Doppler ultrasound, and D = pulmonary artery, mitral, or aortic diameter, assuming there is a circular cross section.

From a practical point of view, an aortic approach seems to be the most favorable, because aortic blood flow velocity can be assessed easily and reliably by suprasternal Doppler insonation in almost all people. Cardiac output can then be calculated from the estimated flow velocity, systolic ejection time, heart rate, and aortic cross section. The assumption of a circular cross section is valid in most patients, so cardiac output calculation can be based on the aortic diameter, which can be determined individually by echocardiography or taken from a nomogram using the patients' personal data (sex, age, height, weight).

Continuous Determination of Cardiac Output

Based on the methodological assumptions described above, a cardiac output can be continuously monitored if blood flow velocity is determined continuously. For this, we used a transesophageal (TE) Doppler ultrasound device (ACCUCOM, Datascope) consisting of an esophageal and a suprasternal probe and a computer-assisted terminal which allows entry of the patients' data (sex, age, height, weight, aortic diameter, CVP, blood pressure) and displays the values calculated for cardiac output, cardiac index, and systemic vascular resistance.

A continuous wave (cw) Doppler system (2.5 MHz) is mounted on the tip of the esophageal probe. The ultrasound beam transmitted is reflected by the bloodstream within the descending aorta. The insonation angle is 10°. This device enables continuous recording of changes in aortic blood flow velocity. The suprasternal Doppler ultrasound device (2.5 MHz) is used for the initial calibration of the system by measuring blood flow velocity in the ascending aorta as a reference for the continuously measured aortic blood flow velocity determined by transesophageal Doppler ultrasound. Alternatively, a known value of actual cardiac output determined by thermodilution, echocardiography, or angiography can be used as a reference value. An updated value of cardiac output representing the mean of the calculations for 12 heart beats is displayed on the monitor every 15 s.

In practice, the esophageal Doppler ultrasound probe was positioned in the esophagus as illustrated in Fig. 1. The position of the ultrasound probe was changed until an optimal signal was obtained. Additional esophageal probes were removed in order to prevent interactions. After entering the patients' personal data into the terminal, the flow velocity in the ascending aorta was measured as a reference using the suprasternal Doppler ultrasound

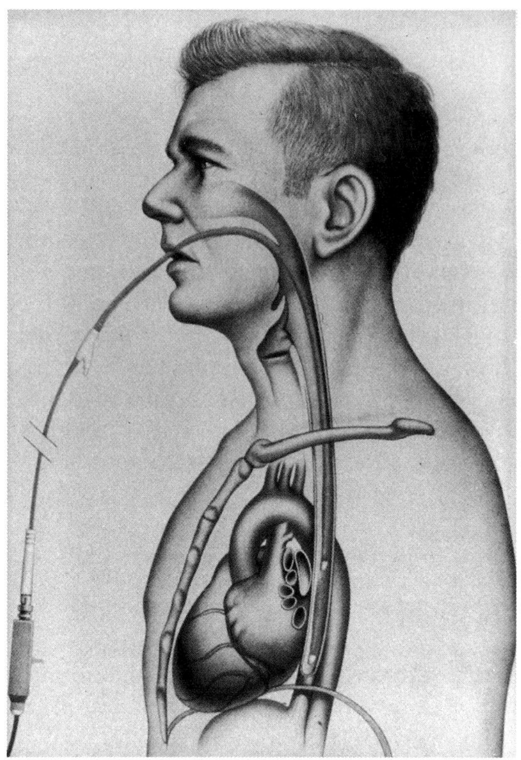

Fig. 1. The esophageal Doppler ultrasound probe in situ

device. Finally, the cardiac output is calculated continuously and displayed on the terminal four times per minute.

Validation Studies

To validate the cardiac output values calculated continuously by transesophageal Doppler ultrasound, a comparison was made to the results obtained simultaneously by thermodilution. The transesophageal Doppler ultrasound device was used in 16 intubated and artificially ventilated patients who had also been supplied with a balloon-tipped pulmonary artery catheter that included a thermistor element for thermodilution measurements of cardiac output. In all 16 patients we were able to obtain proper transesophageal and suprasternal signal levels. Cardiac output determinations were repeated ten times and the means were taken as definitive values (Hande et al. 1989). The results are displayed in Fig. 2, where the calculated differences between the cardiac output values determined simultaneously by thermodilution and transesophageal Doppler ultrasound are plotted on the y-axis against their corresponding means on the x-axis (Altman and Bland 1983). The mean standard deviation of all cardiac output measurements by thermodilution was used

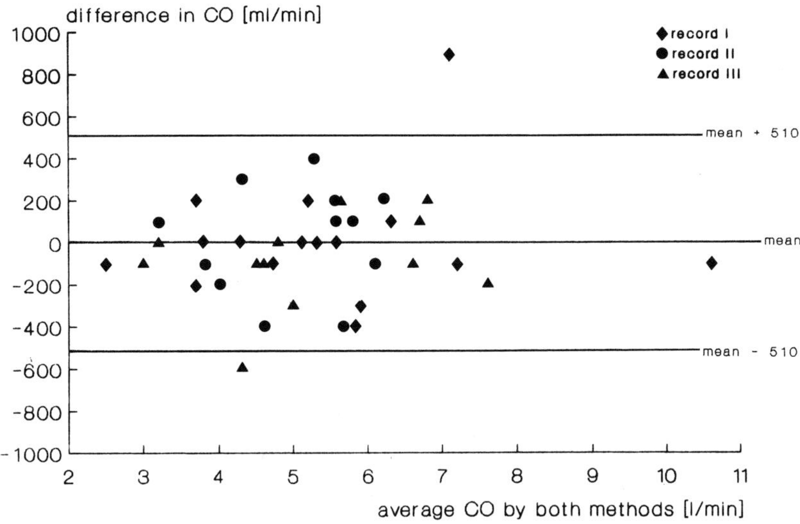

Fig. 2. Plot of the calculated differences between cardiac output values determined simultaneously by thermodilution and transesophageal Doppler ultrasound (*y*-axis) against the corresponding means of both methods (*x*-axis). Record *I, t* = 0 h; record *II, t* = 1 h; record *III, t* = 24 h

as a confidence interval. It was shown that, as well as there being a close correlation between the cardiac output values estimated by both methods, nearly all measurements were within this confidence interval.

For the purpose of investigating short-term and long-term reproducibility, these measurements were repeated after 1 h and 24 h (12 patients). Again, a very close correlation between the measurements taken by both methods was found (Fig. 2).

Conclusion

Although the validation studies revealed very good results and transesophageal Doppler ultrasound proved to be a practicable and reliable method for continuous determination of cardiac output in intubated and artificially ventilated patients, some methodological and practical problems have to be discussed (Table 1). The aortic cross section is assumed to be circular and its diameter is used for the calculation of cardiac output by Doppler ultrasound. Possible changes in aortic diameter due to wall distensions [12] in systole were not considered. In all cases in the validation study aortic diameters were taken from a nomogram. In some cases an estimate was made by echocardiography, but we did not find any large discrepancies from the nomographic values. Aortic dilatation may lead to large errors in calculation of cardiac output when nomographically established diameters are used.

Table 1. Problems related to CO monitoring by transesophageal Doppler ultrasound

---

Methodological
- Aortic diameter
- Assumption of a flat blood flow velocity profile
- Underestimation of CO at increasing insonation angles
- Suprasternal reference measurement

Practical
- Dislocation of the probe
- Interaction with additional esophageal probes
- Anatomical changes within the esophagus (strictures, stenoses, varices)

Another important factor is the underestimation of aortic blood flow that may be caused by an increase in the insonation angle at the descending aorta. An angle of 10° was assumed for calculation of cardiac output using the esophageal probe.

A flat-shaped velocity profile is another assumption of the Doppler ultrasound method, a condition that is given best just distal to the aortic valve and that can not be assumed easily in the descending aorta [3]. This factor is of great relevance, especially when pulsed-wave Doppler ultrasound devices are used and the exact site of the sample volume is not known [4]. Cw Doppler ultrasound systems are affected less.

In some cases the insonation of the ascending aorta required for calibration of the system may be impaired for anatomical reasons or if there is significant aortic insufficiency and so may not lead to proper signal levels.

More practical problems are related to possible dislocation of the esophageal probe and interactions with other esophageal tubes. Anatomical variations and pathological changes of the esophagus may prevent the use of the esophageal Doppler ultrasound probe. Another disadvantage compared to calculating cardiac output by the thermodilution method using pulmonary artery catheters is the lack of additional hemodynamic information such as central venous pressure (CVP) and pulmonary artery pressure (PAP).

Finally, it must be pointed out that the Doppler ultrasound device presented seems to be usable only in intubated patients at the moment because of the size of the probe. Further development may result in a reduction of its present diameter of 7 mm that will allow a use in conscious man as well.

Taking these considerations into account, transesophageal Doppler ultrasound may not only be a useful method for the continuous and non invasive monitoring of cardiac output in critically ill patients with little need of personal interaction [6, 14] but also an ideal tool for undertaking hemodynamic studies when continuous monitoring of cardiac output is required. For example, we examined the effect of changes in positive end-exspiratory pressure (PEEP) during artificial ventilation on cardiac output in intubated patients, these studies showing that there was a decrease in cardiac output when PEEP was increased (Fig. 3).

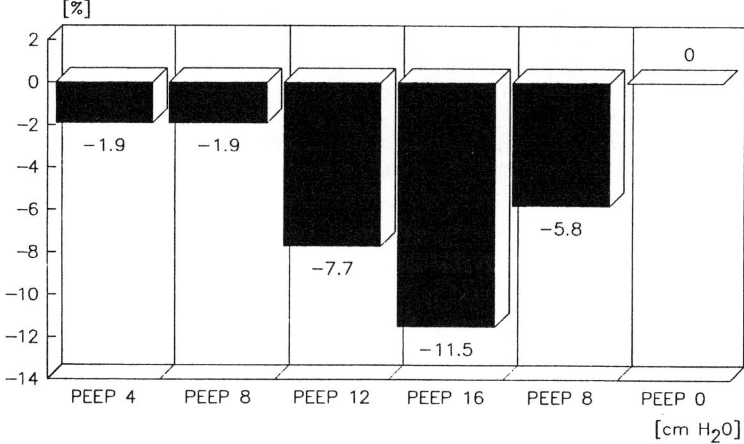

Fig. 3. PEEP-induced changes in CO measured by transesophageal Doppler ultrasound in 16 patients, expressed as percentage decrease from the initial value

References

1. Altman DG, Bland JM (1983) Measurement in medicine: the analysis of measurement comparison studies. Statistician 32:307–317
2. Darsee JR, Walter PF, Nutter DO (1987) Transcutaneous Doppler method of measuring cardiac output – II. Noninvasive measurement by transcutaneous Doppler aortic blood velocity integration and M-mode echocardiography. Am J Cardiol 46:613–18
3. Farthing S, Peronneau P (1979) Flow in the thoracic aorta. Cardiovasc Res 13:607–620
4. Fisher DC, Sahn DJ, Friedman MJ, Larson D, Valdez-Cruz LM, Horovitz S, Goldberg SJ, Allen HD (1983) The effect of variations on pulsed Doppler sampling site on calculation of cardiac output: an experimental study in open-chest dogs. Circulation 67:370–376
5. Foote GA, Schabel SI, Hodges M (1974) Pulmonary complications of the flow-directed balloon-tipped catheter. N Engl J Med 290:927–931
6. Freund PR (1987) Transesophageal Doppler scanning versus thermodilution during general anesthesia. Am J Surg 153:690–694
7. Ganz W, Donoso R, Marcus HS, Forrester JS, Swan HJC (1971) A new technique for measurement of cardiac output by thermodilution. Am J Cardiol 27:392–396
8. Goldberg SJ, Sahn DJ, Allen HD, Valdez-Cruz LM, Hoenecke H, Carnahan Y (1982) Evaluation of pulmonary and systemic blood flow by 2-dimensional Doppler echocardiography using fast fourier transform spectral analysis. Am J Cardiol 50:1394–1400
9. Haude M, Gerber T, Brennecke R, Erbel R, Meyer J (1989) Noninvasive determination of cardiac output by transesophjageal Doppler ultrasound – clinical application and validation. In: Proceedings of the 1988 computers in cardiology conference
10. Haude M, Gerber T, Erbel R, Brennecke R, Meyer J (1988) Bestimmung des Herzzeitvolumens mittels Thermodilution und kontinuierlicher transösophagealer Doppler-Ultraschallmessung – eine Vergleichsuntersuchung bei intubierten Patienten. Biomed Tech 33 (Suppl 2):121–122
11. Huntsman LL, Stewart DK, Barnes SR, Franklin SB, Colocousis JS, Hessel EA (1983) Noninvasive Doppler determination of cardiac output in man: clinical validation. Circulation 67:593–602
12. Merillon JP, Motte G, Fruchaud J, Masquet C, Gourgon R (1978) Evaluation of the elasticity and the characteristic impedance of the ascending aorta in man. Cardiovasc Res 12:401–406

13. Rahimtoola SH, Swan HJC (1965) Calculation of cardiac output from indicator-dilution curves in the presence of mitral regurgitation. Circulation 31:711−718
14. Seyde WC, Stephan H, Rieke H (1987) Noninvasive determination of cardiac output by Doppler ultrasound. Experiences and results by using the ACCUCOM. Anaesthesist 36:504−509
15. Swan HJC, Ganz W, Forrester J, Marcus H, Diamond G, Chonette D (1970) Catheterization of the heart in man with the use of a flow-directed balloon-tipped catheter. N Engl J Med 283:447−451

Monitoring of Cardiac Function During Anesthesia with Two-Dimensional Transesophageal Echocardiography

M. K. CAHALAN

Introduction

Echocardiography is the most widely applicable noninvasive cardiovascular imaging technique in use today. Recent advances in this technique have extended its use into the operating room, making it possible for anesthesiologists and surgeons to acquire monitoring and diagnostic information in the form of remarkably revealing images of cardiovascular anatomy and physiology. Patients and physicians should benefit from these images because they offer more information and less risk than alternative techniques. This chapter will summarize the basic principles, techniques, advantages, and disadvantages of transesophageal echocardiography pertinent for intraoperative use.

Basis Principles and Applications of Echocardiography

Piezoelectric crystals are the transducers and receivers of the sound waves used in echocardiographic studies. These quartz crystals vibrate, when electrically stimulated to produce ultrasound — sound at frequencies above the level detectable by the human ear (> 20000 Hz). Conversely, when struck by ultrasound, the crystals produce an electrical signal. Typically, an echocardiographic study involves intermittent pulses of ultrasound at $2.5-5$ MHz. When ultrasound strikes the interface of tissues of different densities — for example, the pericardium and the heart — a portion of it is reflected. The greater the difference in densities, the greater the portion of ultrasound reflected. For example, air in the left ventricle (LV) reflects a much greater portion of the transmitted ultrasound than blood, and is translated as a brighter signal on the display screen. The longer the sound wave takes to bounce back to the transducer, the greater is its distance from the transducer. This provides information on the location of the tissue. (Sound is assumed to travel at 1540 m/s in all tissues of the body at 37°C.) No ionizing radiation of any type is used in echocardiography, and no adverse effects of ultrasound have been demonstrated in humans.

The first echocardiograms were single-plane views of cardiac structures traced on moving photosensitive paper, and were called motion or M-mode studies. Today, M-mode echocardiograms are still used for viewing rapidly

Transesophageal Echocardiography
Edited by R. Erbel et al.
© Springer-Verlag Berlin Heidelberg 1989

moving structures such as valve leaflets, because M-mode transducers can produce up to 1000 images/s. However, M-mode echocardiograms reveal only a small portion of the heart at one time, making orientation and interpretation of spatial relationships difficult. By using multiple crystals (linear or phase-darray transducers) or rapidly moving a single crystal (mechanical transducer), multiple views can be obtained and collated into a two-dimensional (2-D) image. Although 2-D techniques produce only about 30 images/s, definition in two dimensions provides an enormous advantage in recognizing anatomic and pathologic landmarks. Images are displayed in "real time" on a monitor screen or recorded on video tape for later review. When viewing them, one has the illusion of continuous movement, similar to movies. By altering the position or angle of the ultrasound beam relative to the heart, the operator produces multiple cross-sectional images of the heart which together reveal the external and internal anatomy and function of the heart and great vessels. The relative and absolute size of the chambers and vessels are noted, the extent and pattern of regional and global contraction estimated, and the anatomic or pathologic abnormalities delineated.

Although 2-D echocardiography exquisitely defines anatomic structures, it rarely provides direct imaging of blood flow. Contrast echocardiography and Doppler techniques are needed for this purpose. When 3—5 ml of normal saline is injected into a peripheral or central vein, the microbubbles contained in the saline provide adequate contrast in the right side of the heart for delineation of blood flow. These bubbles collapse in the pulmonary circulation, but even if they cross into the systemic circulation via intracardiac shunts, they are too small and in too low a concentration to harm a patient. Experimental microbubble preparations are now under study which cross the pulmonary circulation and delineate blood flow in the left heart (Keller et al. 1987). These preparations appear safe in animals and have the advantage that they transit the coronary circulation after leaving the left ventricle. Echocardiographic visualization of this contrast in the myocardium should provide at least a qualitative evaluation of myocardial blood flow.

Doppler echocardiography provides an alternative method for imaging blood flow. Quantitative tools have been recently introduced to assess the Doppler shift while simultaneously producing 2-D echocardiograms. The Doppler shift is the apparent shift in frequency of a wave when the source of the wave (in this case, the reflected wave) is moving in relation to a stationary listener or observer. The classic example is the change in pitch of a train whistle as the train approaches and then passes the observer. When the ultrasound beam strikes a moving object, the reflected sound returns to the transducer with a slightly altered frequency. This shift in frequency is proportional to the speed of the object, for instance, a red blood cell. However, a point by point examination of blood cell velocities is very time-consuming, and does not reveal the instantaneous distribution of flow velocities throughout the cross-sectional image. For these reasons, color-coded Doppler flow imaging was developed. This new technology, usually referred to as "color Doppler," simultaneously presents real-time images of intracardiac blood flow and structure in two dimensions: continuous color maps of flow superimposed on monochromatic cross-sectional echocardiograms (Omoto 1984). Color Doppler greatly increases the speed and ease of evaluation of valvular function and intracardiac shunts. Thus, it is a technology ideally suited for operating room applications. Unfortunately, color Doppler provides only qualitative estimates of blood flow velocities and with current technology cannot provide meaningful data on coronary blood flow.

However, 2-D echocardiography provides other important information on the presence and extent of ischemic heart disease. Since Tennant and Wiggers first described the association of segmental wall motion abnormalities (SWMA) and ischemia, others have proven that ischemic segments of human and animal heart do not exhibit normal inward wall motion or thickening during systole. Although focal myocarditis and certain rare infiltrative disorders and tumors of the myocardium may also produce SWMAs, they are much less common causes than ischemic heart disease. The presence of an akinetic (noncontracting) or dyskinetic (paradoxically moving) segment of the LV may indicate an old infarction. However, the development of a new SWMA during examination, e.g., during a stress test, is likely to be caused by myocardial ischemia. Nearly all patients having transmural infarctions will have SWMAs. The extent of the abnormalities detected by echocardiography correlates with overall ventricular function and patient prognoses, but usually results in overestimates of the extent of infarction.

Precordial 2-D echocardiography provides reliable estimates of ventricular filling and ejection, wall thickness, and mass. Such quantitative data can be used to calculate end-diastolic volume, ejection fraction, systolic wall stress, and correlates of contractility, such as velocity of circumferential fiber shortening. Echocardiography is thus the premier clinical tool for assessment of ventricular function. However, no echocardiographic parameter is an ideal measure of ventricular function, because all available measures are critically dependent on cardiac loading conditions, valvular function, and, often, heart rate. Newer indices of ventricular function are emerging which appear to be independent of loading conditions, but these require volume and intraventricular pressure determinations, such as end-systolic pressure-volume indices.

Transesophageal Echocardiography

With the introduction in West-Germany of a phased-array transducer which could be positioned in the esophagus, intraoperative 2-D echocardiography became a practical diagnostic tool for anesthesiologists (Schlüter et al. 1982). At the Medical Center of the University of California, San Francisco, we use a commercially available 5.0-MHz transducer system (Hewlett-Packard, Andover, MA) consisting of 64 piezoelectric elements mounted on the tip of a gastroscope. The transducer is 42 mm long, 13 mm wide, and 11 mm thick. With appropriate phasing of the elements by an ultrasonograph, a 90° sector for real-time imaging is obtained.

Once the transducer is inserted through the mouth and advanced approximately 35−40 cm, all four cardiac chambers can be viewed. The juxtaposition of the left ventricular outflow track, aortic valve, and mitral valve also can be observed. Advancing the transducer another 2−5 cm (and angling it forward) allows cross-sectional images of the left ventricle, including a short-axis view at the level of the papillary muscles. If the heart is not enlarged, a cross-sectional view of both ventricles can frequently be obtained. In studies of more than 1500 patients, we have obtained high resolution echocardiograms 97% of our patients. Three suspected complications have been noted. In one patient the entire esophageal stethoscope was buried in the esophagus and not removed until the third postoperative day. In a second patient, upper gastrointestinal bleeding (about one liter) was noted after coronary artery surgery. This bleeding ended spontaneously and its exact site was not determined. In the third patient, a splenic injury was noted during abdominal aortic aneurysmectomy. It was not thought to be due to surgical retraction. An incidental splenectomy was performed because heparinization was planned. In all three cases, insertion and manipulation of the echocardiographic probe were accomplished without difficulty.

As a precaution, we do not perform transesophageal echocardiographic monitoring in patients with a history of swallowing complaints or esophageal disease. One published report describes two patients who suffered temporary unilateral vocal cord paralysis after transesophageal echocardiographic monitoring during "sitting" craniotomies (Cucchiara et al. 1984). Both these patients were positioned with nearly full neck flexion. The authors of this report believe (personal communication), that the recurrent laryngeal nerve was injured when the larynx, endotracheal tube, and shaft of the gastroscope were compressed between the chin and vertebral column. These authors now use a smaller gastroscope and have reported no further complications. The controls of the smaller gastroscope allow positioning of the transducer along only one axis, which is adequate for intraatrial air monitoring but occasionally inadequate for left ventricular monitoring.

In our experience, inserting and positioning the ultrasound transducer usually requires less than 60 s. We monitor the short-axis view of the left ventricle at the level of the papillary muscles and have done so for up to 12 h. In approximately 8%−10% of patients, this view cannot be obtained because of horizontal displacement of the heart by the contents of the abdomen. Other views, such as a four-chamber view, must then be monitored, but changes in left ventricular filling and segmental contraction are not as easily assessed. Quantitative estimates of left ventriular filling and ejection that are consistent to within 10% can be produced by the same observer, and estimates consistent to within 15% can be produced by different observers, using a computer-assisted video review system.

These measurements are valid estimates of left ventricular filling and ejection, but the analysis necessary is too time-consuming to be of practical value in the operating room. In contrast, we use qualitative estimates of left ventricular filling and ejection in real time to guide our administration of fluids and inotropes. Marked changes in filling and ejection can occur before, simultaneously with, or in the absence of changes in blood pressure or filling pressures. A video processing computer (Cine View, Freeland Medical, Indianapolis, IN, or Frame Grabber, Microsonics, Purchase, NY) converts the echocardiographic images from one cardiac cycle into a digital code and then plays the images over and over again in a loop for comparison with other loops captured at other times during surgery. This juxtapositioning of images greatly facilitates the evaluation of changes in left ventricular filling and ejection.

Similarly, SWMAs can be detected by the anesthesiologist and are a reliable sign of intraoperative myocardial ischemia. We observed 50 patients at high risk for intraoperative myocardial ischemia while undergoing coronary artery or major vascular surgery (Smith et al. 1985). At predetermined intervals, we recorded echocardiograms and multilead ECGs, both of which were evaluated by "blind" observers. All patients had postoperative ECGs and cardiac isoenzyme studies. Intraoperatively, six patients had ST-segment changes characteristic of myocardial ischemia, while 24 had new SWMAs. No patient experienced and ST-segment change before or in the absence of a corresponding wall motion abnormality. In three of the six patients who experienced ST-segment change, echocardiographic changes occurred minutes before the ECG change. Three of the 50 patients suffered intraoperative myocardial infarctions, and all three had a SWMA develop and persist in the corresponding area of the myocardium. Only one of these patients had intraoperative ST-segment changes characteristic of ischemia. However, detection of SWMAs may be influenced by artifacts. For example, median sternotomy and pericardiotomy alter the translational and rotational motion of the heart within the chest, and thereby induce artifactual changes in ventricular septal endocardial motion. Consequently, a valid system for assessing SWMAs during cardiac surgery must compensate for this translational and rotational movement, and then evaluate both endocardial motion and segmental thickening. Unfortunately, no currently available automated wall motion analysis system adequately manages these problems for transesophageal cross-sectional images.

Transesophageal echocardiography can also detect the small quantities of intravascular air which may enter the circulation. Moreover, 2-D transesophageal echocardiography provides a nearly ideal examination of the intraatrial septum, and, during contrast studies, can reliably diagnose atrial septal defects. Thus, 2-D transesophageal echocardiography is the first intraoperative monitor that can identify patients at risk of experiencing paradoxical emboli. Cucchiara et al. (1984) monitored 12 patients during suboccipital craniotomy in a sitting position using 2-D transesophageal echocardiography and precordial nonimaging Doppler. All eight cases of Doppler-detected air were visualized by the transesophageal echocardiograms. In two of the cases, air was noted first on the echocardiogram. In two more cases, a questionable Doppler change was noted, and the presence of air was verified by the echocardiogram. For one severe episode of embolization, air could be seen crossing from the right to left atrium and passing to the left ventricle and aorta. The precordial Doppler monitor did not detect this event, because it does not image the heart and thus, cannot localize an air embolism within the atria. A recent study in animals confirms that transesophageal echocardiography is more sensitive for detection of venous air embolism than monitoring the precordial Doppler, pulmonary artery pressure, end tidal carbon dioxide concentration, or arterial oxygen tension (Glenski et al. 1986).

Intraoperative transesophageal echocardiography functions primarily as a monitoring tool for the anesthesiologist, but primarily as a diagnostic tool for surgeons and cardiologists. Together with color Doppler, it is an ideal technique for evaluation of mitral and aortic diseases because of the proximity of the transesophageal transducer to the left atrium, mitral valve, aortic valve, and aorta. For instance, Kyo et al. (1987) report its value for immediate evaulation of mitral and tricuspid valvuloplasty, prosthetic valve function, closure of intracardiac shunts, and the adequacy of pericardectomy for relief of constrictive pericarditis. In our experience color Doppler evidence indicative of persistent mitral regurgitation after valvuloplasty has prompted our surgeons to reinstitute the cardiopulmonary bypass and replace the mitral valve. Our belief is that in so doing we have avoided the necessity of reoperation in the early postoperative period. However, not all repairs or diagnostic problems can be evaluated by transesophageal echocardiography. For instance, no commercially available transesophageal probe is small enough for use in infants, and none yet adequately images the coronary arteries. For these applications, epicardial echocardiography should be considered.

Conclusion

Clearly, intraoperative echocardiography can provide information vital for patient care. Unlike traditional monitors, transesophageal echocardiography reveals direct information on cardiac filling and ejection. Such information may result in earlier and more reliable detection of hypovolemia, air embolism, myocardial ischemia, and left ventricular failure. In addition, color Doppler, a recent advance in the electronic processing of the echocardiograms, vividly displays real-time maps of intracardiac blood flow velocities, quickly revealing valvular dysfunction or intracardiac shunts. Although current transesophageal probes are too large for use in infants and small children, epicardial probes can be used during congenital heart surgery to reveal diagnostic information which may improve the surgical plan and prevent the need for reoperation. Thus, intraoperative echocardiography represents a significant advance for surgical patients with heart disease. Because of its safety, speed, and diagnostic accuracy, intraoperative echocardiography should play an increasingly important role in cardiovascular anesthesia and surgery.

References

Cucchiara RF, Nugent M, Seward JB, Messick JM (1984) Air embolism in upright neurosurgical patients: detection and localization by two-dimensional transesophageal echocardiography. Anesthesiology 60:353–355

Glenski JA, Cucchiara RF, Michenfelder JD (1986) Transesophageal echocardiography and transcutaneous O_2 und CO_2 monitoring for detection of venous air embolism. Anesthesiology 64:541–545

Hiratzka LF, McPherson DD, Lamberth WC Jr, Brandt B III, Armstrong ML, Schroder E, Hunt M, Kieso R, Megan MD, Tompkins PK (1986) Intraoperative evaluation of coronary artery bypass graft anastomoses with high-frequency epicardial echocardiography: experimental validation and initial patient studies. Circulation 73:1199–1205

Keller MW, Feinstein SB, Watson DD (1987) Successful left ventricular opacification following peripheral venous injection of sonicated contrast agent: an experimental evaluation. Am Heart J 114:570–575

Kyo S, Takamoto S, Matsumura M, Asano H, Yokote Y, Motoyama T, Omoto R (1987) Immediate and early postoperative evaluation of results of cardiac surgery by transesophageal two-dimensional Doppler echocardiography. Circulation 76:113–121

Omoto R (1984) Color atlas of real-time two-dimensional Doppler echocardiography. Shindan-To-Chiryo, Tokyo

Schlüter M, Langenstein BA, Polster J, Kremer P, Souquet J, Engel S, Hanrath P (1982) Transesophageal cross-sectional echocardiography with a phased array transducer system. Technique and initial clinical results. Br Heart J 48:67–72

Smith JS, Cahalan MK, Benefiel DJ, Byrd B, Lurz FW, Shapiro W, Roizen MF, Bouchard A, Schiller NB (1985) Intraoperative detection of myocardial ischemia in high risk patients: electrocardiography versus two-dimensional transesophageal echocardiography. Circulation 72:1015–1021

Other Suggested Reading

Cahalan MK, Litt L, Botvinick EH, Schiller NB (1987) Advances in noninvasive cardiovascular imaging: implications for the anesthesiologist. Anesthesiology 66:356–372

Clements FM, deBruijn NP (1987) Perioperative evaluation of regional wall motion by transesophageal two-dimensional echocardiography. Anesth Analg 66:249–261

DeBruijn NP, Clements FM (1987) Transesophageal Echocardiography. Boston, Martinus Nijhoff

Systolic Pressure-Dimension Relationships and Diastolic Dimensions for Monitoring of Left Ventricular Function

H. Heinrich

Introduction

Left ventricular function is determined by preload, afterload, contractility, and heart rate. The best description of the interactions of these main determinants on left ventricular function is the pressure-volume diagram. However, in clinical practice, use of the pressure-volume diagram was, and still is, restricted to the catheter laboratory and to experimental conditions, the main problem for clinical use being the difficulty involved in determining the left ventricular volume.

The purpose of our studies was to use transesophageal echocardiography as a tool for the measurements of left ventricular dimensions, which are used instead of ventricular volumes, in order to realize essential parts of the pressure-volume diagram for monitoring left ventricular function. Instead of left ventricular pressures, we measured the radial artery pressure.

The End-Systolic Pressure-Volume Relationship

The measure of contractility on the pressure-volume diagram is the steepness of the maxima curves. The original pressure-volume diagram of Otto Frank shows different curves for isometric, isotonic, and auxotonic contractions (Frank 1897). An increase in contractility increases the steepnesses of the maxima curves, and negative inotropic interventions decrease the slopes of the curves. In contrast to Frank, the Japanese Suga pointed out that the maxima curves can be approximated to a single straight line, the slope of which responds to inotropic changes, as do the maxima curves (Suga et al. 1973).

This simplified maxima curve is called the end-systolic pressure-volume curve (Fig. 1). This relationship was, and still is, the subject of extensive studies. Suga and others showed that at a constant contractility the end-systolic pressure-volume points were always on the the same line, regardless of differences in end-diastolic volumes between different heart beats (Suga et al. 1973). This is not, however, perfectly true (Jacob and Weigand 1966; Kissling et al. 1985), the end-systolic pressure-volume relationship being merely less sensitive to preload changes.

Afterload, which is determined by the left ventricular pressure, is incorporated into the endsystolic pressure-volume relationship and does not change the slope. Furthermore, transient changes of left ventricular pressures and

Transesophageal Echocardiography
Edited by R. Erbel et al.
© Springer-Verlag Berlin Heidelberg 1989

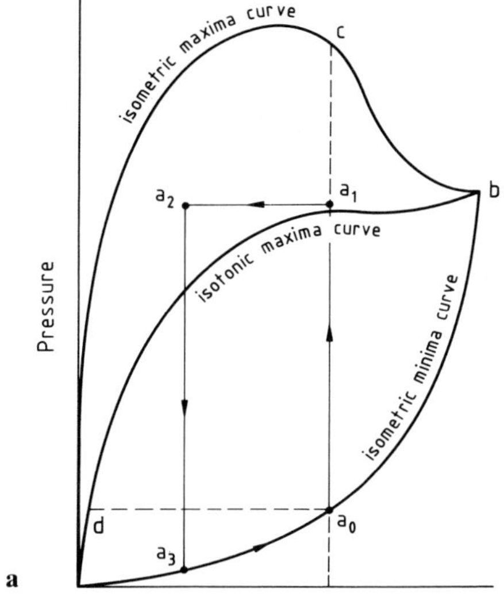

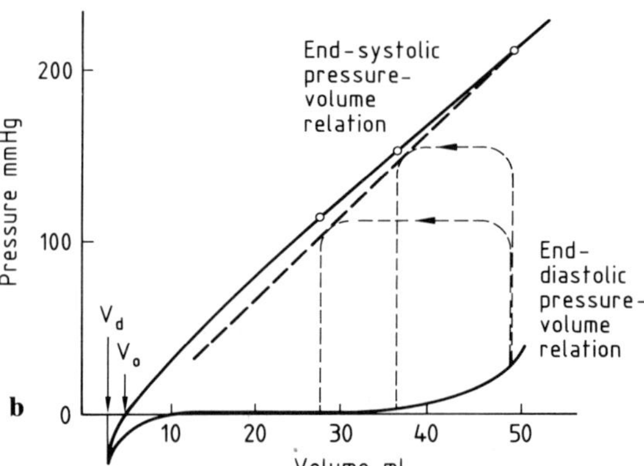

Fig. 1a, b. The pressure-volume diagram and end-systolic pressure-volume relationship. The original pressure-volume diagram of Otto Frank (1897). Note the different curves for isometric and isotonic maxima. The auxotonic maxima curve is not depicted. The end-systolic pressure-volume relationship (Suga et al. 1973). The different maxima curves are *approximated* to a single straight line. (From Sagawa 1984)

volumes are needed to get at least two different pressure-volume points, these being necessary for the determination of the slope because the pressure-volume line does not pass through the origin of the pressure-volume diagram.

Determination of the Peak Systolic Pressure-Diameter Relationship

Method. We measured left ventricular diameters by transesophageal two-dimensional (2-D) and M-mode echocardiography. A cross section of the left ventricle at the midpapillary muscle level was visualized. The maximum anterior-posterior diameter was continuously displayed on a second screen. In order to avoid respiratory artifacts, the capnogram was recorded as a guide and measurements were taken only in end expiration. For later off-line evaluation, all recordings were stored on video tape and evaluated by a computer assisted device (Fig. 2).

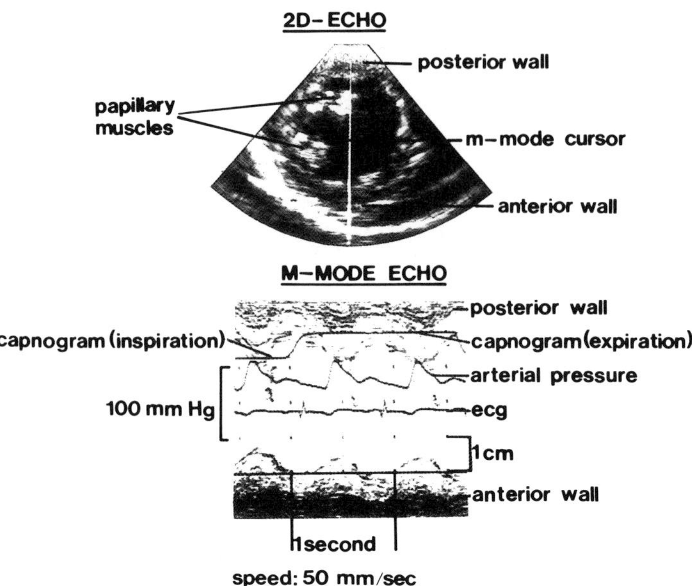

Fig. 2. Method for determination of the systolic pressure-diameter relationship

Protocol. The patients investigated were 10 healthy individuals undergoing minor surgical procedures. After induction of anesthesia (midazolam 0.1 mg/ kg; fentanyl 0.005 mg/kg; vecuronium 0.1 mg/kg; normoventilation N_2O/O_2, FIO_2 0.3) and endotracheal intubation, the gastroscope was introduced (echoscope 3.5 MHz, Diasonics). Following a resting period of 10 min to let the hemodynamic effects of endotracheal intubation subside, 0.2 mg nitroglycerin was injected intravenously for transient load manipulation. This part of the study was named control 1. After restabilization of arterial pressure and heart rate and a resting period of 5 min, nitroglycerin was again injected. This was named control 2. After restabilization of arterial pressure, an infusion of dobutamine at a rate of 5 µg/kg · min was started. After an infusion period of 5 min, nitroglycerin was again injected.

Data Evaluation. For determination of the peak systolic pressure-end-systolic diameter relationship, the relationship between pressures and diameters during the decrease of arterial pressure was determined by the least squares method. End-systolic diameters were measured as the smallest diameters in systole by the trailing edge-leading edge method. Peak systolic pressures and end-systolic diameters during the period of restabilization of arterial pressure were not used.

Results

We found a close linear relationship during the pressure decrease after nitroglycerin administration. Values taken during restabilization of arterial pressure were shifted to the left of the regression line, thus reflecting the increase in contractility by homeometric autoregulation (Fig. 3).

The slopes of this relationship were equal at control 1 and control 2. With dobutamine, the slopes increased in all patients (Fig. 4). The calculated diameter at the theorethical Zero pressure remained constant (Fig. 5).

Discussion

Our results can be summarized as follows: The end-systolic pressure-volume relationship can be approximated by the peak systolic pressure-end-systolic diameter relationship. This relationship is reproducible and the slope responds as the original relationship does. The precondition for measurement without autonomic blockade is to measure only during a transient pressure decrease after the injection of nitroglycerin. The mode of altering load is a combination of reduced preload and afterload (Heinrich et al. 1987a).

Our principle of measuring during the early period of hemodynamic changes after load manipulation was confirmed by Kass in experiments on dogs (Kass et al. 1986). These authors changed load by transient occlusion of

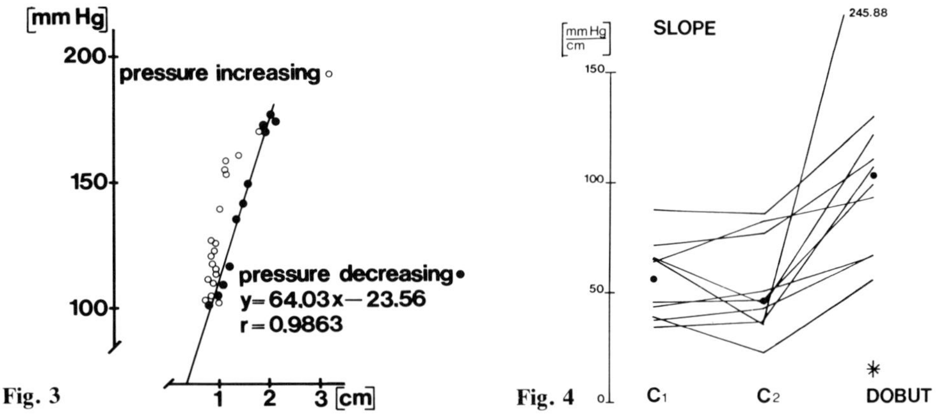

Fig. 3. Systolic pressure-diameter relationship. A linear relationship between peak systolic pressures and end-systolic diameters was found during the pressure decrease after the intravenous injection of nitroglycerin. Values taken later on, during normalization of arterial pressure, were shifted to the left, indicating the enhanced contractile state with sympathetic activation

Fig. 4. Slopes of the systolic pressure-diameter relationship. No differences between control 1 (C_1) and control 2 (C_2), but increase of the slope with dobutamine 5 µg/kg min in all patients (paired Wilcoxon test, $p < 0.05$)

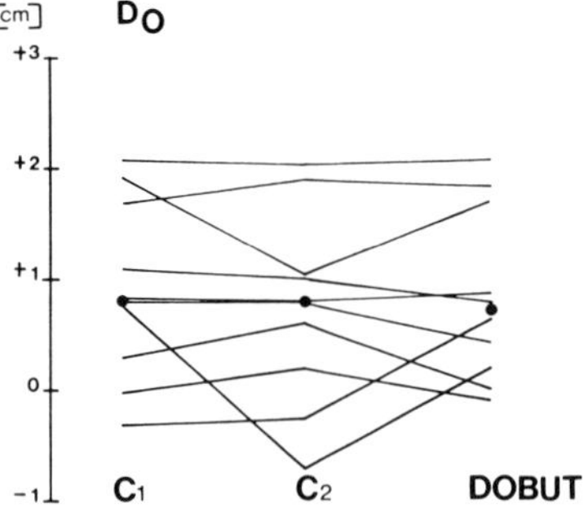

Fig. 5. Theoretical diameter at zero systolic pressure (D_0). No differences between the controls and dobutamine, i.e., the position of the regression line remains stable

the vena cava. They found a linear relationship during the decrease of left ventricular pressure. Values obtained later on, during the release of caval occlusion, were shifted to the left, indicating an enhanced myocardial contractile state. Measurements taken during the first few seconds of a decrease in arterial pressure avoid being affected by contractility changes through homeometric autoregulation, because the reaction time of the sympathetic nerves (which alone are activated: Glick and Braunwald 1965) is relatively slow (Warner and Cox 1962), and the Bowditch treppe caused by the subsequent tachycardia develops only gradually (Koch-Weser and Blinks 1963). The other direction for a transient change in arterial pressure − an increase in arterial pressure − does not work without autonomic blockade because an increase in arterial pressure activates the very fast vagus nerve (Warner and Cox 1962). The resulting bradycardia immediately increases contractility (post-tachycardia potentiation) and thus falsifies the contractility measurements (Heinrich et al. 1988).

However, because changing the arterial pressure can be hazardous for many patients, it would be desirable to estimate the slope of the peak systolic pressure-diameter relationship from a single pressure/diameter point, the so-called end-systolic quotient.

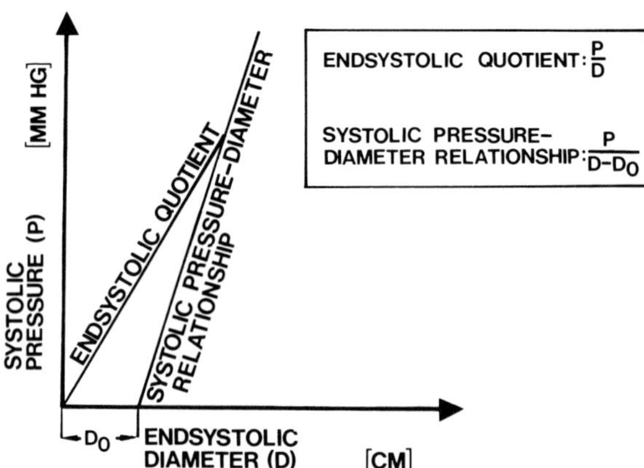

Fig. 6. Systolic pressure-diameter relationship and end-systolic quotient. Whereas the slope of the systolic pressure-diameter relationship does not change with the systolic pressure, the end-systolic quotient is expected to change with the peak systolic pressure (decrease with decreasing pressure, increase with an increase in systolic pressure)

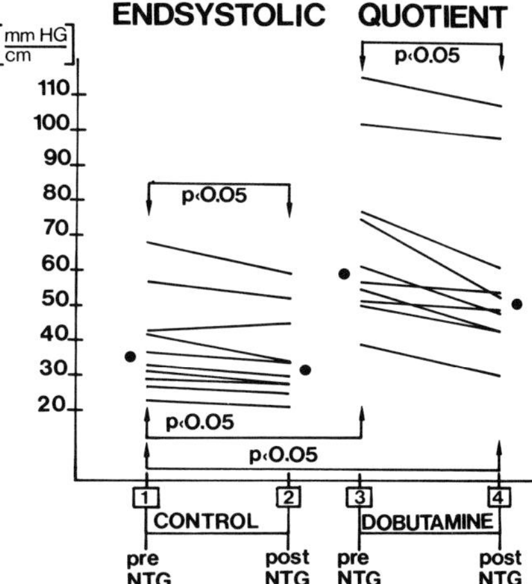

Fig. 7. End-systolic quotient in different inotropic states and under different loading conditions. The quotient is less sensitive to changes in afterload than to changes in the contractile state

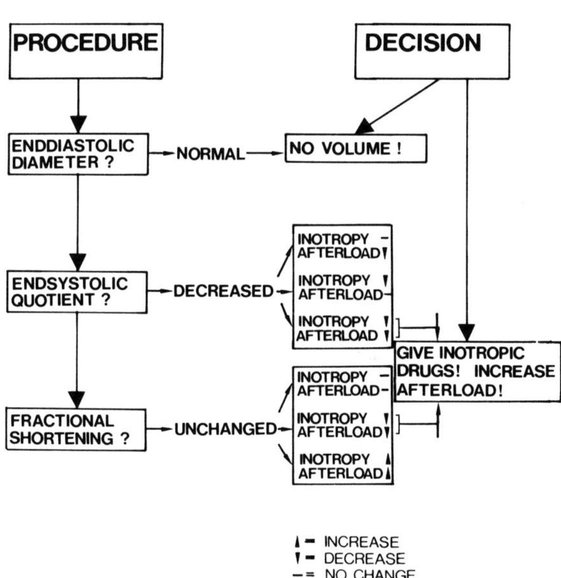

Fig. 8. Example of an algorithm for evaluating the cause of a case of acute hypotension. As a first step, the preload (end-diastolic diameter) is checked. Because the end-diastolic diameter is normal, the first decision is: "hypotension is not caused by low intravascular volume, no volume is necessary!" The second step is to measure the end-systolic quotient, which is found to be decreased. Because of the afterload sensitivity of the quotient, a decrease means either "unchanged inotropy and low afterload," "low inotropy and unchanged afterload," or "low inotropy and low afterload." Then, fractional shortening is measured, which changes in the same direction as the end systolic quotient with inotropic changes, but in the opposite direction with changes in afterload. Fractional shortening is found to be "unchanged." Comparison of the three possibilities for "unchanged fractional shortening" with the possible causes of a "decreased end-systolic quotient" reveals the combination of "low inotropy and low afterload" as the only possible solution. Consequently, the therapeutic decision is to give a positive inotropic drug and increase afterload

The End-Systolic Quotient

The relationship between the true linear correlation and the so-called end-systolic quotient is depicted in Fig. 6. Obviously, the quotient is afterload dependent, since it must change if afterload changes. The question is, how clinically relevant is this afterload dependence. We calculated the end-systolic quotient in the patients mentioned above before and at the lowest peak systolic pressure after nitroglycerin administration with and without dobutamine. We found the expected afterload dependence of the quotient. The quotient decreased after nitroglycerin administration. However, the decrease in the quotient with nitroglycerin was much lower than the increase of the ratio after dobutamine (Fig. 7). Thus, it can be stated that moderate changes in the myocardial contractile state have much more influence on the quotient than marked changes in the loading conditions (Heinrich et al. 1987 b).

Returning to the pressure-volume diagram, the systolic pressure-diameter relationship (contractility) in combination with the end-diastolic diameter (preload) and peak systolic pressure (afterload) realizes essential parts of the diagram in a clinically practical way. During intraoperative monitoring, these measures of preload, afterload, and contractility may help anesthesiologist to make therapeutic decisions.

Particularly, the combined use of these easy-to-obtain parameters (left ventricular dimensions by echocardiography and peripherally measured peak systolic pressure) enables immediate diagnosis and quick reaction to hemodynamic instability.

An example algorithm in a case of acute hypotension is shown in Fig. 8.

Limitations

The systolic pressure-diameter diagram, of course, has specific limitations. The peak systolic pressure does not reflect left ventricular pressures if a stenosis of the conducting system is present, such as in aortic stenosis. End-systolic and end-diastolic diameters are not a substitute for left ventricular volumes of severe wall motion abnormalities occur. In these cases, cross-sectional areas would probably better reflect volume. In addition, normalization for interindividual comparison of the slope has not yet been established.

References

Frank O (1897) Die Wirkung von Digitalis (Helleborein) auf das Herz. Sitzungsberichte der Gesellschaft für Morphologie und Physiologie zu München H2: 14−43

Glick G, Braunwald E (1965) Relative role of the sympathetic and parasympathetic nervous system in the reflex control of heart rate. Circ Res 16:363−375

Heinrich H, Fösel TH, Fontaine L, Spilker D, Winter H, Ahnefeld FW (1987 a) Assessement of contractility changes in humans by transesophageal echocardiography − the peak-systolic pressure end-systolic diameter relationship (PSPESDRS). Int J Clin Monit Comput 4:243−248

Heinrich H, Fontaine L, Wilder-Smith O, Winter H, Ahnefeld FW (1987b) Usefulnes of the endsystolic quotient and of fractional shortening for assessment of contractility changes under different loading conditions. Anesthesiology 67 [Suppl:]A209

Heinrich H, Fontaine L, Winter H (1988) Ist die Bestimmung der systolischen Druck-Durchmesserbeziehung durch passagere Druckanhebung mit Methoxamin ohne autonome Blockade möglich? Anaesthesist 37 (Suppl):109

Jacob R, Weigand KH (1966) Die endsystolischen Druck-Volumenbeziehungen als Grundlage einer Beurteilung der Kontraktilität des linken Ventrikels in situ. Pflügers Arch 289:37−49

Kass DA, Yamazaki T, Burkhoff D, Maughan WL, Sagawa K (1986) Determination of left ventricular end-systolic pressure-volume relationships by the conductance (volume) catheter technique. Circulation 73:586−595

Kissling G, Takeda N, Vogt M (1985) Left ventricular end-systolic pressure-volume relationships as a measure of ventricular performance. Basic Res Cardiol 80:594−607

Koch-Weser J, Blinks JR (1963) The influence of the interval between beats on myocardial contractility. Pharmacol Rev 15:601−652

Sagawa K (1984) End-systolic pressure-volume relationship in retrospect and prospect. Fed Proc 43(9):2399−2401

Suga H, Sagawa K, Shoukas AA (1973) Load independence of the instantaneous pressure-volume ratio of the canine left ventricle and effects of epinephrine and heart rate on the ratio. Circ Res 32:314−322

Warner HR, Cox A (1962) A mathematical model of heart rate control by sympathetic and vagus efferent information. J Appl Physiol 17:349−355

Assessment of Diastolic Function by Transesophageal Pulsed Doppler Echocardiography: Effect of Different Loading Conditions on Mitral Inflow Velocities During Coronary Bypass Surgery

M. D. ABEL and R. A. NISHIMURA

Introduction

The clinical manifestations of congestive heart failure can be related to a low cardiac output and elevated ventricular filling pressures. In the past, the pathogenesis of heart failure has been attributed to abnormalities of systolic function. More recently, however, it has been demonstrated that abnormalities of diastolic function may play an important role in the production of these signs and symptoms (Dodek et al. 1972; Dougherty et al. 1984). Diastolic filling of the heart has been relatively difficult to study because of its inherent complexity, in part related to the multiplicity of interrelated factors that contribute to this aspect of cardiac function (Mirsky 1984).

The advent of Doppler echocardiography has provided a means by which intracardiac blood velocity can be assessed noninvasively (Nishimura et al. 1985). It has been proposed that by examining the velocity of blood flow through the mitral valve during diastole, abnormalities of diastolic function can be detected (Rokey et al. 1985; DeMaria and Wisenbaugh 1987). Many of the studies examining transmitral flow have suggested that characteristic flow patterns exist in various pathologic states (DeMaria and Wisenbaugh 1987). These abnormalities include a lowering of the initial blood velocity across the mitral valve (E) and a decrease in the ratio of E to A (the velocity at atrial contraction) in disease entities such as coronary artery disease, hypertrophic cardiomyopathy, aortic stenosis and long-standing hypertension (DeMaria and Wisenbaugh 1987; Labovitz and Pearson 1987). However, even though different mitral velocities are found in these disease entities, their presence is by no means universal in a given condition and the interpretation of the various velocity patterns remains to be elucidated. Part of the explanation for the great variability in transmitral velocity patterns amongst patients with a given disease process may be the diverse loading conditions imposed upon the heart. It is hypothesized that changes in preload and afterload might alter mitral inflow velocity in the absence of changes in the intrinsic myocardial properties.

The following discussion is based upon results of a recent study in which the mitral flow velocity curves were obtained under differing loading conditions (Nishimura et al. 1989 b)

Transesophageal Echocardiography
Edited by R. Erbel et al.
© Springer-Verlag Berlin Heidelberg 1989

Loading Studies

The purpose of this study was to examine the changes in the mitral inflow velocity curves by varying the loading conditions of the left ventricle. Ten patients undergoing myocardial revascularization with left ventricular ejection fractions greater than 40% were selected. Patients with left main coronary artery stenosis were excluded. All patients were monitored with an arterial line and pulmonary artery catheter. The mitral inflow velocity was obtained with a transesophageal pulsed Doppler echocardiogram with the sample volume positioned at the tips of the mitral leaflets (Appleton et al. 1988). Transesophageal echocardiography affords an excellent view of the mitral valve inflow region as well as providing a stable image over extended periods of time. Hemodynamic and Doppler mitral inflow data were recorded during maneuvers designed to alter left ventricular loading conditions as follows.

Intravenous nitroglycerin was utilized to provide a reduction in preload of the left ventricle. Nitroglycerin was given to decrease the systolic blood pressure and pulmonary capillary wedge pressure by at least 20% compared with their respective control values. As compared to the control state, there was a significant decrease in the E velocity and prolongation of the deceleration time. In addition, the A velocity also decreased, so that the E : A ratio was unaffected.

An intravenous infusion of phenylephrine was given to produce an increase in afterload by raising the systolic blood pressure 20% above its control value. There was a variable effect on the pulmonary artery capillary wedge pressure. Infusion of the vasopressor resulted in a decrease in the E velocity compared to the control situation. In addition, there was a prolongation of the deceleration time as well as an increase in the A velocity. This resulted in a decrease in E : A ratio.

After allowing the various hemodynamic indices to return to baseline, 0.5−1.0 L 0.9% saline was rapidly infused to produce an increase in preload, defined by a 20% increase in the pulmonary artery capillary wedge pressure. This increase in preload resulted in an increase in the E velocity and a decrease in the deceleration time. The effect on the A velocity was more variable but generally this too was increased. The E : A ratio showed no singificant trend.

Discussion

These findings provide a conceptual framework for interpretation of the various mitral inflow velocity profiles. The transmitral velocity should be looked upon as representing the relative changes in the left atrial to left ventricular pressure gradient during ventricular filling (Nishimura et al. 1989a). The transmitral velocity curves begin when the left ventricular pressure drops below the left atrial pressure at mitral valve opening. This is due to continued relaxation of the myocardium, as well as to the diastolic suction effect of the left ventricle, resulting in forward blood velocity across the mitral valve (E velocity). The left ventricular pressure will then begin to increase due to the viscoelastic forces of the myocardium, concomitant with a fall in the left atrial pressure. As the left ventricular pressure increases and the left atrial pressure decreases, there will be a fall in the mitral velocity. This decrease in velocity if measured by the deceleration time. At atrial contraction, there is again a rise in left atrial pressure above the left ventricular pressure, which causes an increase in velocity across the mitral valve (A velocity).

In the presence of a decreased preload, ther will be a lower left atrial pressure relative to the left ventricular pressure at mitral valve opening. This will result in a decreased "driving pressure" across the mitral valve and thus the E velocity will be decreased. Since the lower filling pressure will result in a decrease in the height of the rapid filling wave, there will be a prolonged positive gradient between the left atrium and left ventricle and so the deceleration time will be increased. The height of the atrial velocity will decrease due to the fact that there is a lower left atrial volume at atrial contraction.

In the presence of an increase in afterload, there will be a prolongation of myocardial relaxation. This results in a decrease in the rate of fall of the left ventricular pressure. This will result in a decreased "driving pressure" across the mitral valve and a reduced E velocity. Myocardial relaxation continues further into the diastolic filling period, prolonging the deceleration time. There will be less ventricular filling in early diastole, and thus there will be a greater contribution from atrial contraction and hence the A velocity will be increased.

In the presence of an increase in preload, there is a higher left atrial pressure at mitral valve opening. This results in an increase in "driving pressure" across the mitral valve, producing an increase in the E velocity. The increase in preload causes a right shift along the diastolic pressure-volume relationship of the ventricle, resulting in a rapid deceleration of the initial E velocity and a reduction in the deceleration time.

Conclusions

Diastolic left ventricular function, as assessed by the transmitral velocity profile, must take into account the influence of loading conditions. In a patient with low E and A velocities and a prolonged deceleration time, a low filling pressure (preload) might be the explanation. If there is a low E velocity and prolonged deceleration time with a large A velocity, then this most likely represents an "abnormality of relaxation." This is the type of mitral velocity curve that is seen in patients with hypertrophic cardiomyopathy, hypertension, and aortic stenosis, as well as various coronary ischemic syndromes and can be emulated by increasing afterload in "normal" patients. When there is a high E velocity and a rapid deceleration time, this represents "restriction to filling." This is seen in any type of abnormality that produces a large rapid filling wave such as dilated cardiomyopathy, restrictive cardiomyopathy, and ischemic cardiomyopathy with high filling pressures and can be mimicked by increasing preload in "normal" patients. An understanding of the physiologic principles governing various velocity curves allows a clearer interpretation of these curves in various disease entities. Caution needs to be exercised, however, in reaching a definitive conclusion about diastolic function without some attempt to vary loading conditions of the left ventricle.

References

Appleton CP, Hatle LK, Popp RL (1988) Relation of transmitral flow velocity patterns to left ventricular diastolic function: new insights from a combined hemodynamic and Doppler echocardiographic study. J Am Coll Cardiol 12:426−440

DeMaria AN, Wisenbaugh T (1987) Identification and treatment of diastolic dysfunction: role of transmitral Doppler recordings (editorial). J Am Coll Cardiol 9:1106−1107

Dodek A, Kassebaum DG, Bristow JD (1972) Pulmonary edema in coronaryartery disease without cardiomegaly. Paradox of the stiff heart. N Engl J Med 286:1347−1350

Dougherty AH, Naccarelli GV, Gray EL, Hicks CH (1984) Congestive heart failure with normal systolic function. Am J Cardiol 54:778−782

Labovitz AJ, Pearson AC (1987) Evaluation of left ventricular diastolic function: clinical relevance and recent Doppler echocardiographic insights. Am Heart J 114:836−851

Mirsky I (1984) Assessment of diastolic function: suggested methods and future considerations. Circulation 69:836−841

Nishimura RA, Miller FA Jr, Callahan MJ, Benassi RC, Seward JB, Tajik AJ (1985) Doppler echocardiography: theory, instrumentation, technique, and application. Mayo Clin Proc 60:321−343

Nishimura RA, Abel MD, Hatle LK, Tajik AJ (1989a) Assessment of diastolic function of the heart: background and current applications of Doppler echocardiography. Part II: clinical studies. Mayo Clin Proc 64:181−204

Nishimura RA, Abel MD, Hausmanns PR, Warnes CA, Tajik AJ (1989b) Mitral flow velocity curves as a function of differing loading conditions: evaluation by intraoperative transesophageal Doppler echocardiography. J Am Soc Echocardiography 2:79−87

Rokey R, Kuo LC, Zoghbi WA, Limacher MC, Quinones MA (1985) Determination of parameters of left ventricular diastolic filling with pulsed Doppler echocardiography: comparison with cineangiography. Circulation 71:543−550

Are Changes in Pulmonary Capillary Wedge Pressure an Indicator for Myocardial Ischemia? Wedge Pressure Related to Electrocardiogram and Transesophageal Echocardiographic Wall Motion Analysis

M. E. R. M. van Daele

The pulmonary capillary wedge pressure (PCWP) is often monitored during both cardiac and general surgery in patients who are considered to be at significant risk for perioperative cardiac complications. The precise meaning of a change in the PCWP, however, is often unclear since PCWP is influenced by many factors such as volume loading, diastolic myocardial compliance, systolic contractility, and pericardial properties.

In clinical practice, the PCWP is used primarily as an index for left ventricular preload, changes in which in theory reflect any change in cardiac function. The real index for preload, however, is the end-diastolic fiber length, or its correlate the left ventricular end-diastolic volume. The end-diastolic volume is determined by two factors: end-diastolic pressure and diastolic compliance of the left ventricle. As the PCWP indirectly assesses only one of these, it is not surprising that several studies have demonstrated a poor correlation between the PCWP and end-diastolic volume, concluding that PCWP may often be misleading when used as an index of preload [1−3].

PCWP is also used as an indicator of intraoperative myocardial ischemia [4], based on the assumption that myocardial ischemia results in a decrease in myocardial compliance and thereby in an increase in PCWP. However, the correlation between evolving myocardial ischemia and an increase in PCWP has not been extensively studied in humans during anesthesia. Despite studies demonstrating significant increases in PCWP when myocardial ischemia was induced by percutaneous transluminal angioplasty (PTCA) [5, 6], exercise testing [7], or cardiac pacing [8, 9], it remains unknown whether such results may be extrapolated to the insidious onset of myocardial ischemia which may occur during anesthesia in patients with coronary artery disease. It is also not clear what the value of PCWP as a monitor to detect the early onset of myocardial ischemia is.

A limitation of previous studies assessing the value of PCWP in monitoring for ischemia is the lack of a standard method to define presence or absence of ischemia. The electrocardiogram is not ideal, especially in the operating theatre when, for practiacal reasons, only one or two leads are monitored. For example, Kaplan [4] monitored simultaneously the PCWP and a two-lead (leads II and V5) ECG in 40 patients undergoing coronary artery bypass grafting. Ten patients had abnormal PCWP tracings associated with increased PCWP without ST-segment depression on the ECG, three had ST-segment depression without PCWP changes, while only five had both changes in PCWP

Transesophageal Echocardiography
Edited by R. Erbel et al.
© Springer-Verlag Berlin Heidelberg 1989

and the ECG. It was suggested that PCWP changes alone my be the more sensitve indicator of ischemia because the changes in the PCWP tracings were similar to those reported during stress testing and catheterization. But it remains uncertain whether the patients with PCWP changes alone really had myocardial ischemia.

With the advent of transesophageal echocardiography, a device became available for intraoperative monitoring of left ventricular regional wall motion abnormalities (RWMA), the earliest sign of myocardial ischemia. Wall motion analysis by transesophageal echo may also not be the ultimate standard method but has been reported to be the most sensitive technique currently available [10]. Therefore, it may be interesting to correlate PCWP changes to new RWMA.

Leung et al. [11] monitored for RWMA in a series of 40 patients undergoing coronary artery bypass grafting and found 49 episodes of RWMA in 20 patients: 17 prebypass, 22 postbypass and 10 in the intensive care unit (ICU). Only 10% of all RWMA were preceded by an acute rise in PCWP, suggesting that such an elevation is not an early marker of regional myocardial ischemia.

In order to obtain more insight into the relative sensitivity of techniques used to monitor for myocardial ischemia in the anesthetized patient, we recently conducted a study [12] in which we simultaneously monitored (1) left ventricular short-axis view by transesophageal echocardiography, (2) PCWP, and (3) a standard 12-lead ECG, at five set intervals during and following induction of anesthesia in 68 patients prior to coronary artery bypass grafting. Regional wall motion was graded by two independent observers, blind to the ECG data, according to the criteria described by Smith et al. [10].

Diagnoses of myocardial ischemia by transesophageal echo cardiography and ECG correlated closely, transesophageal echo cardiographs appearing to be the more sensitive technique; in 11 patients we diagnosed an episode of RWMA, eight of which had 1 mm or more ST-segment depression on one or more ECG leads. In all eight patients with both RWMA and ST-segment depression, the RWMA was apparent either before or simultaneously with the ST-segment depression. No patients had ECG changes before RWMA or ECG changes alone.

Changes in PCWP, however, correlated poorly with both RWMA and ECG changes. Although new RWMA were associated with an increase in PCWP of 3.2 ± 4.9 mmHg v 0.0 ± 2.2 mmHg when no new RWMA was apparent ($p < 0.01$), the wide variation in PCWP in both ischemic and nonischemic groups resulted in many false-positive and false-negative results when an increase in PCWP was used to diagnose myocardial ischemia.

In our experience, PCWP is not a reliable early indicator of myocardial ischemia in the anesthetized patient. Transesophageal wall motion analysis appears to be the method of choice, especially when a standard 12-lead ECG cannot be obtained for practical reasons.

References

1. Beaupre PN, Cahalan MD, Kremert PF, Roizen MF, Cronnely R, Robinson S, Lurz MA, Alpert R, Hamilton WK, Schiller NB (1983) Does pulmonary artery occlusion pressure adequately reflect left ventricular filling during anesthesia and surgery? Anesthesiology 59:A3
2. Hansen RM, Viquerat CE, Matthay MA, Wiener-Kronish JP, deMarco T, Bathia S, Marks JD, Botvinck EH, Chatterjee K (1986) Poor correlation between pulmonary arterial wedge pressure and left ventricular end-diastolic volume after coronary artery bypass graft surgery. Anesthesiology 64(6):764−770
3. Calvin JE, Driedger AA, Sibbald WJ (1981) Does the pulmonary capillary wedge pressure predict left ventricular preload in critically ill patients? Crit Care Med 9(6):437−443
4. Kaplan JA, Wells PH (1981) Early diagnosis of myocardial ischemia using the pulmonary arterial catheter. Anesth Analg 60:789−793
5. Wijns W, Serruys PW, Slager C et al. (1986) Effects of coronary occlusion during percutaneous transluminal angioplasty in humans on left ventricular chamber stiffness and regional diastolic pressure-radius relations. J Am Coll Cardiol 7:455−463
6. Bertrand ME, Lablanche JM, Fourrier JL et al. (1988) Left ventricular systolic and diastolic function during acute coronary balloon occlusion in humans. J Am Coll Cardiol 12(2):341−347
7. Carroll JD, Hess OM, Hirzel HO, Krayenbuehl HP (1983) Exercise-induced ischemia: the influence of altered relaxation on early diastolic pressures. Circulation 67(3):521−528
8. Mann T, Goldberg S, Mudge GH, Grossmann W (1979) Factors contributing to altered left ventricular systolic and diastolic properties during angina pectoris. Circulation 59:14−20
9. Iskandrian AS, Bemis CE, Hakki AH et al. (1986) Ventricular systolic and diastolic impairment during pacing-induced myocardial ischemia in coronary artery disease: simultaneous hemodynamic, electrocardiographic and radionuclide angiographic evaluation. Am Heart H 112:382−391
10. Smith JS, Cahalan MK, Benefiel DJ, Byrd BF, Lurz FW, Shapiro WA, Roizen MF, Bouchard A, Schiller NB (1985) Intraoperative detection of myocardial ischemia in high risk patients: electrocardiography versus two-dimensional echocardiography. Circulation 72:1015−1021
11. Leung J, O'Kelly B, Browner W et al. (1988) Are regional wall motion abnormalities detected by transesophageal echocardiography triggered by acute changes in supply and demand? Anesthesiology 69:A801
12. van Daele M, Sutherland G, Mitchell M et al. (to be published) Do changes in pulmonary capillary wedge pressure adequately reflect myocardial ischemia during anesthesia? A correlative perioperative haemodynamic, electrocardiographic and transesophageal echocardiographic study

Transesophageal Echocardiography Versus Epicardial Echo

Monitoring During Noncardiac Surgery

K. Wenda, G. Ritter, N. Wittlich, and R. Erbel

Circulatory reactions and pulmonary impairment are well-known phenomena during total hip replacement. Usually blood pressure decreases and pulmonary arterial pressure increases slightly directly after insertion of the stem of the prosthesis. Although the impairment is mostly transient, in some cases cardiac arrest and even intraoperative death have occurred. Pulmonary histology of a patient who died intraoperatively directly after the insertion of the prosthesis showed pulmonary fat embolism. Whether bone marrow is displaced out of the femoral cavity by the prosthesis was discussed widely until it was proved for the first time by transesophageal echocardiography (Heinrich et al. 1985). In intraoperative transesophageal echocardiography the right heart is full of contrast directly after the insertion of the prosthesis. We showed the same effect with intramedullary nailing (Fig. 1) (Wenda et al. 1988) and after release of the tourniquet after insertion of a knee prosthesis. The contrasts correlate with a rise in intrafemoral pressure during the surgical procedure. Intraoperative recordings revealed that during total hip replacement the intrafemoral pressure always increases to over 1000 mmHg independent of the venting technique (drainage of bore hole). In osteosynthesis by intramedullary nailing the intrafemoral pressure increases during the drilling process, usually up to 600 mmHg and in some cases to over 1000 mmHg. Two echocardiographic phenomena after the pressure elevation can be distinguished: "snowflakes" are always to be seen after elevation of the intrafemoral pressure, for example after reposition of fractures of long bones, after drilling in the femoral cavity and after insertion of a prosthesis. With considerable elevation of the intrafemoral pressure, large emboli of up to 5 cm can be

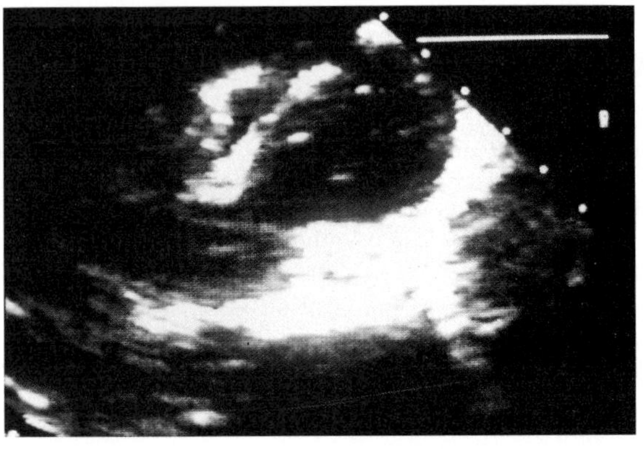

Fig. 1. Intraoperative transesophageal echocardiography during intramedullary nailing: passage of a 4-cm embolus through the tricuspid valve

Transesophageal Echocardiography
Edited by R. Erbel et al.
© Springer-Verlag Berlin Heidelberg 1989

seen during their passage through the right heart. Our results, raised the question how bone marrow emboli of such size can pass through the vessels of the bone. Indeed, there was a discrepancy between the lumen of the veins and the size of the emboli.

For clarification of the substrate of the emboli, a study was performed in sheep. After application of a particular pressure on the femoral cavity, the vena cava was investigated sonographically through a laparotomy and blood was taken proximally from the vein. After pressure elevation of over 200 mmHg, sonographic "snowflakes" appeared in the vena cava. There was no difference in the sonographic appearance after applying pressure with sodium chloride solution, bone marrow, or air, so the substrate of the snowflakes cannot be distinguished by sonography. Much more productive were the observations after applying pressure of over 400 mmHg, when the passage of large emboli in the vein could be observed. With regard to thrombogenesis, it is of great importance that with artificial ventilation the flow in the vein and the movement of the emboli stopped completely during the inspiration phase. To our surprise, macroscopic examination of blood taken from the proximal vein revealed "mixed emboli," composed of a core of bone marrow and surrounding thrombotic apposition. Obviously, the bone marrow induces aggregation of thrombocytes and thrombotic material.

Histological examination of the lungs of the sheep revealed bone marrow in the branches of the pulmonary artery, which explains the pulmonary impairment after the elevation of intrafemoral pressure associated with surgical procedures. In conclusion, intraoperative echocardiographic investigations in man prooved that bone marrow is displaced into the circulation with surgical procedures, and mean that surgical procedures that avoid an increase of intrafemoral pressure are required.

At present we are investigating the effectiveness of supracondylar suction drainge during intramedullary nailing to avoid passage of bone marrow into the circulation.

Total hip replacement involves the highest rate of thrombosis of any operation. Currently, we are investigating whether a more subtle surgical procedure preventing the increase of the intrafemoral pressure diminishes the rate of thrombosis during total hip replacement.

References

Heinrich H, Kremer P, Winter H, Wörsdörfer O, Ahnefeld FW (1985) Transösophageale zweidimensionale Echokardiographie bei Hüftendoprothesen. Anaesthesist 34:118−123
Wenda K, Ritter G, Degreif J, Rudigier J (1988) Zur Genese pulmonaler Komplikationen nach Marknagelosteosynthesen. Unfallchirurgie 91:432−435

Feasibility and Value of Transesophageal Echocardiography in Anesthetized Children

J. LAM, B. V. D. BURG, D. C. G. BASART, A. NIJVELD, J. L. SCHULLER, O. DANIELS, and C. A. VISSER

Introduction

The value of transesophageal echocardiography (TEE) in adults is now well established (Visser et al. 1988). The experience with this modality in children, however, is still very limited. This is mainly due to the relatively large size of the presently commercially available transducers on the one hand, and to the better images usually obtained in infants and children on the other hand. Transthoracically inaccesible structures may, however, exist, e.g., retrosternal conduits. TEE may also be used in the operating room for monitoring purposes.

The present study was undertaken to determine a) the minimum body weight for TEE application, b) the additional diagnostic value of TEE, and c) its potential pediatric applications.

Patients and Methods

Twenty-one patients were studied, 15 boys and six girls (Table 1). TEE was performed with all but one patient under general anesthesia. Before and after TEE, transthoracic echocardiography (TTE) was performed. The majority of patients (18) were studied with a commercially available Hewlett-Packard 5 MHz transducer, the other three with a commercially available Toshiba 3.75 MHz transducer. Patients with a body weight above 25 kg were studied

Table 1. Patient characteristic and TEE application

	Operating room	Catheter laboratory or intensive care unit
No. of patients	10	11
Ages (years)	5−16	6−15
No. < 12 years	5	5
Bodyweights (kg)	17−65	21−65
No. < 30 kg	4[a]	4[b]

[a] 17, 20, 20, 28 kg
[b] 21, 27, 27, 29 kg

Transesophageal Echocardiography
Edited by R. Erbel et al.
© Springer-Verlag Berlin Heidelberg 1989

routinely, but patients with a body weight below 25 kg only underwent TEE when it was anticipated that results might affect management during surgery or balloon valvuloplasty.

Results

The probe could be inserted, in all 21 patients, and standard views displaying the intracardiac anatomy were obtained. In all cases this included the short-axis view of the aortic root, the biatrial, four-chamber and long-axis views, or comparable views in cases with a univentricular heart. In all cases color flow mapping was performed during TEE, and in all cases there was excellent visualization of the aortic root, atrial anatomy, and right ventricular anterior wall. The short-axis view of the left ventricle was obtained only in a minority of cases. When the body weight was above 30 kg, the ease of manipulation was comparable to that in adults; when the body weight was below 30 kg, manipulation was hampered; in particular, the short-axis view of the left ventricle was more difficult to obtain. In the first period of the study the pulmonary artery including the bifurcation was not systematically looked for, but it was visualized in six of the last seven patients. The pulmonary valve was clearly demonstrated in only one patient, who underwent repair of a tetralogy of Fallot (Fig. 1). The surgical patients are summarized in Table 2. The two patients undergoing a Fontan operation both had a body weight of 20 kg. One was diagnosed as having a univentricular heart with moderate hypoplasia of the mitral valve. As obstruction through the mitral valve was anticipated after complete separation of the systemic and pulmonary circulation, TEE was performed to monitor mitral valve flow. In case of flow impairment, the Fontan repair could be reversed and changed to a more palliative type of surgical treatment. The patient, however, came off the bypass without problems. In the other patient undergoing a Fontan operation, TEE was performed a few

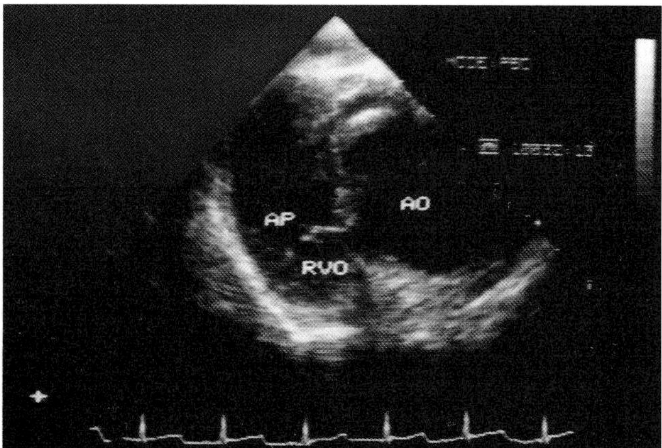

Fig. 1. 14-year-old boy with tetralogy of Fallot. Pulmonary artery view also demonstrating the pulmonary valve, *AO*, aorta; *AP*, pulmonary artery; *RVO*, right ventricular outflow tract

Table 2. Surgical cases

Fontan operation (2)
Ascending aorta replacement
Homograft implantation in aortic position
Repair of tetralogy of Fallot
Ventricular septal defect closure
Atrial septal defect closure
Mitral valve repair
Repair of double outlet right ventricle
Resection of discrete subaortic stenosis

---

weeks after this operation during a reoperation because of cardiac tamponade (see below). The patient undergoing repair of a double outlet right ventricle had a body weight of 17 kg. Because the surgeon was concerned about obstruction due to the constructed intracardiac tunnel, TEE was performed. Both the tunnel from the right ventricle towards the pulmonary artery and from the left ventricle towards the aorta were clearly visualized. The patient was studied with TEE again after a few days because of recurrent pericardial effusion. Despite the low body weight, the two TEE examinations were well tolerated.

TEE and Surgical Management

In two cases, TEE proved to be extremely important. In the above-mentioned case with a cardiac tamponade, a few weeks after the Fontan operation severe myocardial dysfunction was revealed during surgical exploration, presenting as low output state. Initially, it was thought that the cause was related to the type of repair, but TEE showed that contractility improved after starting the cardio-pulmonary bypass and deteriorated when the bypass was stopped. This prompted the surgeon to insert an intra aortic balloon pump, despite the small body size, and the patient finally recovered. The other patient revealed severe residual mitral regurgitation after repair of a prolapsing mitral valve with anulus dilatation. This was considered to be an indication to replace the valve with a St. Jude mechanical prosthetic valve. In two other patients, additional surgery might in retrospect, have been considered. One patient with replacement of the ascending aorta and resuspension of the native aortic valve had persistent, severe aortic regurgitation at the end of the procedure as judged by TEE; this progressed during follow-up studies. In retrospect for this case, there was the option of also replacing the aortic valve. In another patient with aortic regurgitation due to a bicuspid valve combined with a tetralogy of Fallot with a subarterial ventricular septal defect (VSD), this regurgitation had increased at the end of surgery, also progressing during follow-up studies. It is conceivable that suturing the VSD patch could have caused some damage to the aortic valve. In that case, retrospect in there was the option, of opening up the ascending aorta and inspecting the aortic valve.

TEE in the Catheter Laboratory or Intensive Care Unit

The nonsurgical patients who underwent TEE are summarized in Table 3. In this group, four patients were studied for diagnostic purposes. One of these, a 13-year-old boy with a body weight of 37 kg underwent the procedure without anesthesia, but this caused considerable discomfort.

Value of TEE During Interventions

In the cases of aortic balloon valvuloplasty, information was obtained concerning the position of the balloon and guide wire. In one case, the guide wire was trapped in the mitral valve apparatus. This was seen on the two-dimensional image, and color flow mapping revealed mitral regurgitation throughout that period. This is important, as false positioning of a guide wire may be fatal (Scholler et al. 1988). Regarding the evaluation of the effect of dilatation, information could be obtained about the aortic valve using the short-axis view, which showed the anatomy before and after the dilatation, as described by Cyran et al. (1988). No major changes in valve morphology or

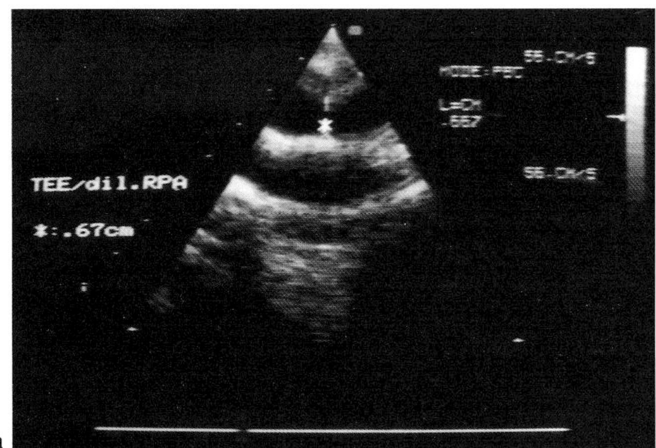

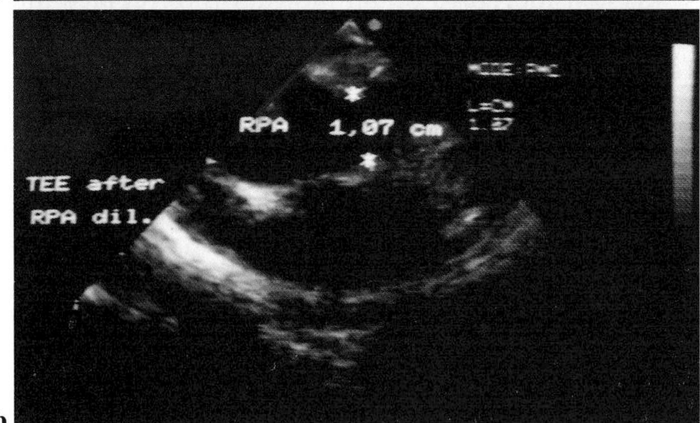

Fig. 2 a, b. 16-year-old boy. Pulmonary artery view. Balloon dilatation of peripheral pulmonary artery stenosis proximal in right pulmonary artery (*RPA*) after unsuccessfull-debanding. Diameter of stenosis before dilatation (0.67 mm); diameter of stenosis after dilatation (1.07 mm)

Table 3. Cases studied in the catheter laboratory of intensive care unit

Balloon dilatation	7
Aortic valve	4
Pulmonary valve	1
Peripheral pulmonary artery	2
Diagnostic studies	4

function after dilatation were seen. Follow-up Doppler studies performed the next day did not reveal a major gradient reduction. Although in this series the aortic valvuloplasties were unsuccessful, possible it is theoretically to use TEE to guide the procedure by chosing the optimal balloon-size, and increasing balloon size when no changes in valve morphology are noted after dilatation with a smaller balloon. Todt et al. (1988) described a case in which a supravalvular pulmonary stenosis was treated with balloon dilatation under TEE monitoring after incomplete debanding. We applied TEE in a 16-year-old boy in whom a stenosis persisted in the proximal part of the right pulmonary artery after debanding. Turbulent flow was clearly demonstrated across the stenotic area. Two-dimensional echocardiographic measurements performed before and after dilatation demonstrated an increase in diameter of the stenotic area from 0.67 cm to 1.07 cm (Fig. 2). A ventilation-perfusion scan clearly showed an increase in flow through the right lung.

Transthoracic Versus Transesophageal Echocardiography

The additional diagnostic information which was obtained with TEE in 21 patients is summarized in Table 4. In four patients, a total of seven anomalies was detected, and in one case, the position of a VSD was better identified. One patient, a 15-year-old girl, was scheduled for balloon dilatation of a stenotic pulmonary valve, but TEE revealed an additional secundum type atrial septal defect (ASD). The dilatation was not performed because of this finding and the patient was treated surgically. During surgery, both the pulmonary valve stenosis and the ASD were confirmed. In another patient who was

Table 4. Additional diagnostic information provided by TEE (all patients) compared with TTE

Secundum type atrial septal defect
L-R shunt through foramen ovale
Conduit flow after Fontan operation
Mitral regurgitation (2)
Tricuspid regurgitation
Aortic regurgitation
Better localization of ventricular septal defect

scheduled for VSD closure, a small left to right shunt through the foramen ovale was detected. The VSD was thought to be perimembranous, but TEE revealed it to be located in the membranous septum. One patient with atrial fibrillation after a Fontan operation underwent TEE to rule out a thrombus in the left atrium appendage prior to cardioversion. This patient had an atrioventricular conduit because of a hypoplastic tricuspid orifice, and conduit flow was clearly shown. This patient also had mitral and aortic regurgitation and tricuspid regurgitation through the hypoplastic native tricuspid valve. All these features were not shown with TEE. One patient, a 16-year-old girl, underwent dilatation of a stenotic peripheral pulmonary artery. TEE revealed concomitant mitral regurgitation which could not be confirmed with TTE later on.

Complications

In one patient, some bloodstains were seen on the probe after removal. This was the patient with severe myocardial dysfunction and a body weight of 20 kg. No other complications related to TEE were observed.

Conclusions

TEE is feasible in anesthetized children with a body weight of approximately 20 kg or more. Also, in congenital heart disease, additional diagnostic information can be obtained, particularly in bigger children. Moreover, an important indication is the application during surgery. The technique may be of value during interventions. The applications will unquestionably further expand when smaller transducers become available.

Acknowledgements. The authors are indebted to Dr. M.A. Taams for performing TEE in the patient illustrated in Fig. 2, and to A.N. Kimmings for doing the literature research.

References

Cyran SE, Kemball TR, Schwartz DC, Meyer RA, Steed RD, Kaplan S (1988) Evaluation of balloon aortic valvuloplasty with transoesophageal echocardiography. Am Heart J 115:460–462

Scholler GF, Keane JF, Perry SB, Sanders SP, Lock JE (1988) Balloon dilatation of congenital aortic valve stenosis. Circulation 78:351–360

Todt H, Erbel R, Pop T, Bednarczyk I, Drexler J (1988) Dilatation einer supravalvular pulmonalisstenose bei TE echocardiographischem monitoring. Kissing Balloon Technik. Z Kardiol, 77:385–388

Visser CA, Koolen JJ, van Wezel HB, Dunning AJ (1988) Transesophageal echocardiography: technique and clinical applications. J Cardiother. Anaeasthesiol 2:pp 74–91

Assessment of Regional Myocardial Perfusion Using Contrast Echocardiography During Coronary Artery Surgery*

S. H. Johnson, J. S. Kabas, J. Kisslo, and P. K. Smith

Introduction

Coronary artery bypass grafting (CABG) has reached a prominent status in the treatment of coronary artery disease. The main objective of CABG is increasing coronary blood flow to ischemic myocardium in order to preserve and improve ventricular function. Objective measurements of the completeness of myocardial revascularization during and immediately after CABG have been limited by an inability to assess regional myocardial perfusion. The combination of intraoperative two-dimensional (2-D) echocardiography with the use of intravascular echocardiographic contrast agents (contrast echocardiography makes ultrasonic imaging an attractive method to assess regional myocardial perfusion during surgical revascularization. In addition, this method has shown promise in studying transmural changes in myocardial blood flow and in the quantitation of myocardial perfusion. The intraoperative application of this procedure to coronary artery surgery could allow immediate assessment of the completeness of surgical myocardial revascularization.

Contrast echocardiography began with the observation that dye injected into the ascending aorta during echocardiography produced significant image enhancement (Gramiak and Shah 1968). This enhancement was attributed to ultrasonic reflection from gaseous microbubbles present in the contrast dye (Meltzer et al. 1980). Other authors identified this contrast effect with other agents and cardioplegic solutions were utilized for contrast enhancement intraoperatively to identify perfusion deficits prior to bypass grafting (Ziskin et al. 1972; Kemper et al. 1983; Goldman and Mindich 1984). Initially, contrast echocardiography was used to evaluate intracardiac anatomy, shunts, and valvular pathology (Kerber et al. 1974; Reid et al. 1983; Valdez-Cruz and Sahn 1984). These studies employed contrast solutions containing microbubbles created by hand agitation. Investigation of microbubbles created by this technique revealed large diameters of 15 μm or greater, which could become trapped in the coronary microvasculature for as long as 200 s (Kort and Kronzon 1982; Feinstein et al. 1984). Contrast agents with large microbubbles were also found to cause transient ECG changes and impairment of left ventricular function (Gillam et al. 1985; Lang et al. 1987). These findings limited the usefulness of contrast solutions created by this method.

* Supported by National Heart, Lung, and Blood Institute Grant Nos. K04-HL02051 and R01-HL41087, North Carolina Affiliate of the American Heart Association Grant No. 1988-89-A-04, and by a grant from the Warren W. Hobbie Charitable Trust of Roanoke, Virgina

Transesophageal Echocardiography
Edited by R. Erbel et al.
© Springer-Verlag Berlin Heidelberg 1989

In order to safely evaluate myocardial perfusion, contrast agents needed to be developed which could pass through the coronary microvasculature in physiologic times. Keller applied high-frequency ultrasonic energy to various agents, a process now known as sonication, to produce smaller and more uniform microbubbles. In vitro testing with scanning laser and Coulter counter methods documented the average diameter of these microbubbles to be less than 10 μm. Sonicated Renografin, a frequently employed contrast agent, produces microbubbles with an average diameter of 4.5 ± 2.8 μm and a half-life of 102 s (Keller et al. 1986). Further investigation showed that these microbubbles had flow characteristics similar to red blood cells and could pass unimpeded through the coronary microvasculature (Feinstein et al. 1984). These observations led to numerous perfusion studies with sonicated Renografin both in the laboratory and in the clinical setting. Intracoronary injection of these microbubble solutions was found to produce a rapid increase in myocardial echogenicity followed by a gradual return to baseline intensity as the microbubbles were washed from the myocardium. These studies were found to cause minimal adverse hemodynamic or electrocardiographic effects, and subsequently, numerous myocardial perfusion studies were performed utilizing contrast echocardiography (Feinstein 1986; Moore et al. 1986). Recent investigations report that this technique effectively estimates coronary flow reserve and identifies myocardium at risk for ischemic damage and myocardial infarction (Armstrong et al. 1982, 1983, 1984; Kaul et al. 1984, 1987; Ten Cate et al. 1984; Taylor et al. 1985). In addition, this method has been utilized during interventional cardiac catheterization to evaluate nonsurgical revascularization without untoward effects (Lang et al. 1986).

After documentation of the safety and usefulness of contrast echocardiography, it seemed logical to apply this technique to surgical revascularization. The purpose of this investigation is to demonstrate the efficacy and safety of contrast echocardiography in the evaluation of myocardial perfusion during CABG.

Methods

Adult males at Duke University Medical Center and the Asheville Veterans Administration Medical Center between the ages of 40 and 75 were enrolled in the study after Institutional Review Board approval and individual patient consent. All patients in the study had CABG performed for the treatment of coronary artery disease and had stable hemodynamics, normal renal and neurologic function, and no history of allergy to contrast dye or iodinated products. Patients were specially selected based upon the good quality of distal coronary arteries to minimize the possibility of technical anastomotic problems.

All patients underwent routine CABG with reversed saphenous vein grafts and internal mammary arteries to improve myocardial perfusion. Precise indications for surgical therapy varied in specific cases and were not controlled in the study population. Routine invasive monitoring of systemic and pulmonary artery pressures, central venous pressure, and cardiac output was established prior to surgery. The ECG was continuously monitored. After median sternotomy, patients were heparinized and placed on partial cardiopulmonary bypass at 37°C. Adequate venous drainage was accomplished with two-stage venous return cannulae to ensure retrograde ascending aortic flow during the study.

Myocardial perfusion studies with contrast echocardiography were performed at three specific intervals: (1) ascending aortic injection of contrast agent prior to bypass grafting; (2) direct injection of contrast into each saphenous vein graft after the completion of both proximal and distal anastomoses (no internal mammary arteries were studied) and (3) ascending aortic injection of contrast after completion of bypass grafting. These studies were performed with the following objectives: (1) to document the safety of contrast study during CABG; (2) to identify underperfused myocardium before bypass grafting; (3) to demonstrate perfusion area and patency of each saphenous vein graft; and (4) to document improvement in global myocardial perfusion after bypass grafting.

The echocardiographic contrast agent was prepared under sterile conditions prior to each injection. The method of preparation has been previously described (Keller et al. 1986). Commercially available Renografin 76 was purchased in a sterile form. A gas-sterilized Branson sonicator (Heat Systems-Ultrasonics, Inc.) was mounted in the operating room using a specially designed clamp. The probe of the sonifier was placed in an inverted syringe containing 8 ml Renografin. Sonication for 30 s produced a highly echogenic, gaseous microbubble suspension with an average microbubble diameter of 5.0 µm. Immediately after removal of the syringe, the sonicated Renografin was used for contrast injection.

Transesophageal or epicardial 2-D Echo, using a 3.5 or 5.0-MHz probe, was performed prior to and for 100 s following each contrast injection with an Aloka 880 scanner (Asheville Veterans Administration Medical Center) or a Hewlett-Packard 500 scanner (Duke University Medical Center). Reference short-axis imaging of the left ventricle at midpapillary level was performed initially and optimal gain settings established, which remained fixed throughout the study. Images were visually interpreted in real time and stored on a Panasonic AG-6300 VHS recorder for future analysis. Both echocardiographic and external landmarks were used to keep imaging planes consistent.

Results

Saphenous vein graft injection with sonicated Renografin produced a rapid increase in regional myocardial echocardiographic enhancement which progressively diminished and returned to baseline intensity as the contrast was washed from the heart by native coronary and graft flow. The areas of revascularized myocardium defined by contrast enhancement correlated well with the size and distribution of the native coronary artery. These findings are illustrated in Fig. 1, which displays short-axis images of the left ventricle during contrast injection in a bypass graft to the posterior descending coronary artery. A return to baseline intensity occurred in every injection within 20 s.

Significant improvement in image enhancement quality occurred during the initial study period. This was due, in part, to improved techniques in preparation, handling, and injection of the contrast agent. Initial saphenous vein graft studies were performed with 1 ml contrast injected through a 20-gauge needle. In vitro preparations revealed significant microbubble disruption after passing through small bore needles. Therefore, to improve image quality, the injection needle size was increased to 18 gauge. In addition, the amount of contrast injected in each vein graft was increased from 1 ml to 3 ml.

Ascending aortic injections with 4 ml contrast agent provided only minimal myocardial enhancement, both before and after CABG. Therefore,

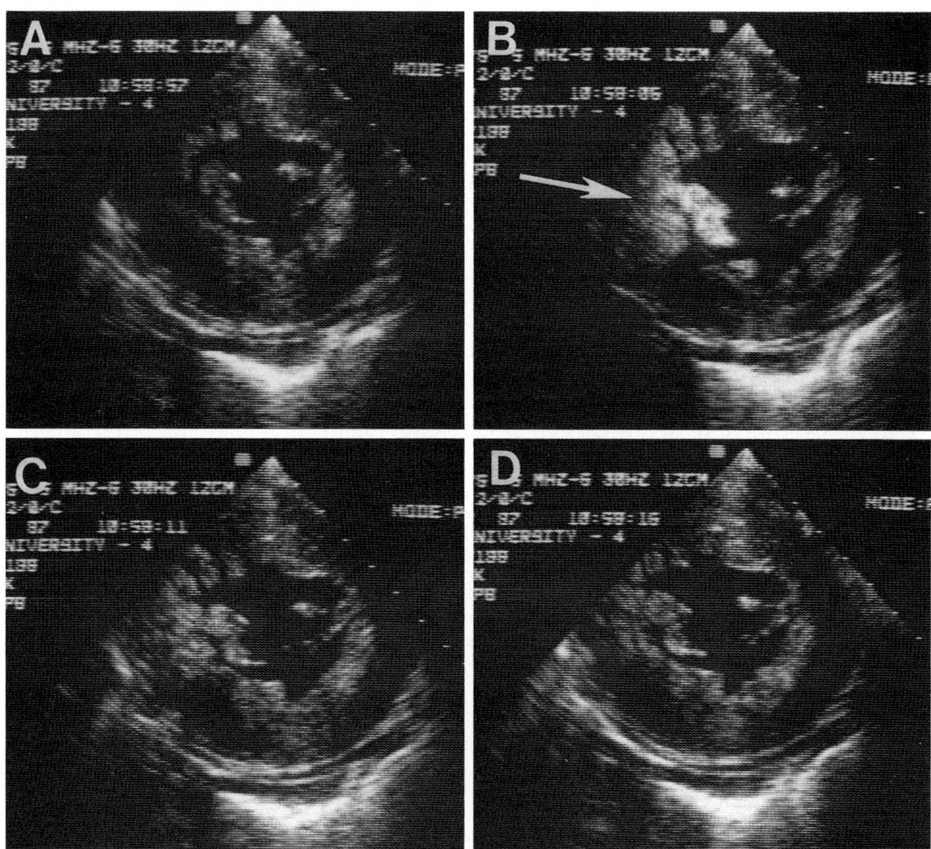

Fig. 1 A–D. Sequential left ventricular short-axis echocardiographic images during contrast injection of a posterior descending artery bypass graft. The septum is on the *left* and the anterior left ventricle is on *top*. **A** Reference image prior to contrast injection. **B** Peak image enhancement in the posterior-septal region (*arrow*). **C, D** Contrast is washed from the myocardium as the image returns to baseline intensity

preoperative perfusion deficits could not be defined and augmentation of global short-axis myocardial perfusion after surgical revascularization could not be documented.

A total of 44 saphenous vein injections and 30 ascending aortic injections were performed in 18 patients. The surgical procedure, with experience, was only minimally prolonged (approximately 10 min). There were no hemodynamic changes and no patient required postoperative inotropic support. In addition, ECG monitoring revealed no ischemic or conduction changes during injection. Postoperatively, there were no renal, infectious, hemorrhagic, or clinically apparent neurologic complications.

Discussion

This investigation applied contrast echocardiography intraoperatively to assess the results of CABG. This technique proved useful in assessing individual bypass graft function by defining the completeness of revascularization, the area of contrast enhancement, and the rate of contrast washout. Therefore, the real-time assessment of end-organ perfusion was documented. These observations would permit immediate and specific operative revision if poor enhancement or prolonged washout were found. This technique could prove invaluable in assessing technically difficult anastomoses, where endarterectomy or embolectomy is performed, and the distal circulation is questionable. No revisions of bypass grafts were performed in this study; however, patients were specifically selected to reduce the likelihood of technical complications. The study caused no perioperative complications and only minimally prolonged the surgical procedure, documenting the safety and feasibility of multiple contrast echocardiography studies.

Reproducible contrast enhancement was not produced by ascending aortic injections. This failure was due in part to the self-imposed limitation to 4 ml contrast agent. In this dosage, microbubble concentration was not high enough to cause significant myocardial contrast enhancement. Future studies with greater doses of contrast agent or the use of other contrast agents with a higher microbubble concentration may provide satisfactory enhancement. This would then allow for the determination of perfusion deficits before CABG and the documentation of reperfusion after myocardial revascularization.

This study should be considered preliminary because although an excellent qualitative assessment of myocardial revascularization was achieved, *quantitation* of myocardial perfusion (the ultimate goal of contrast echocardiography) is not yet possible. This is due, in part, to the nonideal characteristics of the echocardiographic contrast agent. The size and concentration of microbubbles present in the contrast agent significantly influences contrast enhancement. Although the majority of microbubbles in sonicated Renografin are less than 10 μm in diameter, a large variability in the range of size exists (1−50 μm). Small microbubbles have a short half life, which is not long in comparison to the coronary capillary transit time. Therefore, the concentration of microbubbles can change over the course of myocardial contrast washout. Also, ultrasonic reflectivity is proportional to the sixth power of the microbubble radius (Powsner et al. 1986). The minority of large microbubbles (> 10 µm) may be trapped in the coronary microvasculature and cause excessive echocardiographic enhancement. These factors account for significant variability which precludes accurate and reproducible quantitation of myocardial perfusion using sonicated Renografin as a contrast agent.

Both transesophageal and epicardial echocardiographic probe positions are applicable in contrast echocardiography. Transesophageal methods are attractive because the probe remains out of the sterile field and can be continuously recorded during the procedure. However, the number of visual planes is limited and the short-axis view is not complete with currently available transesophageal probes. However, this method does allow for excellent regional study of myocardial perfusion. Epicardial echocardiography provides an excellent short-axis view of the left ventricle and has numerous imaging planes available. Its main disadvantage is that the probe must be sterilized and brought into the operative field.

In conclusion, our initial experience with contrast echocardiography suggests that its intraoperative use is safe and provides immediate qualitative assessment of saphenous vein bypass grafts. Graft patency and graft blood flow distribution can be evaluated, allowing for immediate correction if necessary. Furthermore, information obtained during bypass grafting may lead to improved interpretation of the long-term results of CABG. In the future, the development of stable albumin microspheres would facilitate studies and possibly allow for intraoperative *quantitative* assessment of myocardial blood flow. In addition, contrast echocardiography could be applied to other cardiovascular procedures such as aortic valve replacement and congenital cardiac surgery where the coronary perfusion may be compromised. The simplicity, safety, and potential benefit of contrast echocardiography could result in its becoming an important asset in cardiac surgery.

References

Armstrong WF, Mueller TM, Kinney EL, Tickner EG, Dillon JC, Feigenbaum H (1982) Assessment of myocardial perfusion abnormalities with contrast-enhanced two-dimensional echocardiography. Circulation 66:166−173

Armstrong WF, West SR, Mueller TM, Dillon JC, Feigenbaum H (1983) Assessment of location and size of myocardial infarction with contrast-enhanced echocardiography. J Am Coll Cardiol 2:63−69

Armstrong WF, West SR, Dillon JC, Feigenbaum H (1984) Assessment of location and size of myocardial infarction with contrast-enhanced echocardiography. II. Application of digital imaging techniques. J Am Coll Cardiol 4:141−148

Cheirif J, Zoghbi WA, Raizner AE et al. (1988) Assessment of myocardial perfusion in humans by contrast echocardiography. I. Evaluation of regional coronary reserve by peak contrast intensity. J Am Coll Cardiol 11:735−743

Feinstein SB, Shah PM, Bing RJ et al. (1984) Microbubble dynamics visualized in the intact capillary circulation. J Am Coll Cardiol 4:595−600

Feinstein SB, Ong K, Staniloff HM et al. (1986) Myocardial contrast echocardiography: examination of intracoronary injections, microbubble diameters, and video-intensity decay. Am J Physiol Imaging 1:12–18

Gillam LD, Kaul S, Fallon JJ et al. (1985) Functional and pathologic effects of multiple echocardiographic contrast injections on the myocardium, brain, and kidney. J Am Coll Cardiol 6:687–694

Goldman ME, Mindich BP (1984) Intraoperative cardioplegic contrast echocardiography for assessing myocardial perfusion during open heart surgery. J Am Coll Cardiol 4:1029–1034

Gramiak R, Shah PM (1968) Echocardiography of the aortic root. Invest Radiol 3:356–366

Kaul S, Pandian NG, Okada RD, Pohost GM, Weyman AE (1984) Contrast echocardiography in acute myocardial ischemia. I. In vivo determination of total left ventricular "area at risk". J Am Coll Cardiol 4:1272–1282

Kaul S, Glasheen W, Ruddy TD, Pandian NG, Weyman AE, Okada RD (1987) The importance of defining left ventricular area at risk in vivo during acute myocardial infarction: an experimental evaluation with myocardial contrast two-dimensional echocardiography. Circulation 75:1249–1260

Keller MW, Feinstein SB, Briller RA, Powsner SM (1986) Automated production and analysis of echo contrast agents. J Ultrasound Med 5:493–498

Kemper AJ, O'Boyle JE, Sharma S et al. (1983) Hydrogen peroxide contrast-enhanced two-dimensional echocardiography: real-time in vivo delineation of regional myocardial perfusion. Circulation 68:603–611

Kerber RE, Kioschos JM, Lauer RM (1974) Use of ultrasonic contrast method in the diagnosis of valvular regurgitation and intracardiac shunts. Am J Cardiol 34:722–727

Kort A, Kronzon I (1982) Microbubble formation: in vitro and in vivo observations. J Clin Ultrasound 10:117–120

Lang RM, Feinstein SB, Feldman T, Neumann A, Chua KG, Borow KM (1986) Contrast echocardiography for evaluation of myocardial perfusion: effects of coronary angioplasty. J Am Coll Cardiol 1:232–235

Lang RM, Borrow KM, Neumann A, Feinstein SB (1987) Echocardiographic contrast agents: effect of microbubbles and carrier solutions on left ventricular contractility. J Am Coll Cardiol 9:910–919

Meltzer RS, Tickner EG, Sahines TP, Popp RL (1980) The source of ultrasound contrast effect. J Clin Ultrasound 8:121–127

Moore CA, Smucker ML, Kaul S (1986) Myocardial contrast echocardiography in humans. I. Safety – a comparison with routine coronary arteriography. J Am Coll Cardiol 8:1066–1072

Powsner SM, Keller MW, Saniie J, Feinstein SB (1986) Quantitation of echo-contrast effects. Am J Physiol Imaging 1:124–128

Reid CL, Kawanishi DT, McKay CR, Elkayam U, Rahimtoola SH, Chandraratna PAN (1983) Accuracy of evaluation of the presence and severity of aortic and mitral regurgitation by contrast 2-dimensional echocardiography. Am J Cardiol 52:519–524

Taylor AL, Collins SM, Skorton DJ, Kieso RA, Melton J, Kerber RE (1985) Artifactual regional gray level variability in contrast-enhanced two-dimensional echocardiographic images: effect on measurement of the coronary perfusion bed. J Am Coll Cardiol 6:831–838

Ten Cate FJ, Feinstein S, Zwehl W et al. (1984) Two-dimensional contrast echocardiography. II. Transpulmonary studies. J Am Coll Cardiol 3:21–27

Valdez-Cruz LM, Sahn DJ (1984) Ultrasonic contrast studies for the detection of cardiac shunts. J Am Coll Cardiol 3:978–985

Ziskin MC, Bonakdarpour A, Weinstein DP, Lynch PR (1972) Contrast agents for diagnostic ultrasound. Invest Radiol 7:500–505

Intraoperative Echocardiography in Congenital Heart Disease: An Overview

G. R. Sutherland, J. Quaegebeur, M. E. R. M. van Daele, O. F. W. Stumper, and J. Hess

Introduction

Intraoperative epicardial cross-sectional imaging has now been available for some 8 years [1−5] without gaining widespread acceptance as an essential aid to the cardiac surgery of congenital heart disease. Despite the high-quality imaging of cardiac morphology obtained by direct epicardial scanning, the epicardial two-dimensional image alone may provide little important additional diagnostic information when compared to the preoperative findings. As the primary morphologic diagnosis is seldom incomplete in such cases after combined preoperative cardiac catheterisation and echo studies, most cardiac surgeons consider additional prebypass intraoperative ultrasound studies as an unnecessary prolongation of surgical time. In recent years, the use of intraoperative contrast echocardiography to assess the results of surgical repair has, after a period of initial surgical enthusiasm [6, 7], largely been abandoned. The reason for this was that in clinical decision making, intraoperative contrast echo proved to be an unreliable technique; it must be analysed over only the initial heartbeats following injection and the findings are dependent on a number of variables: (a) the amount of contrast medium injected, (b) the velocity with which the agent is injected, (c) the precise site of injection, and (d) the haemodynamics at that particular moment. In addition, although an intraoperative contrast study may prove the existence of a significant intracardiac shunt, it usually fails to localise its site and also fails to distinguish between one or multiple residual defects.

However, there is now renewed interest in intraoperative echocardiography. This has been created by two new developments in cardiac ultrasound: (1) The introduction of color flow mapping as an adjunct to cross-sectional imaging and (2) the introduction of transoesophageal echocardiography. The reasons why colour flow mapping should be an advantage are: (a) it can determine both the site and direction of normal and abnormal intracardiac flows, (b) it readily distinguishes between laminar and turbulent flow, (c) it facilitates the identification of both the precise number and site of atrial and ventricular septal defects, (d) it can aid in the assessment of both valvular insufficiency and either valvular or subvalvular stenosis, and (e) it can indicate various other haemodynamic changes associated with abnormal cardiac morphology. Unlike contrast echocardiography, the colour flow map can be continuously recorded in real time over an unlimited number of heartbeats. On-line analysis of the colour map normally provides a rapid assessment of

Transesophageal Echocardiography
Edited by R. Erbel et al.
© Springer-Verlag Berlin Heidelberg 1989

the optimal sampling site for pulsed wave and continuous wave Doppler measurements. In effect, the colour flow map should provide the surgeon with the equivalent of intraoperative angiography to complement the high resolution structural imaging information and spectral Doppler information.

An alternative approach to the standard epicardial intraoperative study (described above) has now been provided by the introduction of cardiac imaging from the oesophagus. In theory, this approach incorporating both high-resolution imaging, pulsed Doppler interrogation and colour flow mapping, has many potential advantages when compared to the epicardial approach. The most important practical advantage is that information can be obtained without invading the surgical field or interfering with the surgical procedure. Furthermore, transoesophageal echocardiography may provide more detailed information on cardiac structures adjacent to the oesophagus (e.g., atria, atrial septum, atrioventricular valves), which are not always well visualised from the praecordium. The transoesophageal approach may also obtain imaging and colour flow information from other areas that are "masked" from the epicardial view by interposed prosthetic material.

Recent reports have suggested that the integrated use of either intraoperative epicardial [8] or transoesophageal [9] high-resolution cross-sectional imaging combined with colour flow mapping, and pulsed and continuous Doppler measurements, could both further improve the accuracy of preoperative diagnosis and, more importantly, permit the immediate, precise evaluation of the results of surgical repair before closure of the chest.

From 1. January 1988 to 1. January 1989, we have performed complete epicardial echocardiographic studies in virtually every case of congenital heart disease ($n = 143$) undergoing surgical correction in the Thoraxcentrum. The studies were carried out both immediately before and after cardiopulmonary bypass. In a few appropriate cases, epicardial and transoesophageal examinations were combined. The information and opinions contained in this chapter are based on the initial 1-year surgical experience, but included in this evaluation is also information gained in the outpatient clinic on the role of transoesophageal echocardiography in the evaluation of complex congenital heart disease in adolescents and adults.

Who Should Record and Interpret the Study?

Having performed intracardiac corrective surgery in complex congenital heart disease, every surgeon has a keen interest in evaluating the immediate results of his work. This could lead to the problem of surgical bias in interpretation if the surgeon is left alone to perform the postbypass ultrasound examination and interpret the results in isolation. At our institution, all the intraoperative studies in patients undergoing surgery for congenital heart disease are performed by a surgeon in conjunction with an experienced echocardiographer with an understanding of congenital cardiac malformations. At present, this would appear to be the optimal situation, as the information obtained during a full intraoperative study (especially the colour flow mapping information) is too complex to allow on-line interpretation, considering the currently limited experience which most cardiac surgeons have with this technique. Furthermore, even the most experienced echocardiographer will make frequent mistakes (both false-positive and false-negative errors) if these complex intraoperative colour flow maps are reviewed only on-line. Subsequent detailed frame-by-frame analysis is required before a final opinion is given to the cardiac surgeon. Only by observing these rules will surgical trust be obtained and mistakes in interpretation of the ultrasound information reduced to a minimum. In our experience, intraoperative echocardiography in congenital heart disease is without any doubt the most difficult aspect of the whole field of cardiac ultrasound − in no other area are flow maps so complex − and immediate, correct diagnostic decisions are required.

Finally, it is not sufficient for the echocardiographer to simply identify the existence of a residual lesion, as not all of these require reoperation. Here again, the surgeon's decision to accept any residual lesion or recommence bypass to effect further surgery may have to be in part guided by the experience of the echocardiographer in evaluating the colour flow map.

The Aims of Intraoperative Echocardiography in Congenital Heart Disease

As nowadays most of the cardiac surgery performed on patients with congenital heart disease is corrective surgery, the major aim of intraoperative echocardiography should be to provide the surgeon with an additional aid to achieve better and safer surgery. Surgical mortality in this complex cardiac surgery is already remarkably low. In the best series, the overall bypass mortality is 5% − 8%. To improve on this figure might be difficult, but a significant part of the mortality is due to the presence of major unsuspected residual or acquired lesions following bypass. The identification of these at the end of the operation and their subsequent correction during a second period of bypass prior to the patients transfer to the postoperative care area might lead to a further reduction in surgical mortality.

The Ultrasound Techniques Involved

A complete epicardial intraoperative study consists of two distinct parts: (1) the preoperative epicardial study and (2) the postoperative epicardial study following decannulation.

The Precardiopulmonary Bypass Study

The information derived from the precardiopulmonary bypass epicardial investigation should confirm both the morphologic and haemodynamic diagnoses, and rule out any unsuspected additional malformation. This high-resolution intraoperative cross-sectional scanning frequently contributes to a more precise understanding of detailed anatomy and morphology of the malformation than was available from either the praecordial ultrasound study or angiography. This may provide information which influences the surgical procedure (e.g. the relationship of an atrioventricular valve and subvalvular apparatus to a ventricular septal defect in cases where possible abnormal chordal implantation is suspected). It may also be of value in defining the most appropriate surgical approach (i.e. transatrial vs transpulmonary approach for closure of ventricular septal defect). In addition, the prebypass cardiac dimensions and ventricular performance are readily assessed (Table 1).

The intraoperative haemodynamic situation prior to bypass, with the chest open and the patient under anaesthesia, may differ substantially from the presurgical situation with the chest closed. The former can be rapidly evaluated by colour flow mapping. Specific abnormal features of the haemodynamic situation can then be quantified by means of pulsed and continuous wave Doppler investigation (e.g. pressure gradient across intracardiac shunts, stenoses). In our experience, when a comparison was made with the presurgical information, valuable new haemodynamic or morphologic insights were added in approximately onefifth of the cases in this series by the intraoperative prebypass study. In addition, although most of the information obtained from the prebypass study is already known, the prebypass findings (especially the colour flow maps) are essential for the interpretation of the subsequent postbypass study, as the findings of both have to be correlated before decisions can be made about the results of surgery.

The Postcardiopulmonary Bypass Study

The most important aim of the postcardiopulmonary bypass study is to exclude any important residual lesion, the presence of which might be life-threating or require further surgery in the first hours or days after surgery. (Secondary aims are to check on ventricular function and to exclude postbypass hypovolaemia). If any defects are present, the postbypass study has to

Table 1. Role of intraoperative ultrasound in congenital heart disease prior to commencement of bypass

1. To check preoperative diagnosis
2. To obtain base-line morphologic and haemodynamic information for comparison with the postbypass study
3. To determine or modify the operative approach (e.g., transatrial transpulmonary approach to ventricular septal defect closure)

Table 2. Role of intraoperative ultrasound in congenital heart disease after bypass

1.	Check the repair
2.	Gradient estimation
3.	Exclude significant residual shunts
4.	Left ventricular function check
5.	Hypovolaemia check

provide enough information to evaluate precisely the haemodynamic effects of both residual and surgically acquired lesions (Table 2). The findings have to be judged against a combination of factors: (a) the background findings of the prebypass investigation, (b) the possible long-term sequelae of residual defects (e.g. small residual ventricular septal defects may close spontaneously with time), and (c) the risks of a further period of cardiopulmonary bypass the need for definitive surgical repair.

The four most frequent residual problems following corrective surgery for congenital heart disease are: (1) residual intracardic shunts, (2) residual outflow tract obstruction, (3) valve regurgitation, and (4) impaired myocardial function. The routine postbypass imaging and colour flow mapping study is designed to confirm or exclude the presence of any such lesions. In any case where doubt exists following the combined imaging and colour flow studies, a contrast echo study can, in selected cases, contribute additional information (e.g. in differentiating between a small residual ventricular septal defect from a right ventricular outflow tract obstruction, both of which may be poorly defined on the cross-sectional image, and both of which have virtually identical colour flow mapping abnormalities within the right ventricular outflow tract).

The information obtained from the postcardiopulmonary bypass study has to be immediately and thoroughly discussed with the surgeon, especially in cases where the findings suggest that bypass should be resumed and further definitive repair attempted. In such a situation, there must be complete certainty in the results of the ultrasound examination, and the surgeon must have complete trust in the cardiologist interpreting the study. Unfortunately, the correct surgical decision to recommence bypass to effect further repair is not always as clear-cut as in the situation where the postbypass study demonstrates a residual atrial shunt following a Fontan procedure, or where a large second muscular ventricular septal defect is noted following the closure of what was suspected to be an isolated non-restrictive perimembranous ventricular septal defect. Much more experience has yet to be gained on both the advantages and pitfalls of intraoperative ultrasound in complex congenital lesions before any definitive conclusions can be drawn on its precise advantages and disadvantages.

The Epicardial Study

In children undergoing cardiac surgery for the correction of congenital heart disease, the pre- and postcardiopulmonary bypass epicardial studies are performed using multiple transducers, as no current generation single transducer can derive all the ultrasound information required in paediatric cases. We currently use a 5-MHz phased array transducer for optimal cross-sectional imaging of cardiac morphology, and a 3.75-MHz transducer for combined colour flow mapping and pulsed wave Doppler studies. In a subset of patients, either a 2.5-MHz duplex transducer or a continuous wave "pencil probe" is added to the ultrasound armamentarium for continuous wave Doppler quantification of high velocity jets.

The transducers and wires are packed in long sterile bags prior to connection to the ultrasound machine. A small amount of sterile gel is applied to the transducer tip prior to placement in the sterile bag, as this improves the transmission of ultrasound and hence the image quality. After sternotomy and pericardiotomy, but prior to cannulation for cardiopulmonary bypass, a complete echocardiographic investigation is performed after the pericardium has been opened.

Warm saline solution is poured into the pericardial sac to enlarge and improve the contact area between the transducer and the beating heart; this has the additional benefit of reducing any mechanical irritation of the heart which could cause arrhythmias. A continuous electrocardiogram is recorded via the auxilliary input of the machine and displayed on the video monitor of the ultrasound apparatus. Potential sources of electrical interference which create ultrasound artefacts such as diathermy should be switched off. The whole study is continuously recorded on video tape to allow subsequent slow-motion or frame-by-frame analysis.

The complete paediatric intraoperative study at our institution is performed and interpreted by a combination of the surgeon and cardiologist. Each pre- and postbypass study routinely consists of three parts:

1. A high-frequency (5 MHz) cross-sectional imaging study is done. Whenever possible, standard scan planes similar to those recorded from the praecordial approach should be used in order to facilitate interpretation and allow comparison with the prior praecordial examinations. In addition, many new and useful non-standard scan planes may be recorded from the epicardium which provide new and useful insights into the morphology of the underlying lesions. This part of the study is carried out to confirm the pre-operative diagnosis and obtain more precise information concerning the topographic anatomy and the morphology of the defect or malformation. Cardiac dimensions and ventricular performance can be readily assessed. M-mode tracings can be recorded which help in the precise evaluation of ventricular function and dimensions. A 5 MHz color flow map may be recorded.

2. Changing to the 3.75-MHz probe, optimal scan positions are chosen in order to perform colour flow mapping. Emphasis is placed on determining

the site and morphology of intracardiac shunts, the nature of valvular reguritations and the location of any areas of abnormal turbulent flow.

3. Subsequently, the quantification of blood flow velocities (pressure gradients) can be achieved by locating the pulsed wave Doppler sampling volumes or the continuous wave Doppler into the area of turbulence or maximum velocity as depicted in the colour map.

The postbypass study, following completion of the repair, should not be performed until the haemodynamic parameters (e.g. heart rate, systolic blood pressure) have returned to as near normal as possible, and all cannulae are removed. This latter point is of particular importance in neonates and infants, since the large diameter of cannulation tubes, relative to the vessel diameter, is likely to produce unpredictable intracardiac flow patterns, and hence pose problems in the exact interpretation of the findings. The same transducers should then be used in the same sequence and manner as described above for the prebypass study. A rapid on-line visual assessment should be made, and an initial impression of the results may be given to the surgeon if he wishes. Then, while the surgeon completes haemostasis and commences chest closure, the echocardiographer should immediately review the tape using careful frame-by-frame analysis. Normally, this can be completed in 5−10 min, and then the final conclusions can be discussed with the surgeon prior to chest closure.

Transoesophageal Studies

Compared with epicardial studies, an intraoperative investigation from the transoesophageal approach has (despite major inherent limitations) several potential advantages (Table 3).
The major advantages in practice are:

1. Ultrasound information can be obtained without interference with the surgical field. This means that the study can be performed without prolongation of surgical time, and that any potential risks of direct bacterial contamination of the operating field are excluded.

2. The scanning planes obtained by transoesophageal echo can contribute additional information relevant to the surgical repair, when compared to that obtained from an epicardial study. This is especially relevant concerning the morphology of atrial structures and atrioventricular valves. If prosthetic material casts ultrasound shadows when using the praecordial approach, then the transoesophageal approach can circumvent the problem by looking from „behind" the prosthetic material.

3. Although the image quality and the colour flow maps obtained by transoesophageal echo may be good, they are still markedly inferior to epicardial images because most transoesophageal probes have only half the number of ultrasound crystals present in the modern praecordial probes.

Table 3. Epicardial vs transoesophageal echocardiography in the intraoperative setting

Epicardial	TEE
1. Multiple imaging planes available	1. Limited imaging planes
2. Better image quality than TEE	2. Good image quality
3. Both PW and CW can be used to recorded velocity waveforms on line	3. No CW routinely available (poor alignment of PW/CW to intracardiac flows)
4. Good visualisation of all intracardiac structures	4. Poor visualisation of cardiac apex, anterior trabecular septum and right ventricular outflow tract
5. Possible in even smallest neonate (but limited image planes because of large transducer size)	5. Not possible at present in small children
6. Invades operative field (two or more transducers may be required)	6. Does not invade operative field
7. Flow masking by prosthetic material	7. Flow masking by prosthetic material
8. Multiple transducers of varying frequency can be used	8. Only one transducer can be used
9. Possible arrhythmogenicity	9. Very rarely arrhythmogenic
10. Possible interference with pacing wires, etc.	10. Interference with lines, anaesthetic management
11. No probe temperature problem due to short exposure	11. Possible oesophageal damage

PW, pulse wave; CW, continuous wave; TEE, transoesophageal echocardiography

4. The epicardial window is only available during surgery. In comparison, the transoesophageal echo can easily be used if problems arise after surgery and the findings can be easily correlated with the immediate postbypass information.

At present, the use of transoesophageal echo in surgery for congenital heart disease is limited to children older than 5 years, since the current range of transoesophageal transducers remain too large (15 mm max. diameter) to allow a completely safe introduction of the probe into smaller children. However, the development of smaller paediatric transoesophageal transducers is now underway. A further current limitation of the transoesophageal approach in the evaluation of complex congenital malformations is that the number of planes which can be scanned is limited both by transducer properties and by the spatial constraints of transducer manipulation within the oesophagus. A relatively small multiplanar or rotating oesophageal ultrasound device will have to be developed to image the multiple planes which can be scanned from the epicardial approach. Thus, at present, a complete diagnostic transoesophageal intraoperative study can rarely be achieved in the majority of complex cardiac malformations. This is especially true in cases where the malformations include abnormalities of the anterior rabecular septum, the muscular outlet septum and the right ventricular outflow tract, as all three are normally "blind areas" to any transoesophageal approach. Thus, in our experience the transoesophageal approach remains second best to the epicardial study in the majority of complex lesions in terms of both image quality and the planes which can be scanned.

In clinical practise, the transoesophageal probe is introduced after complete preparation for surgery by the anaesthesist. Prior to introducing the probe, all other catheters in the oesophagus should be removed. The probe is then normally left in place throughout the whole operation, but has to be switched off while not in use in order to avoid any risk of thermal damage to the oesophagus. A cross-sectional imaging study to record multiple imaging sections is followed by a colour flow mapping study and pulsed Doppler measurements where appropriate.

Problems and Limitations Associated with Intraoperative Echocardiography

Analysis Problems

Cross-sectional imaging alone fails to provide complete intraoperative information either before or after the repair. Colour flow mapping is, in our experience, a necessary adjunct to any complete study. However, the use of colour flow mapping provides us with the problem of how to handle and interpret the very complex information obtained by this technique. Intraoperative on-line analysis of a colour flow map from the rapidly beating infant heart is often extremely difficult, even if the study is performed by a very experienced echocardiographer. Real-time analysis leads to many mistakes even in the most experienced hands. Therefore, for the precise analysis of the complex flow maps, an immediate precise "off-line" frame-to-frame analysis by a number of echocardiographers often produces the best results.

Image Masking by Prosthetic Material

Any prosthetic material used for correction of a lesion potentially limits the ultrasound assessment of the haemodynamic situation in the postbypass study. As well as the well-recognised ultrasound shadow which exists behind valve prostheses, virtually every synthetic intracardiac material produces a similar ultrasound shadow which interferes with both imaging and colour flow mapping. Conduits of woven Dacron material or Gore Tex cause the biggest problems. In our experience, even little pledgets of Teflon or suture material can produce shadows in the colour map producing consequent problems in interpretation. Frequently, a combined study using transoesophageal and epicardial echocardiography represents the only possibility to scan all the blind areas behind implanted prosthetic material.

Transducer Design

The most frequently used epicardial transducers are those which are used for the routine praecordial studies. These can limit the number of scanning positions because of their shape and large size, relative to the small dimensions of both the thoracotomy and heart in neonates and infants. Frequently, the optimal imaging planes cannot be scanned and this may result in a less than optimal study. The current commercially available intraoperative high-frequency (i.e. 1.5 MHz) transducers are small, linear array transducers. They, too, are not optimally suited for epicardial use in cardiac surgery of small infants, as, firstly, their size and shape does not allow obtaining views other than from the front of the heart and, secondly, they have a large contact area because of their linear array configuration. In contrast, the ideal clinical transducer would be a phased array or mechanical device with a small contact area, designed to fit between the heart and surrounding tissues. It should be a small, extremely flat device, scanning at an angle. It should have rounded edges to decrease arrhythmogenicity. It should be mounted on a special holding device so that the surgeon can manoeuvre it to inaccessible areas. Such transducers (currently under development) should allow imaging of the heart from areas previously not accessible, such as from the back of the atria (equivalent to a transesohageal image), the lateral borders of the heart, and directly over the aorta and pulmonary artery. Such high-quality multiplane imaging of both the heart and the great vessels from any desired point of view should further increase the diagnostic precision of the intraoperative study.

Arrhythmias

Occasionally, arrhythmias can be caused by epicardial scanning (more often, in our experience, during the post- then the prebypass phase). Mechanical irritation of the heart is normally the cause. The use of saline poured into the pericardial sac (as well as improving ultrasound transduction) helps to minimise mechanical irritation. During our 1-year experience of intraoperative studies in congenital heart disease, we did not provoke any serious arrhythmias. The most commonly encountered rhythm abnormalities were isolated premature ventricular beats or short runs of self-terminating ventricular tachycardia (maximum five beats). Cardioversion due to an ultrasound-provoked arrhythmia was never required.

Infection

The possibility of iatrogenic infection related to intraoperative epicardial scanning is a potential problem. However, both in reviewing our own experience and according to the current information in the literature, there have been no reports of an increase in the frequency of early postsurgical endocarditis. Not only microorganisms introduced into the chest by direct contact with the transducer, but also microorganisms extruded into the atmosphere of the surgical theatre from the cooling fans of the ultrasound machine must be considered.

Costs

Finally, intraoperative echocardiography is an expensive technique; one ultrasound machine remains in the operating theatre for hours in order to perform two studies of only a few minutes duration. The apparatus is therefore used considerably less efficiently than in the outpatient clinic. Nevertheless, we are convinced that the information derived from intraoperative echocardiography will be seen to be of great clinical value in surgery for complex congenital heart disease. Although the impact on surgical technique, postoperative management, and surgical mortality can be estimated only after very large series of patients, we are convinced that intraoperative echo has now come to the cardiac surgical theatre to stay, as an important adjunct to the surgical management of congenital heart disease.

References

1. Spotnitz HM, Malm JR, King DL et al. (1978) Outflow tract obstruction in tetralogy of Fallot: intraoperative analysis by echocardiography. NY State J Med 6:1100–3
2. Spotnitz HM, Malm JR (1982) Two-dimensional ultrasound and cardiac operations. J Thorac Cardiovasc Surg 83:43–51
3. Sahn DJ (1981) Intraoperative applications of two-dimensional and contrast two-dimensional echocardiography for evaluation of congenital, acquired and coronary heart disease in open-chested humans during cardiac surgery. In: Rijsterborgh H (ed) Echocardiology. Martinus Nijhoff, The Hague, pp 8–23
4. Sahn DJ (1982) Application of two-dimensional echocardiography during open heart surgery in humans for evaluation of acquired and coronary heart disease. In: Hanrath P, Bleifeld W, Souquet J (eds) Cardiovascular diagnosis by ultrasound. Martinus Nijhoff, The Hague, pp 294–307
5. Gussenhoven EJ, Essed CE, Villeneuve VH (1982) Two-dimensional echocardiographic diagnosis of atrial and ventricular septal defects. Is it reliable? J Cardiovasc Ultrasonography 1(4):367–372
6. Goldman ME, Mindish BP, Teichholz LE, Burgess N, Staville K, Fuster V (1984) Intraoperative contrast echocardiography to evaluate mitral valve operations. J Am Coll Cardiol 4(5):1035–40
7. Van Herwerden LA, Gussenhoven WJ, Roelandt J, Bos E, Ligtvoet CM, Haalebos MM, Mochtar B, Leicher F, Witsenburg M (1986) Intraoperative epicardial two-dimensional echocardiography. Eur Heart J 7:386–395
8. Takamoto S, Kyo S, Adachi H, Matsumura M, Yokote Y, Omoto R (1985) Intraoperative color flow mapping by real time two-dimensional Doppler echocardiography for evaluation of valvular and congenital heart disease and vascular disease. J Thorac Cardiovasc Surg 90:802–812
9. de Bruyn NP, Clements FM, Kisslo JA (1987) Intraoperative transesophageal color flow mapping: initial experience. Anesth Analg 66:386–390

Transesophageal Echocardiography Adds to Decision Making During Valvular Heart Surgery

K. H. SHEIKH, N. P. DE BRUIJN, J. S. RANKIN, T. STANLEY, F. M. CLEMENTS, and J. KISSLO

Introduction

The first intraoperative, epicardial M-mode echocardiograms were performed in 1972 to assess postoperative valve function in patients undergoing mitral valve commissurotomy and prosthetic valve replacement [13]. It was, however, not until the early 1980s that echocardiography became recognized as a potentially useful intraoperative tool. The first two-dimensional (2-D) intraoperative echocardiogram, reporting echo-guided surgical removal of a foreign body, was from Duke University in 1981 [10]. Subsequently, Spotnitz and Malm [21] first reported epicardial 2-D imaging to be a safe and useful procedure in patients undergoing a variety of cardiac operations. The recent introduction of Doppler color flow mapping has provided the ability to not only assess structure, but also to simultaneously assess blood flow [23].

The development and implementation of both ambulatory and intraoperative transesophageal imaging (TEE) has followed a similar course. The transesophageal approach to cardiac imaging was first introduced in 1976 [6]. With the development of 2-D and Doppler capabilities, it has also become recognized as a valuable diagnostic tool in a variety of clinical settings. In the intraoperative setting, epicardial imaging appears to be superior to TEE in regards to permitting scanning in a greater variety of planes and providing better images of structures in the anterior portion of the heart such as the tricuspid and pulmonic valves [1, 4]. The size of the transesophageal probe prohibits its use in small children. Thus for complex congenital heart disease, epicardial imaging appears to be better suited [24]. However, most adult operations involve the left ventricle and aortic and mitral valves, all of which are imaged quite well from the transesophageal approach. TEE has proven valuable in the assessment of native aortic and mitral valves, prosthetic valves, intracardiac masses, aortic aneurysms and dissection, congenital heart diseases, endocarditis, atrial septal defects and in visualization of proximal coronary segments. TEE also permits alignment of the ultrasound beam more parallel to both antegrade and retrograde flow across the mitral valve, and thus improves the ability to detect regurgitant mitral flow. Furthermore, in contrast to epicardial imaging, TEE permits continuous intraoperative imaging without any interruption of the operative procedure or intrusion into the surgical field. For these reasons, the transesophageal approach may be particularly well suited for routine application in adult cardiac surgery.

Transesophageal Echocardiography
Edited by R. Erbel et al.
© Springer-Verlag Berlin Heidelberg 1989

Methods

Patients. Among nearly 2000 TEE studies performed to date at Duke University Medical Center, over 150 have been performed in patients having cardiac valve operations. This includes patients having both aortic and mitral valve surgery, multiple valve operations, and operations involving combined valve replacement and coronary bypass grafting. The vast majority of operations have been for valve replacement, although the increasing popularity of primary valve repair has resulted in experience with this type of operation as well.

Echocardiographic Studies. Initially, only 2-D TEE images were obtained using a Diasonics 3400R imaging unit (Milpitas, California) and a 3.5-MHz transesophageal probe. Doppler color flow imaging was introduced into routine usage in May 1987, and all subsequent studies have been performed with a Hewlett-Packard 77020CF imaging unit, fitted with a 5-MHz transducer.

Following induction of general anesthesia and endotracheal intubation, the probe is placed in the esophagus, approximately 30–45 cm from the teeth. Initial images are obtained prior to skin incision. Subsequent images are obtained during the operation as warranted, and after removal from cardiopulmonary bypass (CPB), prior to skin closure. Standard images obtained in all patients include a long axis view of the left atrium, left ventricle, mitral and aortic valves, a short axis view of the left ventricle at the papillary muscle level, a four chamber view allowing visualization of the two atrio-ventricular valves and all four cardiac chambers and an interatrial septal view. Additional views are obtained pertinent to the disease entity and at the discretion of the operator as the clinical situation warrants. Doppler color flow imaging is performed with manipulation of the transducer tip to interrogate blood flow in multiple planes.

Echocardiographic Interpretation. Preliminary interpretations of all studies are rendered by the anesthesiologist performing the study during the operative procedure, with consultation from senior cardiology staff available at all times. All operative decisions are based upon this information. During initial application of 2-D and, subsequently, Doppler color flow imaging, all studies were performed under the direction of a senior cardiologist-echocardiographer (J.K.). Unsuspected findings are diagnosed if information obtained by preoperative TEE is conflicting or additional to that known from preoperative evaluation. A minor unsuspected finding is diagnosed if the information is used to assist or modify, but not alter, the planned surgery. A major unsuspected finding is diagnosed if the information significantly changes the planned operation.

Ventricular function is evaluated from left ventricular short axis views. Segmental wall motion is graded by previously established qualitative criteria [3]. Decreased postoperative ventricular function is defined as the presence of new or worsened segmental wall motion or an overall global decrease in ventricular function.

Valvular function is similarly assessed by comparison of pre- and final postoperative images, following removal from CPB. Prior to use of Doppler color flow imaging, valve function and insufficiency was assessed by 2-D visualization of cusp mobility and injection of agitated saline with imaging of the chamber expected to receive regurgitant flow. With the use of Doppler color flow imaging, valvular insufficiency and antegrade turbulence are compared in pre- and postoperative examinations. Given that color flow imaging provides 2-D flow information, valvular insufficiency is estimated visually by integrating *both* the maximum width *and* depth of the color flow jet into the chamber receiving regurgitant flow and graded as none, mild, moderate, or severe [11, 17]. A residual valvular defect is defined as: (a) valvular insufficiency noted to be of moderate degree or greater by either saline contrast or color flow examination; (b) the presence of abnormal antegrade turbulence through a repaired or prosthetic valve or in the left ventricular outflow tract; or (c) abnormal cusp mobility of a repaired or prosthetic valve.

Results and Discussion

Preoperative Utility. We have noted transesophageal echocardiography to add new diagnostic information which either aids or changes the operative procedure in 15%−20% of operations performed for valvular heart disease. In 8%−10% of cases the unsuspected findings are of minor significance, consisting primarily of identification of left atrial thrombi, elongated mitral valve chordae, and atrial septal defects. In these cases, this information may result in modification of the planned surgery. In 5%−10% of cases, the unsuspected findings are of major significance, generally involving identification of unsuspected valvular abnormalities, prompting unplanned valvular surgery. The frequency of unsuspected findings is highest in patients undergoing combined 2-D and Doppler color flow examinations and also in those having mitral valve operations.

Similar results have been reported using combined epicardial and Doppler color flow imaging, in which case 15% of patients undergoing cardiac valve operations have a change in planned surgical therapy based upon echocardiographic results [22]. We have also noted a significant additional impact of epicardial echocardiography with Doppler color flow imaging to the preoperative plan in patients undergoing operations for congenital heart disease, with a 23% incidence of unsuspected findings [24].

There are likely many reasons for detecting unsuspected findings using preoperative TEE. It does not appear, however, that an inadequate preoperative evaluation is one, as over 50% of patients have had preoperative chest echocardiography with Doppler examinations and over 95% have had preoperative cardiac catheterization. All patients are evaluated by several senior staff personnel, including both surgeons and cardiologists, prior to surgery. It appears more likely that the detection of unsuspected findings relates to the nature of the disease entity as well as to the intrinsic limitations of preoperative evaluation techniques and the relative advantages of preoperative TEE.

Certainly, an important advantage of peroperative TEE is that the study is performed immediately prior to the operation. Conditions which can potentially change with time are most likely to be affected by the results of immediately preoperative TEE. Such was the case in two patients with acute aortic dissections who were newly diagnosed with acute cardiac tamponade and acute aortic insufficiency. Ischemic mitral dysfunction may also be very labile and subject to the influences of ongoing ischemia as well as the success of reperfusion therapy [12]. In the patient receiving reperfusion therapy, mitral function assessed at the time of cardiac catheterization may be quite different than that at the time of coronary bypass grafting. We have detected instances of mitral insufficiency at the time of bypass grafting which was not present at the time of cardiac catheterization, prompting mitral valve repair surgery. Conversely, we have also noted patients who have had mitral insufficiency at the time of cardiac catheterization which was negligible at the time of surgery, thus saving the patient from a mitral operation.

Unsuspected findings are also detected by preoperative TEE due to limitations of preoperative cardiac catheterization and echocardiography. Echo-Doppler examinations from the chest approach may be limited by poor sound transmission, limited acoustic windows, and masking of ultrasound signal by prosthetic valves and other intervening echogenic materials. These factors may limit the resolution of chest echocardiography in the assessment of submitral morphology, the native mitral valve, prosthetic valves, and intracardiac thrombi. Structural information, such as the identification of thrombi, submitral morphology, valvular vegetations and aortic root morphology, which can only be obtained echocardiographically may be better obtained by TEE. The ability to place the Doppler signal parallel to blood flow also enhances the ability to properly assess regurgitant lesions. Particularly in regards to mitral valve repair, the assessment of submitral morphology is important as inadequate attention to submitral repair has been cited as a reason for technical failure of this operation [16].

Similarly, intrinsic limitations in cardiac catheterization influence its ability to detect certain abnormalities. As noted above, certain structural abnormalities can only be assessed by echocardiography. Furthermore, while coronary angiography, left ventriculography, and assessment of left ventricular hemodynamics are usually performed during routine cardiac catheterization, unless clinically suspected, aortography, right ventriculography, and assessment of right sided hemodynamics and for subaortic outflow tract obstruction are not routinely performed. With the use of Doppler color flow imaging, aortic insufficiency, tricuspid insufficiency, and subaortic obstruction not detected by cardiac catheterization, can be detected by preoperative TEE.

While it can be argued that many of the findings detected by preoperative TEE would have been detected at the time of surgery, we feel that preoperative knowledge of the findings is important for several reasons. The information provided by TEE saves inspection time, reduces CPB time and provides independent confirmation of structural information to the surgeon under physiologic conditions, prior to cardiac exposure. Furthermore, information about cardiac flows provided by Doppler examination is unique and unavailable at the time of direct inspection.

Postoperative Influence. Postoperative TEE is an important means to assess surgical results and postoperative ventricular function. We have noted inadequate initial surgical results in 5% of cases diagnosed by post-CPB TEE, resulting in immediate further surgery. Frequently, such findings have not been detected by hemodynamic measurements. Assessing surgical results for adequacy is particularly important in mitral valve surgery, given that either postoperative left ventricular outflow obstruction or residual mitral insufficiency prompt repeat cardiopulmonary bypass and further operation in 12%–17% of cases [1, 4, 9, 22]. Left ventricular outflow tract obstruction has been reported as an important complication of mitral valve repair, occuring in 10% of cases and contributing to symptoms of congestive heart failure, syncope, and residual mitral insufficiency [7]. Residual mitral insufficiency following mitral valve repair has been cited as a cause of increased postoperative morbidity and mortality [2, 7, 16].

A variety of methods have been proposed to test postoperative competency of the mitral valve. These include fluid filling of the arrested ventricle, direct palpation of the left atrium for regurgitation, hemodynamic assessments using pulmonary capillary or left atrial pressures, and echocardiographic assessment using either agitated saline or Doppler color flow mapping. Previous studies have emphasized the importance of assessing mitral competency under physiologic conditions and thus techniques such as fluid filling of the arrested left ventricle, left atrial pressure monitoring, direct palpation, and saline contrast injection lack sensitivity in comparison to echocardiography as tests for mitral competency and may be more complex and time consuming [5, 15].

Further testimony to the importance of assessing postoperative results and attempting to leave as little valve insufficiency as possible are the findings of this study indicating a poor prognosis in patients with residual valve insufficiency of moderate degree. Patients with moderate residual defects post-CPB had a 85% postoperative complication rate (congestive heart failure and need for repeat valve surgery) and a 45% mortality rate, compared to 20% and 5% respectively in those without residual defects (p < 0.05 for both). These results confirm previous observations that residual valvular defects, even of moderate degree, carry a higher morbidity and mortality in the postoperative period [2, 16].

Postoperative TEE is useful in identifying patients with decreased ventricular function. Pharmacologic or mechanical ventricular support has been instituted in 10% of cases due to TEE-documented ventricular dysfunction. Patients with persistent decreases in ventricular function carry a poor postoperative prognosis, with a 75% complication rate and a 25% mortality, in comparison to 10% and 5% respectively in those with preserved left ventricular function (p < 0.05 for both). These results are in accord with previous work indicating that postoperative ventricular function abnormalities will be detected in 9%−30% of cases and that such abnormalities identify patients at higher risk for postoperative complications [18, 19].

Safety. We have encountered no complications related to TEE probe placement or imaging in any patient in the current series. The safety of both ambulatory and intraoperative TEE has now been documented in several large retrospective and prospective studies [8, 14, 20]. The only significant complications reported to date have been minor arrhythmias, related to increased vagal tone during positioning of the probe in ambulatory patients.

Conclusions

Intraoperative TEE is a safe and useful tool in patients undergoing cardiac valve operations. Its utility is enhanced with use of combined 2-D and Doppler color flow imaging. Immediately preoperative TEE assists in formulating the surgical plan. Post-CBP TEE assists in evaluating surgical results and in guiding implementation of hemodynamic support. Postoperative residual valve defects or decreased ventricular function identify patients at risk for major complications and mortality. Intraoperative TEE should be encouraged in most patients undergoing cardiac valve operations.

References

1. Bolger A, Czer LS, Friedman A, Kleinman J, DeRobertis M, Chaux A, Maurer G (1988) Intraoperative transesophageal color Doppler imaging: advantages and limitations. J Am Coll Cardiol 11:217A
2. Carpentier A, Chauvaud S, Fabiani JN, Deloche A, Relland J, Lessana A, d'Allaines Cl, Blondeau Ph, Piwnica A, Dubost Ch (1980) Reconstructive surgery of mitral valve incompetence: ten year appraisal. J Thorac Cardiovasc Surg 79:338−348
3. Clements FM, de Bruijn NP (1987) Perioperative evaluation of regional wall motion by transesophageal two-dimensional echocardiography. Anesth Analg 66:248−261
4. Currie PJ, Stewart WJ, Salcedo EE, Agler DA, Lytle BM, Gill CC, Cosgrove DM (1988) Comparison of intraoperative transesophageal and epicardial color flow Doppler in mitral valve repair. J Am Coll Cardiol 11:20A
5. Czer LSC, Maurer G, Bolger AF, DeRobertis M, Resser KJ, Kass RM, Lee ME, Blanche C, Chaux A, Gray RJ, Matloff JM (1987) Intraoperative evaluation of mitral regurgitation by Doppler color flow mapping. Circulation [Suppl. 3] 76:108
6. Frazin L, Talano JV, Stephanides L, Loeb HS, Kopel L, Gunnar RM (1976) Esophageal echocardiography. Circulation 54:102−108
7. Galler M, Kronzon I, Slater J, Lighty GW, Politzer F, Colvin S, Spencer F (1986) Long-term follow-up after mitral valve reconstruction: incidence of postoperative left ventricular outflow obstruction. Circulation 75(1):99
8. Geibel A, Kasper W, Behroz A, Przewolka U, Meinertz T, Just H (1988) Risk of transesophageal echocardiography in awake patients with cardiac diseases. Am J Cardiol 62:337−339

9. Goldman ME, Mindich BP, Teichholz LE, Burgess N, Staville K, Fuster V (1984) Intraoperative contrast echocardiography to evaluate mitral valve operations. J Am Coll Cardiol 4(5):1035−1040

10. Harrison LH, Kisslo JA, Sabiston DC (1981) Extraction of intramyocardial foreign body utilizing operative ultrasonography. J Thorac Cardiovasc Surg 82:345−349

11. Helmcke F, Nanda NC, Hsiung MC, Soto B, Adey CK, Goyal RG, Gatewood RP (1987) Color Doppler assessment of mitral regurgitation with orthogonal planes. Circulation 75(1):175−183

12. Hickey MStJ, Smith R, Muhlbaier LH, Harrell FE, Reves JG, Hinohara T, Califf RM, Pryor DB, Rankin JS (1988) Current prognosis of ischemic mitral regurgitation: implications for future management. Circulation 78(1):51−59

13. Johnson ML, Holmes JH, Spangler RD, Paton BR (1972) Usefulness of echocardiography in patients undergoing mitral valve surgery. J Thorac Cardiovasc Surg 64:922−934

14. Kremer P, Cahalan M, Beaupre P, Schroder E, Hanrath P, Heinrich H, Ahnefeld FW, Bleifeld W, Hamilton W (1985) Intraoperative Überwachung mittels transoesophagealer zweidimensionaler Echokardiographie. Anaesthesist 34:111−117

15. Maurer G, Czer LSC, Chaux A, Bolger AF, DeRobertis M, Resser K, Kass RM, Lee MS, Matloff JM (1987) Intraoperative Doppler color flow mapping for assessment of valve repair for mitral regurgitation. Am J Cardiol 60:333−337

16. Nunley DL, Starr A (1983) The evolution of reparative techniques for the mitral valve. Ann Thorac Surg 37:393−397

17. Perry GJ, Helmcke F, Nanda NC, Byard C, Soto B (1987) Evaluation of aortic insufficiency by Doppler color flow mapping. J Am Coll Cardiol 9:952−959

18. Ren JF, Panidis IP, Kotler MN, Mintz GW, Goel I, Ross J (1985) Effect of coronary bypass surgery and valve replacement on left ventricular function: assessment by intraoperative two-dimensional echocardiography. Am Heart J 109:281

19. Rubenson DS, Tucker CR, London E, Miller DC, Stinson EB, Popp RL (1982) Two-dimensional echocardiographic analysis of segmental left ventricular wall motion before and after coronary artery bypass surgery. Circulation 5:1025−1031

20. Schluter M, Hinrichs A, Thier W, Kremer P, Schroder S, Cahalan MK, Hanrath P (1984) Transesophageal two-dimensional echocardiography: comparison of ultrasonic and anatomic sections. J Am Coll Cardiol 53:1173−1178

21. Spotnitz HM, Malm JR (1982) Two-dimensional ultrasound and cardiac operations. J Thorac Cardiovasc Surg 83:43−51

22. Stewart WJ, Currie PJ, Lytle BW, Gill CC, Cosgrove DM (1988) The role of intraoperative echocardiography during cardiac valvular surgery. J Am Coll Cardiol 11:217A

23. Takamoto S, Kyo S, Adachi H, Matsumura M, Yokote Y, Omoto R, Buckley MJ (1985) Intraoperative color flow mapping by real-time two-dimensional Doppler echocardiography for evaluation of valvular and congenital heart disease and vascular disease. J Thorac Cardiovasc Surg 90:802−812

24. Ungerleider RM, Greeley WJ, Sheikh KH, Philips J, Kisslo JA (1988) Routine intraoperative epicardial pre and post bypass color flow imaging simplifies evaluation of repairs for congenital heart defects. Circulation 78:II−649

Echocardiographic Follow-up After Surgery for Congenital Heart Diseases

W. KASPER, A. GEIBEL, T. HOFMANN, N. TIEDE, G. SPILLNER, V. SCHLOSSER, and H. JUST

Introduction

The diagnostic impact of transesophageal echocardiography in congenital heart diseases of adults is still unsettled. This is especially true after surgery for congenital heart disease. Therefore, in patients who had been operated on because of severe congenital heart disease we studied whether transesophageal echocardiography reveals additional diagnostic information in comparison to transthoracic imaging.

Patients and Methods

Over a period of 54 months a total of 123 patients with congenital heart disease were studied using transthoracic and transesophageal echocardiography. The echocardiographic examination was performed after surgery for congenital heart disease in 26 (21%) of these patients. This patient population formed the basis for this presentation. Twelve patients were studied after closure of an atrial septal defect, four patients after closure of a ventricular septal defect, and four patients after surgery for a tetralogy of Fallot. In five patients echocardiographic studies were performed after surgery for an aortic coarctation and in one patient after closure of a patent ductus arteriosus.

The echocardiographic examinations were performed with a commercially available phased array imaging system with 2.25- and 3.5-MHz probes for the transthoracic approach and 3.5- and 3.75-MHz transducers mounted on the tip of a gastroscope for obtaining transesophageal images. The echocardiographic studies were recorded on video tapes for subsequent evaluation. In transthoracic imaging apical two- and four-chamber views and left parasternal long- and short-axis view were obtained using the subcostal and suprasternal approach. Transesophageal imaging was performed after local anesthesia with lidocaine spray.

Contrast injection to reveal left to right and right to left shunts was done into a left antecubital vein. Contrast effects were generated by the use of 10 ml agitated oxypolygelatin solution, a commercially available plasma substitute (Gelifundol). Each contrast injection was immediately followed by a 10 ml flush injection of a standard 0.9% saline solution.

Transesophageal Echocardiography
Edited by R. Erbel et al.
© Springer-Verlag Berlin Heidelberg 1989

Results

Twelve patients were studied after closure of an atrial septal defect, four men and eight women with a mean age 38 ± 12 years (Table 1). Echocontrast studies were performed in 11 of these patients, and in two patients color flow imaging was also used. Recurrence of a left to right shunt was detected in three patients. Visualization of the atrial septal defect was not possible using the transthoracic approach in any of these patients. However, the atrial septum defect was detected in two patients using the transesophageal technique. In one of these two patients the defect could be visualized only after peripheral contrast injection (Fig. 1). In one additional patient, recurrence of an atrial septal defect was detected with the color flow mapping technique from both the transthoracic and the transesophageal approaches (Fig. 2). A defect of the atrial septum was not detectable in this patient, either by the transthoracic or by the transesohageal approach.

The diagnosis of a left to right shunt at the interatrial level, e.g., a negative contrast phenomenon at the interatrial septum defect, could be made in none of the patients using the transthoracic apporach and in two patients using the transesophageal approach. One patient had a left superior vena cava which could only be visualized using the transesophageal approach (Fig. 3). Its presence could be deduced using the transthoracic approach after a left-sided peripheral contrast injection.

One patient was studied immediately after surgical closure of an atrial septal defect because of a low output syndrome. The transthoracic echocardiogram revealed an echodense mass behind the left and right atria. Further differentiation of this mass was not possible using the transthoracic approach. Transesophageal imaging demonstrated an echodense mass with a liquid area within the structure, which is typical for a hematoma with partial organization (Fig. 4). The mass protruded into the atrial septum and expanded towards the base of the aorta. It seemed to be the cause of an inflow obstruction of the right ventricle.

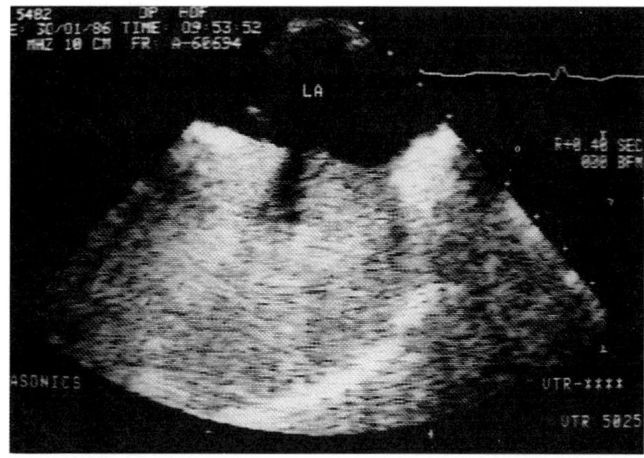

Fig. 1. Transesophageal echocardiogram of a 30-year-old patient with a small sized defect (6 mm) of the atrial septum and a negative contrast phenomenon at the defect. *LA*, Left atrium

Table 1. Patients after closure of an atrial septal defect

Case	Age (years)	Sex	$2D^e$ defect		color defect		NCP 2D defect		Other anomalies	
			TTE	TEE	TTE	TEE	TTE	TEE	TTE	TEE
1	65	m	−	−	nd	nd	−	−	−	−
2	30	m	−	+[a]	nd	nd	−	+	−	−
3	40	m	−	−	nd	nd	−	−	−	−
4	30	f	−	−	nd	nd	−	−	−	−
5	45	f	−	−	nd	nd	nd	nd	−	−
6	28	f	−	−	nd	nd	−	−	−	−
7	48	m	−	+[b]	nd	nd	−	+	TI	TI
8	44	f	−	−	nd	nd	−	−	SVC[c]	SVC[d]
9	33	f	−	−	+	+	−	−	−	−
10	20	f	−	−	nd	nd	−	−	mass	hematoma
11	30	f	−	−	nd	nd	−	−	−	−
12	41	f	−	−	−	−	−	−	−	−

Abbreviations: m, male; f, female; 2D, nd, not done; NCP, negative contrast phenomenon; TTE, transthoracic echocardiography; TEE, transesophageal echocardiography; TI, tricuspide insufficiency; SVC, superior vena cava
[a] 6 mm; [b] 12 mm; [c] Deduced; [d] Identified; [e] 2D, two dimensional

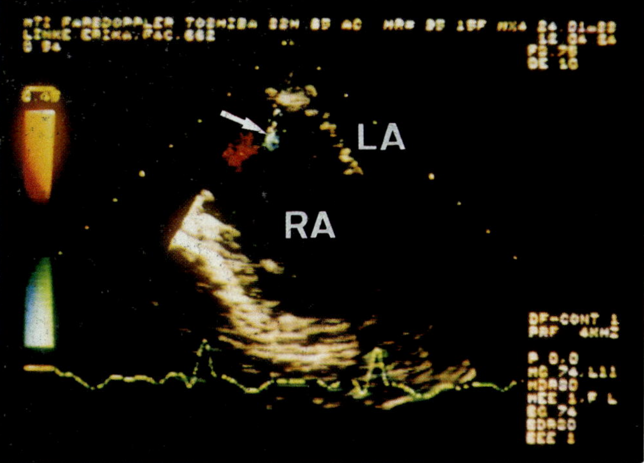

Fig. 2. Transesophageal echocardiogram which showed a small color defect at the atrial septum defect in the vicinity of the superior vena cava. This color defect was also detected from the transthoracic approach. *RA*, right atrium; *LA*, left atrium

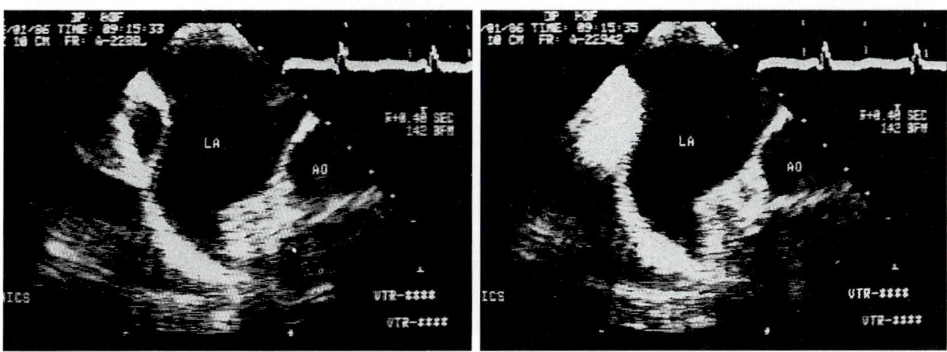

Fig. 3. Transesophageal echocardiogram in a patient with a left superior vena cava before (*left*) and after (*right*) an echocontrast injection. *AO*, aorta; *LA*, left atrium

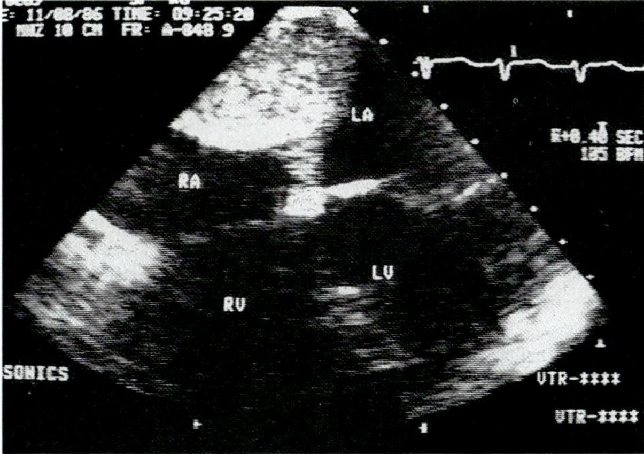

Fig. 4. Transesophageal echocardiogram of a patient with an echodense mass behind the right and left atria after surgery. The liquid areas within that mass were typical of bleeding. *RA*, right atrium; *LA*, left atrium; *RV*, right ventricle; *LV*, left ventricle

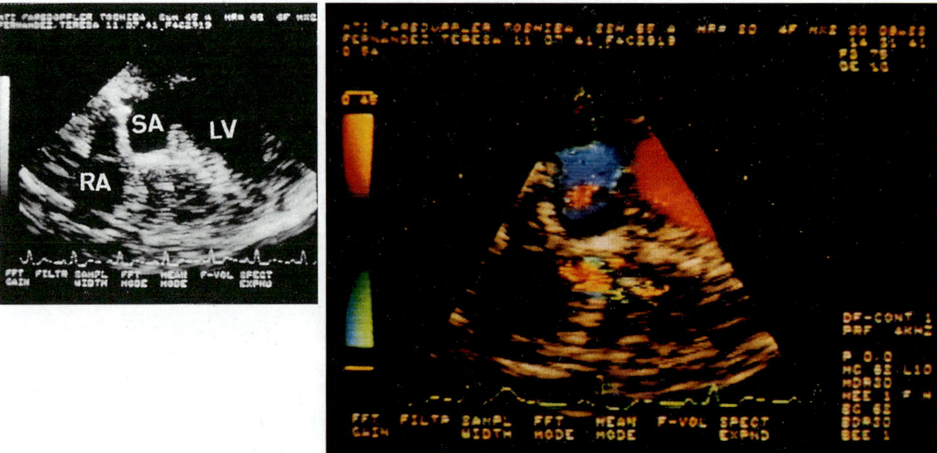

Fig. 5. Transesophageal echocardiogram of a patient after repair of a ventricular septum defect. A large septum aneurysm was present (*left*); the color flow mapping study revealed leaks at the insertion of the patch (*right*). *RA*, right atrium; *LV*, left ventricle; *SA*, septum aneurysm

Two out of four patients who were studied after closure of a ventricular septal defect were found to have a leak in the patch (Table 2). This leakage was detected during color flow imaging study using both the transthoracic and the transesophageal approach (Fig. 5). Four patients were studied after operation of a tetralogy of Fallot (Table 2). Surgical correction was done in three patients and a Blalock anastomosis in one patient. A ventricular septum defect was detected in two of the four patients using both the transthoracic and the transesophageal approach.

Table 2. Patients after closure of a ventricular septum defect (cases 1−4) and operation of a tetralogy of Fallot (cases 5−8)

Case	Age (years)	Sex	2D defect		Color defect		PCP-LV	
			TTE	TEE	TTE	TEE	TTE	TEE
1	44	m	−	−	nd	nd	−	−
2	47	f	−	−	+	+	+	+
3	24	f	−	−	+	+	−	−
4	50	f	−	−	nd	nd	nd	−
5	20	f	−	−	nd	nd	+	+[c]
6	35	m	−	−	+	+	−	−
7	18	m	−	−	nd	nd	−	−
8	39	m	+[a]	+[b]	nd	nd	−	−

Abbreviations: m, male; f, female; nd, not done; PCP, positive contrast phenomenon; LV, left ventricle; TTE, transthoracic echocardiograhy; TEE, transesophageal echocardiography
[a] 36 mm; [b] 38 mm; [c] foramen ovale

Five patients were studied after operation for an aortic coarctation. A patch repair was performed in four patients and a bypass implanted between the left subclavian artery and the descending thoracic aorta in the other patient. A reduction of the lumen of the isthmic portion of the descending thoracic aorta from 22 ± 5 mm to 13 ± 1 mm was seen from the transesophageal view in the patients in whom a patch repair was done. The bypass to the descending thoracic aorta was only visualized using the transesophageal approach. A large hematoma was detected around the descending thoracic aorta at the side of the implantation of the bypass graft. This bleeding was not detected using the transthoracic approach. Dissection of the descending thoracic aorta could not be excluded using the transesophageal approach. This patient suffered from recurrent hemoptysis. At surgery, a communication between the bypass graft and the pulmonary bronchial system was found.

Discussion

There has been increasing interest in transesophageal echocardiography because of its superior imaging quality in comparison to transthoracic echocardiography [1]. However, transesophageal echocardiography has not yet seen wide use in patients with congenital heart disease [2]. Thus, we studied the diagnostic impact of this imaging technique in a subgroup of patients operated on because of severe congenital heart disease. After surgery, most of the patients had inconspicuous echocardiograms from both the transthoracic and the transesophageal approaches. However, in two patients with bleeding complications, in one patient immediately after operation of an atrial septal defect and in the other 9 years after operation of an aortic coarctation, the complications were only correctly identified by transesophageal echocardiography.

Recurrence of a left to right shunt in three patients after closure of an atrial septal defect was detected by transesophageal echocardiography, but only in one patient using the transthoracic approach. In contrast, leakage of the patch on a ventricular septum defect was detected with both the transthoracic and the transesophageal approach.

Thus, it is evident, even in this small group of patients, that transesophageal echocardiography has considerable diagnostic impact in follow-up of patients after operation for congenital heart disease.

References

1.   Schlüter M, Thier W, Hinrichs A, Kremer P, Siglow V, Hanrath P (1984) Klinischer Einsatz der transösophagealen Echokardiographie. Dtsch Med Wochenschr 109:722
2.   Hanrath P, Schlüter M, Langenstein BA, Polster, Engel S, Kremer P, Krebber HJ (1983) Detection of ostium secundum atrial septal defect by transesophageal cross-sectional echocardiography. Br Heart J 49:350

Transthoracic and Transesophageal Echocardiographic Findings After Orthotopic Heart Transplantation*

C. E. ANGERMANN, C. H. SPES, A. R. TAMMEN, H.-U. STEMPFLE, B. M. KEMKES, A. SCHÜTZ, and K. THEISEN

In orthotopic heart transplantation as described by Shumway et al. [11] left and right atria and the great vessels of recipient and donor are anastomosed. Thus, both atrial size and geometry are changed by the procedure, while valvular apparatus and ventricles remain structurally unaltered. In this study, two-dimensional (2D) and Doppler echocardiography were employed to evaluate the morphological and functional changes associated with orthotopic heart transplantation. In addition to the conventional transthoracic approach (TTE), some of the patients were studied by transesophageal echocardiography (TEE), as this technique offers excellent visualization of the intraatrial septum, atrial free walls, and atrioventricular (AV) valves [2, 10, 17]. It should, thus, also provide superior information on the site of atrial anastomoses.

Methods

Study Patients. Thirty-nine patients (32 males, 7 females) with a mean age of 41.2 ± 9.4 years who had undergone orthotopic heart transplant surgery at Munich University were studied. Donors were matched for body weight ± 15%; at intraoperative inspection, all donor hearts had appeared normal from the epicardial surface and from the atrial side of the AV valves. The interval from transplantation to the TTE examination performed for the purpose of this study ranged from 1 to 43 months (20.6 ± 16.5 months). TEE examinations were performed in a subgroup of 14 patients (12 males, 2 females, mean age 46.9 ± 8.7 years, 14.3 ± 7.7 months postoperatively). All patients were in regular sinus rhythm at the time of both studies and none was on anticoagulant therapy.

Transthoracic Echocardiography. The TTE studies were performed with a commercially available system (Toshiba SSH-65A) using a 3.75-MHz transducer (Toshiba PSD-37R) with pulsed wave, continuous wave, and color Doppler capabilities and recorded on video tape. The atria were imaged in various projections; size and shape were assessed and the cavities searched for abnormalities. Mitral or tricuspid regurgitation was diagnosed if a pansystolic flow turbulence directed into the left or right atrium was present on Doppler evalu-

---

* Supported by a research grant from the Wilhelm Sander-Stiftung (AZ 86.015.2)

Transesophageal Echocardiography
Edited by R. Erbel et al.
© Springer-Verlag Berlin Heidelberg 1989

ation. Color flow imaging was employed for assessment of the severity of valve incompetence. Semiquantitation was based on size and shape of the regurgitant jets and graded as mild, moderate, or severe according to maximum regurgitant jet area. Minimal regurgitation with less than 1 cm^2 jet area was excluded from the diagnosis as it was interpreted as a physiological phenomenon related to valve closure rather than as valve incompetence [16]. Thickness, range of systolic movement of mitral and tricuspid leaflets, and end-systolic position of the cusp coaptation points were also analyzed. Mild or moderate systolic superior displacement of one or more mitral or tricuspid leaflet(s) confined to the four-chamber view was considered within the physiologic range of valve motion [5, 6]; echocardiographic mitral or tricuspid prolapse was diagnosed if moderate or severe bowing of one or more leaflet(s) was visible in more than one projection or if a cusp coaptation point was clearly on the atrial side of the valve annulus.

Transesophageal Echocardiography. For the TEE studies an echocardiographic endoscope (Toshiba ESB-37LR connected to the Toshiba SSH-65A system) fitted with a small, side-viewing 3.75-MHz phased-array transducer at its flexible tip was used. With this probe, 2D imaging of a 90-degree horizontal tomographic plane of section as well as pulsed and color Doppler flow imaging are feasible. Patients fasted for at least 6 h and received local pharyngeal anesthesia before the endoscope was inserted. No other medication was given except prophylactic antibiotics in one patient with a history of postoperative bacterial endocarditis. Informed consent was obtained from every patient. TEE was carried out with patients in the supine left lateral position and was tolerated well by all transplant recipients. Video tapes were again carefully evaluated regarding atrial size and configuration, intraatrial abnormalities, and the presence of mitral and/or tricuspid regurgitation or prolapse.

Results

Transthoracic Echocardiography. In all 39 patients atrial geometry was abnormal; the anastomoses of donor to recipient components were found to create a peculiar hour-glass configuration of the new atria with suture lines protruding from the inner boundaries of the atrial walls into the cavities. Atrial size was consistently enlarged. The characteristic echocardiographic appearance of the right and left atrium was best visualized in the apical four-chamber view (Fig. 1). Left ventricular size and function was normal, while the right ventricle appeared to be slightly enlarged in some of the patients.

Mitral regurgitation was diagnosed in 17 of the 39 patients and was, on semiquantative assessment, found to be mild in 15 and moderate in two individuals. Tricuspid regurgitation was present in as many as 37 of the patients though peak systolic pulmonary artery pressure as derived from maximum tricuspid regurgitant flow velocity [15] appeared normal or only slightly elevated. Tricuspid regurgitation was mild in 31 and moderate in six patients.

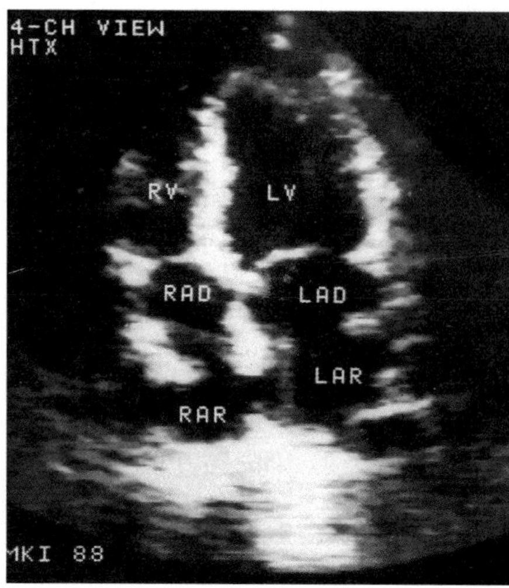

Fig. 1. Two-dimensional apical four-chamber view after heart transplantation. *LV/RV*, left/right ventricle; *LAD/LAR*, donor/recipient part of left atrium; *RAD/RAR*, donor/recipient part of right atrium

Mitral and tricuspid leaflet structure was normal. However, echocardiographic mitral valve prolapse was present in five and tricuspid valve prolapse in two heart transplant recipients.

Transesophageal Echocardiography. The transthoracic findings of enlargement and abnormal shape of the atria were confirmed in all 14 patients examined by TEE. Only by this technique, however, was an asynchronous contraction of the recipient and donor atrial components discernible. Superior imaging of the atrial walls by TEE also revealed that in most patients the

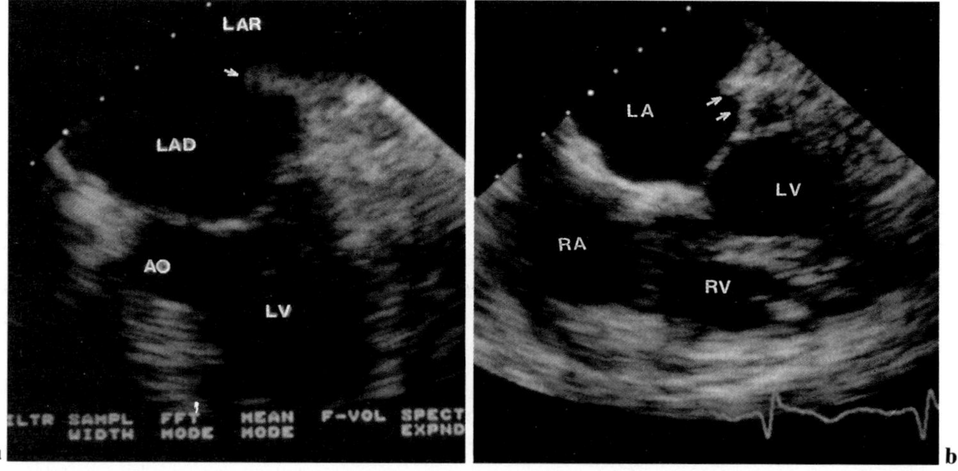

Fig. 2. a Prominent suture (*arrow*) between donor and recipient component of left atrium. **b** Systolic contact (*arrows*) between posterior mitral leaflet and suture. *AO*, aortic root. For further abbreviations, see Fig. 1

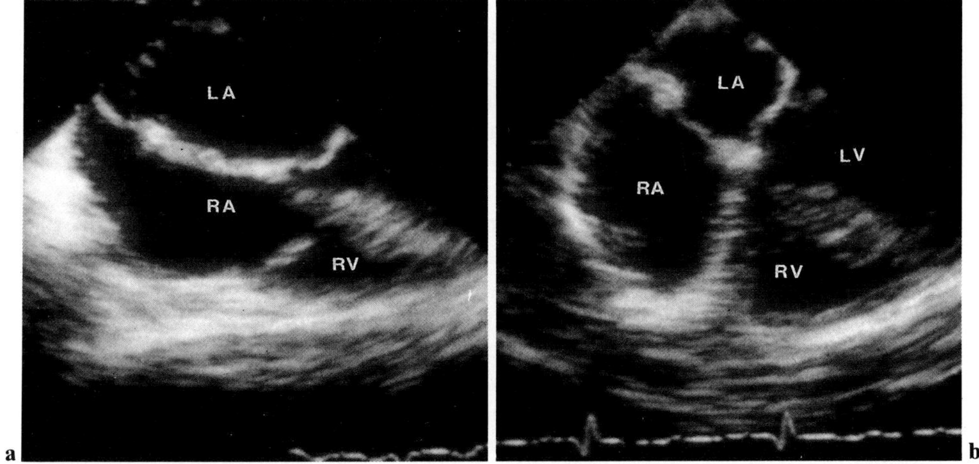

Fig. 3. a Recipient component of atrial septum thinner than donor component. **b** Recipient component of atrial septum thicker than donor component. For abbreviations, see Fig. 1

suture between recipient and donor components was particularly prominent at the left atrial free wall (Fig. 2 a) with a protrusion into the left atrial cavity of less than 10 mm or of 10–20 mm in five patients each, a protrusion of more than 20 mm in one patient, and no visible protrusion in only three patients. In two patients systolic contact between the suture and the posterior mitral leaflet was present (Fig. 2 b). The ratio of recipient to donor atrial septal thickness varied within the group. In seven patients the recipient atrial septum was thinner than the donor component (Fig. 3 a), in four both components had equal thickness, and in three patients the recipient atrial septum

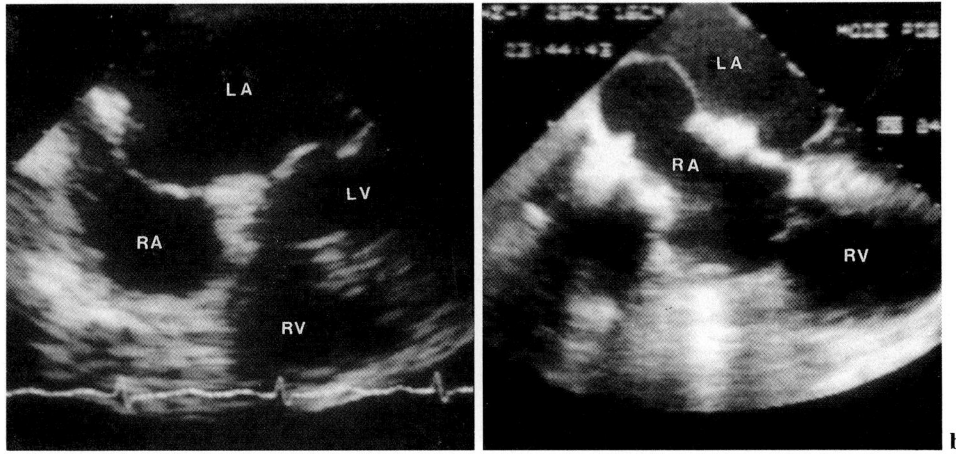

Fig. 4. a Pseudoaneurysm of the donor atrial septal component bulging towards the RA. **b** Pseudoaneurysm of the recipient atrial septal component bulging towards the LA. For abbreviations, see Fig. 1

was thicker than the donor component (Fig. 3b). In addition, several patients showed some phasic excursion of the atrial septum during the cardiac cycle. With reference to Hanley et al. [3], this phenomenon was called pseudoaneurysm if parts of the interatrial septum bulged at least 10 mm beyond the atrial septal plane and if the base of the bulging part was at least 15 mm in diameter. Pseudoaneurysms of the donor part protruding towards the right atrium were found in four patients (Fig. 4a) whereas a pseudoaneurysm of the recipient part protruding towards the left atrium was seen only in one patient who was examined very early after transplantation (Fig. 4b).

Whereas TTE demonstrated no intraatrial abnormalities, left atrial spontaneous echo contrast (SEC) was detected by TEE in four of the 14 patients. One patient also had spontaneous echoes in the right atrium. Moreover, left atrial thrombi were visualized by TEE in two patients with SEC. In each case, the thrombi were attached to the atrial free wall underneath the protruding suture in a niche formed by partial removal of the left atrial appendage during transplantation (Fig. 5a). One of these two patients had suffered from peripheral arterial embolization 2 weeks before the TEE study. Additonally, small mobile structures were detected at the atrial walls of six patients (including three patients with SEC). These structures were located within an atrial septal pseudoaneurysm in four instances and at the left atrial septal suture or atrial free walls in two instances each (Fig. 5b). Though their origin was unclear, their partial association with the presence of SEC suggested that they might also be small thrombi.

In all patients studied by TEE in whom mitral or tricuspid regurgitation was diagnosed by TTE, the findings were confirmed by TEE. However, holosystolic mitral regurgitation was found also in two patients in whom TTE

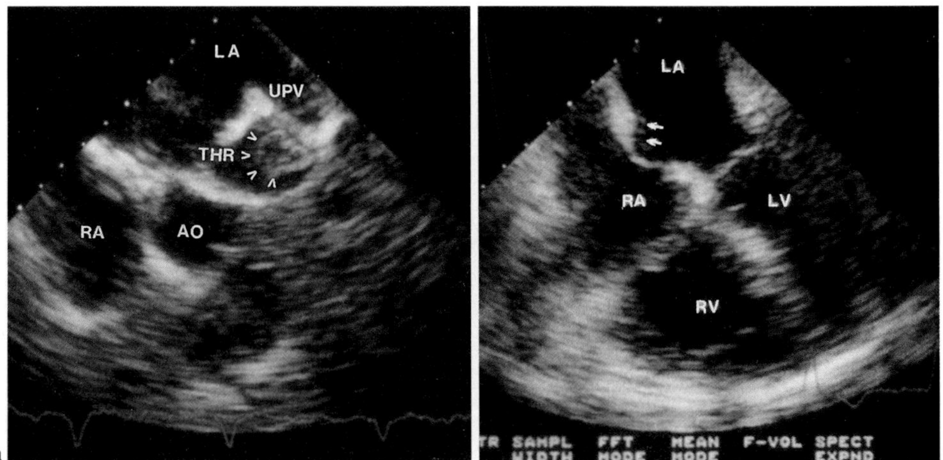

Fig. 5. a Atrial thrombus (*THR*) attached to the left atrial free wall. **b** Small thrombuslike structures (*arrows*) attached to the atrial septum. *UPV*, upper pulmonary vein. For further abbreviations, see Figs. 1 and 2

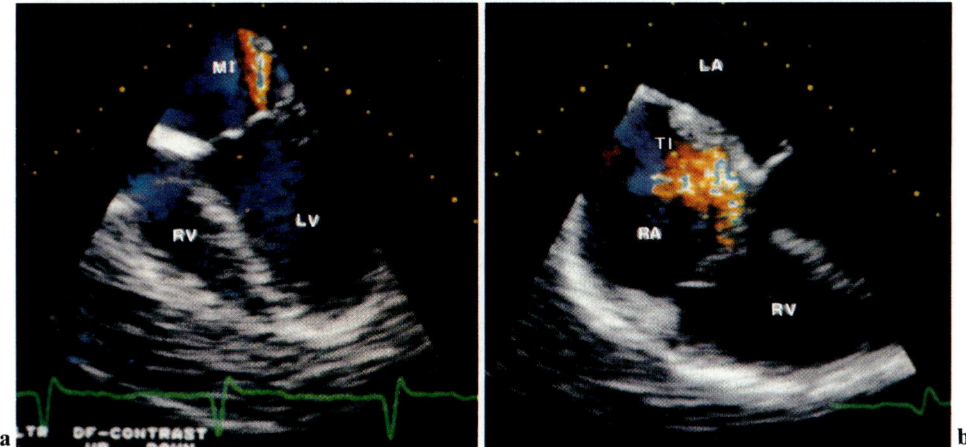

Fig. 6. a Mitral regurgitation (*MI*) with jet directed towards the left atrial free wall. **b** Tricuspid regurgitation (*TI*) with jet directed towards atrial septum. For further abbreviations, see Fig. 1

was negative. All together, mitral regurgitation was diagnosed in nine of the 14 patients by TEE and graded as mild in eight and as moderate in one. Tricuspid regurgitation was present in 12 instances and graded as mild in 11 patients and as moderate in one. TEE allowed clearer visualization of extension and shape of regurgitant jets than TTE and demonstrated that the jet was markedly eccentric in six patients with mitral regurgitation, pointing towards the left atrial free wall (Fig. 6a), and centrally directed in three; in patients with tricuspid regurgitation, the jet was always eccentric and pointed towards the intraatrial septum (Fig. 6b).

As in TTE, thickness and structure of the mitral and tricuspid leaflets appeared normal in all patients. Mitral and tricuspid valve prolapse were diagnosed in three and two patients, respectively, in whom the cusp coaptation points were clearly displaced towards the atrial side of the valve annulus. Only two of the patients with mitral prolapse and one patient with tricuspid prolapse on TEE had the same finding by TTE, while in the two others the transthoracic appearance of the valve motion was normal. All patients with a mitral or tricuspid prolapse on TEE had regurgitation of that valve.

Discussion

Our transthoracic findings confirm an earlier report by Stevenson et al. that orthotopic heart transplantation does not normalize atrial size and leads to abnormal configuration of both atria [12]. Dissociation of the mechanical performance of recipient and donor atria, however, which is a consequence of the persisting independent electrical activity in both components [13], was observed only by the transesophageal approach due to the superior image quality obtained by this technique. An unexpected finding was the relatively high incidence of SEC, which up to now has not been described in transplant patients. In the literature, only a few TTE studies have considered SEC. In two series of patients with valvular heart disease, large left atria, and atrial fibrillation, spontaneous echoes within the left atrial cavity were found in 4% and 32%, respectively [1, 4]. More recently, Daniel et al. reported the superiority of TEE in detecting SEC, as TTE allowed visualization of SEC in only one of 52 patients with mitral stenosis, while by TEE this phenomenon could be documented in over 60% of the same patient group [2]. This is confirmed by the present study, in which SEC could only be visualized by TEE, not by TTE, though identical transducer frequencies were used. Disturbed atrial hemodynamics due to asynchronous atrial contraction as well as the large atrial size after heart transplantation could both contribute to a slow blood flow situation within the atria, which might explain the occurrence of SEC despite normal ventricular function in this group of patients.

Daniel et al. reported also that individuals with mitral stenosis and SEC had a higher incidence of left atrial thrombi than patients without this phenomenon [2]. Our findings, including two atrial thrombi in patients with SEC, a documented arterial embolization in one of these patients, and small structures potentially also of thrombotic origin at the atrial walls of several patients, seem to confirm an increased risk of left atrial thrombus formation and arterial embolization also for transplant recipients with SEC. The niche underneath the left atrial free wall suture seems to be especially at risk for thrombus formation. Less prominent sutures in this area would be desirable; additionally, our data seem to indicate a need for prophylactic antiplatelet therapy in heart transplant recipients. As the number of patients in our preliminary study is small, however, this question will require further investigation.

Stevenson et al. reported mild to moderate mitral regurgitation in 14 (87%) of 16 transplant patients who were examined by transthoracic Doppler echocardiography [12]. In our transthoracic series the incidence was considerably lower, as mitral regurgitation was diagnosed in only 17 (44%) of 39 patients. Apart from mitral valve prolapse in five patients, no morphological or functional abnormalities of the valve or the left ventricle explaining the presence of mitral regurgitation were found. Tricuspid regurgitation was more common than mitral regurgitation and was diagnosed in all but two patients (95%). Pulmonary hypertension, which could have explained this finding [7], was ruled out because systolic pulmonary artery pressure as derived from maximum tricuspid regurgitant flow velocity [15] was normal or only moderately elevated. Though right ventricular enlargement was found in some of the transplant recipients, which represents persistent adaptive changes of the donor heart and may have caused an increase in tricuspid annular size and so relative valve incompetence in individual patients, it fails to explain such a high incidence of tricuspid regurgitation. Neither mitral nor tricuspid regurgitation after orthotopic heart transplantation can thus be accounted for on the basis of valvular or ventricular abnormalities alone.

The only abnormalities which are consistently present in transplant patients and might impair the functional integrity of the mitral and tricuspid apparatus are the hour-glass shaped and enlarged atria. As Perloff and Roberts point out, the left atrium is related to mitral valve competence in terms of contraction and relaxation and in terms of dilatation of its posterior wall [9]. Atrial enlargement can contribute to mitral regurgitation; as the anterior mitral leaflet is in direct fibrous continuity with the aortic root [8], it is little affected by atrial dilatation. Because of the continuity of the atrial endocardium and posterior mitral leaflet, however, any displacement of the posterior atrial wall will exert tension on the posterior leaflet and may so prevent complete closure of the valve [9]. An analogous effect of right atrial size and function on tricuspid valve competence may be postulated as an even greater part of the tricuspid circumference is unsupported by fibrous tissue [14].

As annular size was not assessed quantitatively in our study, a contribution of minor annuloventricular disproportion to mitral and tricuspid regurgitation cannot be ruled out, in particular as Stevenson et al. reported mild mitral annular dilatation and reduced ventricular volume indexes in their transplant patients [12]. However, the transesophageal finding of a prominent and probably rigid circular suture separating donor and receiver components and the visible asynchronous contraction of both suggest that impaired atrial function also plays a role in the genesis of AV-valve incompetence. In addition, the high incidence of atrial septal bulging and even pseudoaneurysms, which was detected only by TEE, points to the possibility of cyclic torsion of the atria during ventricular contraction and relaxation. This hypothesis is supported by the fact that the in situ position of the transplanted organ is characterized by a clockwise rotation. Eccentrically directed jets, which are regularly observed in tricuspid regurgitation and in most instances of mitral regurgitation, as well as bowing of the leaflets may also be due to tension affecting the muscular rather than the fibrous parts of the annuli. No major clinical implications arise from the observation of AV valve incompetence, as the degree is mild in most instances. The transesophageal findings suggest, however, that minor modifications of the operation technique could have a favorable effect on the function of the mitral and tricuspid apparatus.

Conclusion

TEE, which was for the first time used for the evaluation of heart transplant recipients in this study, yielded important information on morphology and function of the transplanted heart which could not be obtained by TTE. The transesophageal findings indicate the need for antiplatelet therapy in heart transplant recipients with atrial SEC and provide potential clues to the pathogenesis of AV valve incompetence.

References

1. Beppu S, Nimura Y, Sakakibara H, Nagata S, Park YD, Izumi S (1985) Smoke-like echo in left atrial cavity in mitral valve disease: its features and significance. J Am Coll Cardiol 6:744−749
2. Daniel WG, Nellessen U, Schröder E, Nonnast-Daniel B, Bednarski P, Nikutta P, Lichtlen PR (1988) Left atrial spontaneous echo contrast in mitral valve disease: an indicator for an increased thromboembolic risk. J Am Coll Cardiol 11:1204−1211
3. Hanlay PC, Tajik AJ, Hynes JK, Edwards WD, Reeder GS, Hayler DJ, Seward JB (1985) Diagnosis and classification of atrial septal aneurysm by two-dimensional echocardiography: report of 80 consecutive cases. J Am Coll Cardiol 6:1370−1382
4. Iliceto S, Antonelli G, Sorino M, Biasco G, Rizzon P (1985) Dynamic intracavitary left atrial echoes in mitral stenosis. Am J Cardiol 55:603−606
5. Krivokapich J, Child JS, Dadourian BJ, Perloff JK (1988) Reassessment of echocardiographic criteria for diagnosis of mitral valve prolapse. Am J Cardiol 61:131−135
6. Levine RA, Stathogiannidis E, Newell JB, Harrigan P, Weyman AE (1988) Reconsideration of echocardiographic standards for mitral valve prolapse: lack of association between leaflet displacement isolated to the apical four chamber view and independent echocardiographic evidence of abnormality. J Am Coll Cardiol 11:1010−1019
7. Nishimura RA, Miller Jr FA, Callahan MJ, Benassi RC, Seward JB, Tajik AJ (1985) Doppler echocardiography: theory, instrumentation, technique and application. Mayo Clin Proc 60:321−341
8. Ormiston JA, Shah PM, Tei C, Wong M (1981) Size and motion of the mitral annulus in man. I. A two-dimensional echocardiographic method and findings in normal subjects. Circulation 64:113−120
9. Perloff JK, Roberts WC (1972) The mitral apparatus. Functional anatomy of mitral regurgitation. Circulation 46:227−239
10. Seward JB, Khandheria BK, Oh JK, Abel MD, Hughes Jr RW, Edwards WD, Nichols BA, Freeman WK, Tajik AJ (1988) Transesophageal echocardiography: technique, anatomic correlations, implementations, and clinical applications. Mayo Clin Proc 63: 649−680
11. Shumway NE, Lower RR, Stofer RC (1966) Transplantation of the heart. Adv Surg 2:265−284
12. Stevenson LW, Dadourian BJ, Kobashigawa J, Child JS, Clark SH, Laks H (1987) Mitral regurgitation after cardiac transplantation. Am J Cardiol 60:119−122
13. Stinson EB, Schroeder JS, Griepp RB, Shumway NE, Dong E (1972) Observations on the behavior of recipient atria after cardiac transplantation in man. Am J Cardiol 30:615−622
14. Tei C, Pilgrim JP, Shah PM, Ormiston JA, Wong M (1982) The tricuspid valve annulus: study of size and motion in normal subjects and in patients with tricuspid regurgitation. Circulation 66:665−671
15. Yock PG, Popp RL (1984) Noninvasive estimation of right ventricular systolic pressure by Doppler ultrasound in patients with tricuspid regurgitation. Circulation 70:657−662
16. Yoshida K, Yoshikawa J, Shakudo M, Akasaka T, Jyo Y, Takao S, Shiratory K, Koizumi K, Okumachi F, Kato H, Fukaya T (1988) Color Dopplker evaluation of valvular regurgitation in normal subjects. Circulation 78:840−847
17. Zenker G, Erbel R, Krämer G, Mohr-Kahaly S, Drexler M, Harnoncourt K, Meyer J (1988) Transesophageal two-dimensional echocardiography in young patients with cerebral ischemic events. Stroke 19:345−348

Perspectives on Transesophageal Echocardiography

Transesophageal Echocardiography:
The View of a Cardiologist

J. R. T. C. ROELANDT

Although this article is subtitled "The view of a cardiologist," it actually represents the pooled experience of a group of investigators at the Thoraxcenter in Rotterdam. We have kept references to a minimum, including only those we feel are key references, as this paper is part of a collection reflecting the current state of the art.

In day-to-day clinical practice, echocardiography combined with Doppler imaging is usually the first cardiac imaging examination performed when cardiac disease is suspected, and the method provides solutions to the majority of the complex diagnostic problems we are presented with. The greatest limitation, however, remains that high quality images cannot be obtained in all patients studied. Small phased array transducers can be fitted on to a flexible gastroscope and allow high quality diagnostic imaging from within the esophagus. Since the clinical introduction of this technique by Dr. P. Hanrath and his colleagues [1], it has been developed from its initial use as an intraoperative monitoring technique into a powerful diagnostic tool in both the routine outpatient and surgical settings [2, 3]. The advantages of the transesophageal approach are:

- No obstruction to ultrasound by chest wall (or intracardiac) structures and lung tissue
- Different imaging planes allow visualization of structures not seen from the precordium
- Higher Ultrasound frequencies provide better resolution and more detailed imaging
- Higher signal-to-noise ratio permits detection of poorly echo-reflective structures
- Reduced target range for pulsed Doppler (color) and allows a higher PRF (pulse repetition frequency) to be used

Within a few years, several new high resolution transducers have been introduced (Table 1), and it is hard to keep up with the pace of new developments.

With the incorporation of simultaneously acquired Doppler and color flow information, the diagnostic potential of the technique has been increased considerably. Its use intraoperativly as a monitoring technique has been extended to surgical decision-making and monitoring of surgical repair. While it was used initially as an alternative approach in out patients with poor precordial images it is now evolving into the ultimate diagnostic technique in a significant number of conditions. These include thoracic aortic pathology, mitral

Transesophageal Echocardiography
Edited by R. Erbel et al.
© Springer-Verlag Berlin Heidelberg 1989

Table 1. Transesophageal Echocardiography Systems (1988)

Manufacturer	Frequency (MHz)	Scan head width/thickness (mm)	Gastroscope Diameter (mm)	Gatroscope Length (cm)
Diasonics/ACMI[a]	3.5	12/16	10.5	110
Oldelft/ACMI	5.6	14/16	10.5	130
Aloka/Olympus	3.5	14/10	9	100
	5	12/10	9	100
	5	7/ 8	6.5	70
Toshiba/Mashida	3.7	10/12	10[c]	105
Vingmed/ACMI[b]	5 and 7.5	15/15	11	100

[a] ACMI, American Cystoscopic Makers, Inc.
[b] Mechanical annular phased array − pulse wave and continuous wave Doppler facilities
[c] Plus fiberoptics

valve prothesis, infective endocarditis and its complications, subaortic obstruction, atrial lesions, and complex congenital heart disease. In virtually all of these conditions, the technique provides a better understanding of both the underlying morphology and its hemodynamic consequences.

Intraoperative Use

Transesophageal echocardiography is particularly well-suited as an intraoperative technique, for both diagnosis and continuous monitoring, since it does not interfere with surgery. It is used in:

− Monitoring of left ventricular function (loading conditions, etc.)
− Detection of wall motion abnormalities (earliest marker of ischemia, early intervention)
− Guidance and assessment of surgery (prosthesis, valve repair, congenital heart disease)
− Assessment effects of anesthetic intervention

For example, in patients at high risk of cardiovascular complications, the transesophageal technique can be used to continuously assess left ventricular function during anesthesia without interfering with the surgical procedure. Monitoring of left ventricular wall motion during the operation permits early detection of ischemia, and allows intervention to prevent myocardial infarction [4]. Transesophageal echocardiography is a more acurate predictor of changes in left ventricular function and ischemia than flow directed wedge catheters (currently the accepted intraoperative technique for monitoring of left ventricular function). Guidance and assessment of surgical intervention including valve replacement, valve repair and the correction of congenital heart defects are possible, and the immediate effects of coronary revascularization can be studied. In noncardiac surgery, the technique allows monitoring of intracardiac air and other emboli passing through the right heart. It also opens a new area of research into the cardiovascular effects of anesthetic drugs, fluid management, and vasodilator and inotropic therapy.

With modern cardioplegia and related surgical techniques, cardiopulmonary bypass time is no longer a limiting factor in cardiovascular operations. Immediate intraoperative evaluation of surgical repair by ultrasound techniques including transesophageal echocardiography allows better results, since the cardiopulmonary bypass can be reinstituted or extended and further surgery performed if necessary. Experience with the use of transesophageal echocardiography and epicardial echocardiography to assist intraoperative decision-making is still limited at present, and the precise advantages and disadvantages of both approaches are still being assessed. However, it is becoming increasingly clear that the information they each provide is often complementary and of clinical importance. There is no doubt that both techniques will achieve wide acceptance in time.

Critical Care Environment

Transesophageal echocardiography is increasingly being used to assess critically ill patients in the emergency unit if an underlying acute cardiac event is suspected in patients with various life-threatening cardiovascular problems.

The technique is valuable in the intensive and postoperative care units when precordial echocardiography becomes impossible or when other diagnostic methods can not be used. It is especially suitable for those on mechanical ventilators. In the coronary care unit, it is becoming an invaluable tool for assessment of patients with shock and hypotension, and it can provide a definitive diagnosis in patients with some complications of myocardial infarction when precordial echocardiography is of insufficient quality. However, certain areas remain blind to the transesophageal approach. These include apical and anterior portions of the trabecular septum. Thus transesophageal imaging is of limited value at present (due to the limited scanning planes) for the diagnosis of anteroapical aneurysm, postinfarct ventricular septal defects and pseudoaneurysms.

Outpatient Use

The clinical indications for transesophageal echocardiography in the assessment of outpatients with suspected cardiac disease continue to evolve. At present, the following are considered as key indications:

1. No precordial (adequate) imaging
2. Thoracic aortic dissection/pathology
3. Intracardiac mass lesions

4. Systemic embolism
5. Mitral prosthesis dysfunction/endocarditis
6. Suspected endocarditis and complications
7. Subaortic lesions (membrane, tunnel, etc.)
8. Specific aspects of congenital heart disease in adolescents and adults

Transesophageal echocardiography is more sensitive than precordial echocardiography for examination of the left and right atria and the interatrial septum, and for detection of intraatrial mass lesions. When combined with color flow mapping techniques, transesophageal echocardiography offers increased sensitivity for detecting regurgitant jets in patients with mitral valve disease. The precordial approach to mitral regurgitant jets is always limited by both the diminishing amplitude of Doppler signals over distance, and poor sound penetration to the area of interest. Flow masking by prosthetic materials (valve prostheses, patches, conduits) can be overcome in order to diagnose abnormalities behind such materials [5]. The technique is excellent for diagnosis of the different types of aortic dissections, and color flow mapping helps to locate entry and reentry tears and to distinguish true from false lumens [6].

Because it provides a complete and reliable preoperative diagnosis within 10 min of clinical suspicion, the method is rapidly becoming the method of choice for the examination of patients suspected of having acute aortic pathology. Because of its higher sensitivity and resolution, transesophageal echocardiography is superior for the diagnosis of complications of infective endocarditis [7]. Valve ring and/or intramural abscesses, mycotic aneurysms, cusp perforation, and complex intracardiac fistulae are readily diagnosed, but only by combining high resolution imaging and color flow mapping. Some specific aspects of congenital heart disease, especially in adolescents and adults, may be better studied from the transesophageal approach. These includes such lesions as complex atrioventricular connections, Fontan and Rastelli circulations, atrial baffle, and left ventricular outflow tract obstruction. Smaller transducers and endoscopes are currently under development to further extent the use of the technique to smaller children and infants.

Future Developments

Transesophageal echocardiographic technology and its applications are in a state of rapid change. Possible future developments are:

- Continuous wave Doppler integration
- Pediatric use (smaller, 7.5 MHz)
- Monitoring during general surgery
- Automated left ventricular detection
- Tissue characterization
- Improved ergonomics?
- Further miniaturization − nasal probe

Both probe miniaturization and increasing the number of scan planes will allow many more views to be examined. This will lead to important new applications. High frequency transducers for increased resolution and integration of continuous wave Doppler facilities would be other major advances. Automatic wall motion analysis and tissue characterization will further extend the monitoring capabilities.

Discussion

Transesophageal echocardiography is a logical extension of standard precordial echocardiography. It represents a major advance in the care of patients with cardiovascular disease. It provides diagnostic information essential for clinical decision-making in patients in whom precordial studies are inadequate and in a large variety of complex cardiac conditions. It offers unique advantages particularly in the acute care environment where other imaging techniques can not be used. In addition, its unique anatomic perspective, from posterior to the heart, sometimes provides clinical information not obtainable by other imaging approaches and technologies. It will undoubtedly become the principal method for analysis of acute cardiac problems since it can be used without delay in the emergency unit and at the bedside in the critical care environment. It is a major diagnostic advance in the evaluation of patients suspected of having an intracardiac source of emboli or infective endocarditis. In a short period of time, it has become the principal method for assessment of mitral valve prostheses and patients suspected of having acute thoracic aortic pathology, the intraperative left ventricular function and wall motion for the early detection of ischemia, and for the assessment of reparative procedures.

Where, within the spectrum of cardiac diagnostic practice, should such a powerful new diagnostic technique be based? It is my opinion that for the present time, transesophageal echocardiographic studies should be restricted to tertiary cardiac referral centers with extensive experience in the use of all routine diagnostic modes of cardiac ultrasound. In addition, such centers should have experienced staff in gastroenterology, thoracic surgery, and anesthesiology departments to collaborate with. In my opinion, current practice dictates that transesophageal echocardiography should not be performed by technicians because of the nature and complexity of the diagnostic problems arising during these studies. It is likely, however, that parts of this technology (e.g., monitoring) will progressively disseminate within the medical services. The educational requirements and consultations that this natural evolution will create are the responsibility of the cardiologist. Training programs must be established to provide the other disciplines with the broad background necessary to cope with this new technical revolution and to apply the new technique in the most cost effective way to improve patient care.

References

1. Schluter M, Langenstein BS, Polster J et al. (1982) Transesophageal cross-sectional echocardiography with a phased array transducer system: technique and initial clinical results. Br Heart J 48:67−72
2. Mitchell MM, Sutherland GR, Gussenhoven EJ, Taams MA, Roelandt TC Jr. (1988) Transesophageal echocardiography. J Am Soc Echo 1:362−377
3. Seward JB, Khandheria BK, Oh JK et al. (1988) Transesophageal echocardiography: technique, anatomic correlations, implementation, and clinical applications. Mayo Clin Proc 63:649−680
4. Smith JS, Cahalan MK, Benefiel DJ et al. (1985) Intraoperative detection of myocardial ischemia in high risk patients: electrocardiography versus two-dimensional transesophageal echocardiography. Circulation 75:1015−1021
5. Taams MA, Gussenhoven EJ, Cahalan MK, Roelandt JRTC, van Herwerden LA, The HK, Bom N, de Jong N (1989) Transesophageal Doppler color flow imaging in the detection of native and Bjork-Shiley mitral valve regurgitation. J Am Coll Cardiol 13:95−99
6. Borner N, Erbel R, Braun B et al. (1984) Diagnosis of aortic dissection by transesophageal echocardiography. Am J Cardiol 54:1157−1158
7. Daniel WG, Schroder E, Nonnast-Daniel B, Lichtlen PR (1987) Conventional and transesophageal echocardiography in the diagnosis of infective endocarditis. Eur Heart J 8 (suppl J):287−292

Intraoperative Transesophageal Echocardiography (TEE): The Surgeon's Perspective

H. OELERT, S. IVERSEN, W. SCHMIEDT, H. JAKOB, and U. HAKE

Out of the various applications of intraoperative echocardiography, the transesophageal approach in particular has become important for surgeons in reconfirming the patient's disease and making appropriate decisions [12]. The usefulness of this method will increase further when technical facilities and surgeons' understanding of echocardiographic imaging enable them routinely to examine patients pre- and postoperatively and to recognize irregularities in their procedures [8].

The distinct advantage of transesophageal echocardiography (TEE) is that it is easy to place the transducer for continuous cardiac monitoring, and that it can be located outside the operative area. The placement is stable, the recording does not interfere with the operation, and all problems of sterility are avoided. Finally, repeated and comparative investigations are possible and may be performed with the chest opened or closed.

Intraoperative TEE has yet to be routinely used during surgical repair of *congenital heart lesions*. Although the retrocardiac position of the transducer should enable residual obstructions and shunts to be detected, intracardiac correction in general takes place during infancy or early childhood when, due to the anatomical dimensions, adequate probes are not available and/or interpretation is difficult. Once these technical problems have been overcome [7], incomplete correction may be avoided. This has already been achieved for surgical treatment of obstructive hypertrophic cardiomyopathy [10] and of postinfarction ventricular septal rupture in adults [4].

Schippers et al. [11] and Engberding et al. (this volume) investigated the potential use of echocardiography in the assessment of thoracic aorta pathology. They found that, in comparison with angiography, which is the standard method in the diagnosis of aortic dissection, only with intraoperative epicardial echocardiography was aortic dissection adequately demonstrated. However, because of its close proximity, echocardiography by the transesophageal approach provides the surgeon with even more information on the whole intrathoracic aorta [6].

Intraoperative TEE has revolutionized *mitral valve* surgery [2, 3, 13]. Combined with color Doppler flow techniques, transesophageal echocardiography is highly sensitive in detecting regurgitant jets in patients with an incompetent native valve or dysfunctioning valve prostheses. In mitral stenosis the degree of mitral valve mobilitiy, subvalvular thickening and shortening, and calcification may be of importance for the surgeon's decision of whether to repair or replace the valve. This information nearly always shows that mitral stenosis due to valvular and subvalvular narrowing as well as mitral valve insufficiency

Transesophageal Echocardiography
Edited by R. Erbel et al.
© Springer-Verlag Berlin Heidelberg 1989

due to prolapse of leaflets caused by elongated or ruptured chordae can be repaired anatomically. Severe calcification and immobilized leaflets, on the other hand, may preclude attempts at reconstructive surgery.

With regard to coronary artery disease, impaired *myocardial performance* before the operation may indicate to the surgeon the need for meticulous myocardial protection, postoperative pharmacological support, or the preparation of an assist device.

Following coronary artery revascularization, two-dimensional echocardiographic indices of left ventricular regional contractile and global systolic function in conjunction with Doppler flow images are becoming of increasing importance in assessing bypass function [5]. Obviously, the state of the myocardium improves following successful bypass grafting in most patients with reduced myocardial function. If it does not, however, continuous TEE has proved indispensable in supervising drug administration as well as mechanical circulatory support and weaning. Examples of how intraaortic balloon counterpulsation can be checked are given in another contribution (Drexler et al., this volume).

With regard to the importance of *preoperative TEE*, we would first like to draw attention to *intraatrial tumors*, which are usually diagnosed as a myxoma. This may in general be true on the left side, but contradictory results have repeatedly been found when operations have been performed based on a previously established diagnosis of a right atrial mass. Figure 1 shows a left atrial tumor prolapsing into the mitral valve orifice during diastole. Surgery confirmed that this tumor was correctly diagnosed as a left atrial myxoma. Figure 2 gives an example of a right atrial mass. Although intermittent prolapse into the tricuspid orifice was demonstrated, no adherence to the right atrial wall or septum could be detected. This, together with a history of recurrent pulmonary embolic episodes and deep vein thrombosis, should draw attention to the possibility of an intracavitary thrombus rather than a cardiac tumor. According to our experience it is unlikely that such a thrombus will cause pulmonary embolism of clinical significance when it escapes or dissolves. Altogether we have seen four patients with this kind of right atrial mass.

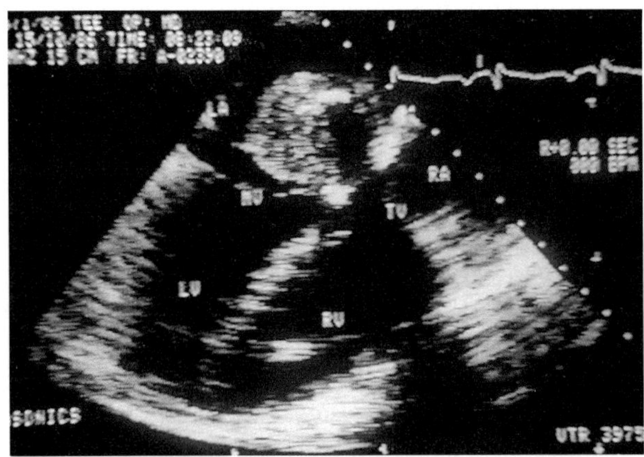

Fig. 1. Left atrial myxoma prolapsing through the mitral valve orifice

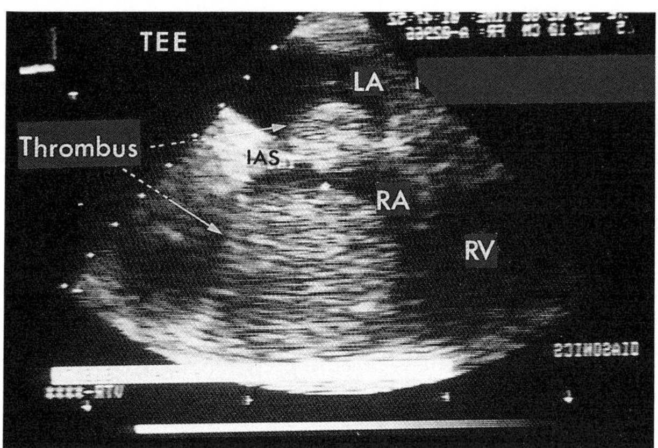

Fig. 2. Right atrial thrombus imitating a tumorous mass

In two who were operated on no residual tumor could be found. The other two were therefore reexamined immediately before operation and were withdrawn from the program when it became obvious that the tumor had vanished. Following this experience we consider it mandatory that patients with a right atrial mass scheduled for operation are reexamined immediately before surgery in order to confirm or exclude the original findings.

While reconstructive measures on or within the heart are usually performed during cardiac arrest, the result can only be assessed while the heart is beating, preferably when it takes over the total work load from the cardiopulmonary bypass. Not only should the functional behavior of heart valves, whether reconstructed or replaced, be ascertained but also myocardial contractility. If results are unfavorable cardiopulmonary bypass can be reinstituted and surgery continued. In the following we will refrain from discussing echocardiographic observation of impaired regional or global myocardial performance in patients with coronary artery disease either before or after operation because of lack of personal experience. Undoubtedly, however, surgeons interest extends to this field when they want to learn more about failure and success of coronary artery revascularization, especially during acute myocardial infarction.

The domain of *intraoperative TEE* in our hands has been the examination of reconstructive procedures on both atrioventricular valves. As well as using color flow mapping, contrast enhancement was achieved by intraventricular injection of agitated gelatine solution (Gelifundol). The injection catheter was placed transmurally into the right ventricular cavity and from there transseptally into the left ventricular cavity, in order to prevent interference with valvular function. In 60 out of 112 patients who underwent mitral valve reconstruction in our institution, the procedure was performed under transesophageal echocardiographic control. Of these patients, 90% underwent successful mitral valve reconstruction while 10% required valve replacement when the repair had failed. Residual mitral incompetence led repeatedly to further efforts at reconstructive measures and, if these failed, to valve replacement.

Special attention must be paid to patients with mitral insufficiency as part of idiopathic *hypertrophic subartic obstruction*. As Cooley et al. [1] have demonstrated, subaortic stenosis can be successfully treated by mitral valve replacement alone. In contrast, resection of the subaortic stenosis never cures but sometimes may improve mitral insufficiency. Reconstructive treatment of the mitral valve in patients promising a good result when tested during cardiac arrest has not necessarily proved to be successful when scrutinized by TEE on the beating heart following termination of cardiopulmonary bypass. However, while a good result can be confirmed and a poor result ought to be prevented, TEE in patients with a residual defect will help one to weigh up the benefits of limited improvement by reconstructive measures against the imponderables of leaving the patient with incomplete resection and/or valve replacement.

Figures 3 and 4 show echocardiographic findings obtained in three patients with a diseased mitral valve. In the first patient mitral valve reconstruction proved to be successful (Fig. 3). In another patient repair of a combined mitral valve lesion failed and resulted in replacement by an artificial substitute. Finally, a third patient who suffered from obstructive hypertrophic cardiomyopathy underwent a standard ventricular septal myotomy-myectomy operation. This, however, because of persistent systolic mitral-septal apposi-

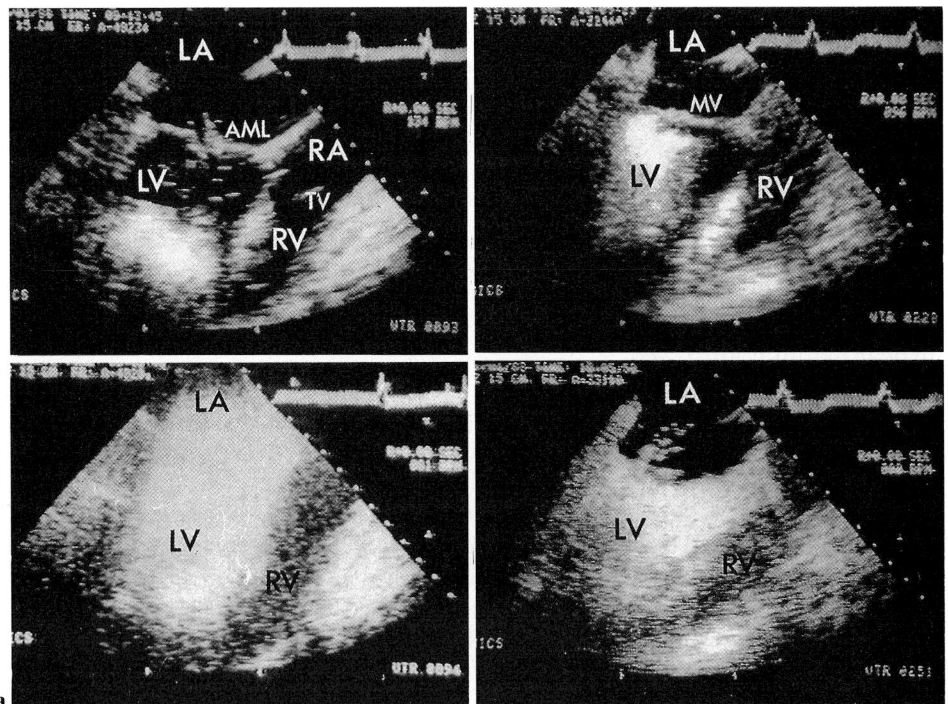

Fig. 3 a, b. Mitral valve insufficiency: TEE **a** before (MI grade III) and **b** after (MI less than grade I) reconstruction

tion, neither relieved left ventricular outflow tract obstruction nor mitral incompetence, which was, instead, worsened. Additional excision of septal musculature from the critical site during a second period of cardiopulmonary bypass resulted in a substantial reduction in the systolic anterior motion of the mitral valve and, hence, decrease of left ventricular outflow obstruction and mitral regurgitation (Fig. 4).

Another factor in TEE of patients with obstructive hyperthrophic cardiomyopathy is the heterogeneity in septal thickness, which can give rise to iatrogenic ventricular septal defects when excessive amounts of muscle are removed. Echocardiographic mapping of septal hypertrophy will allow the surgeon to exclude relatively thin areas of the septum from the myectomy and tailor standard resection to the individual patient's septal anatomy [10].

Right heart failure as well as global disturbances of myocardial contractility in a heart which was contracting well before the operation have been explained by disseminated coronary artery *air embolism* caused by air trapped once left heart cavities have been opened. Transesophageal echocardiography has proved ideal in detecting residual air, especially when it escapes from hidden areas while the lungs are inflated and ventilation resumed. Figure 5 shows a cloud of microbubbles which have emerged from the pulmonary veins once all air already had been evacuated from the heart. Ligation of the left auricle,

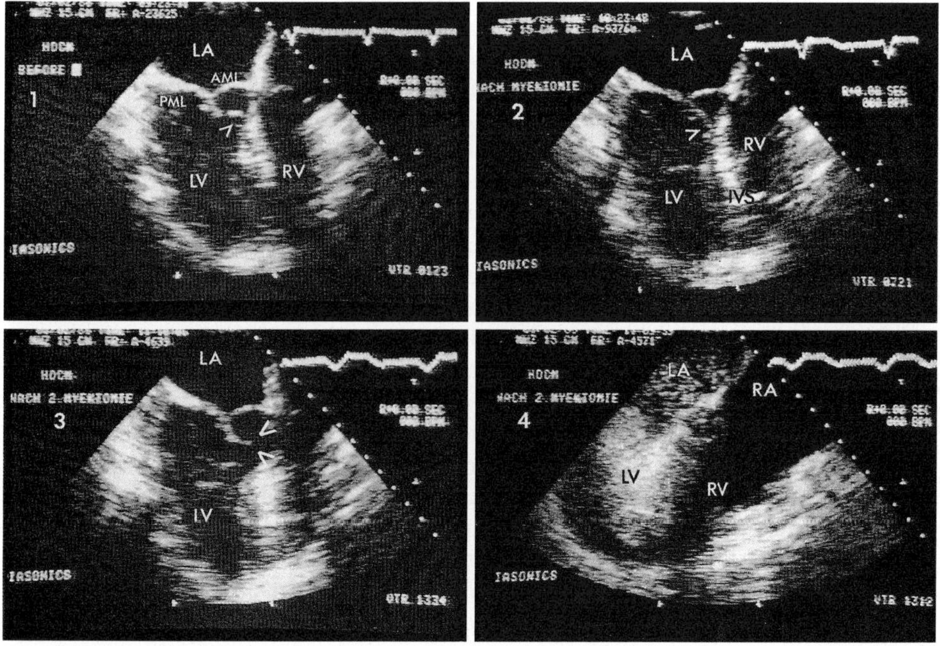

Fig. 4. (*1–4*) TEE demonstrating left ventricular outflow tract obstruction and mitral valve insufficiency. (*1*) before operation; (*2*) after primary myectomy, SAM still visible; (*3*) after secundary myectomy, SAM not longer present; (*4*) contrast injection into LV precluding artificial VSD

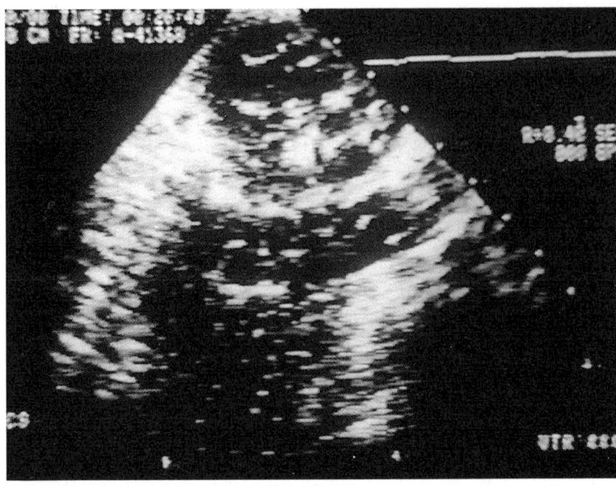

Fig. 5. Microbubbles in the left atrium emerging from the pulmonary veins at termination of cardio-pulmonary bypass

needle puncture of the pulmonary veins and left ventricular apex, and venting of the ascending aorta should prevent patients from suffering postbypass air embolism.

One final advantage of TEE during open heart surgery is the ability to measure changes in left ventricular dimensions and function during the various phases of the operation. This is not only relevant for the administration of drugs during induction of anesthesia and when coming off bypass, but also for volume overload and depletion in an unstable circulatory state. In patients who underwent bypass graft surgery, Matsumoto et al. [9] found no significant changes in the cardiac output, ejection fraction, or velocity of circumferential fiber shortening. However, end-diastolic stiffness showed a considerable increase during sternal wall closure. Consequently, when in some patients a decrease in cardiac output was most marked after sternal closure, this could be attributed less to a decrease in contractility than to a diastolic mechanical restriction of, and hence decrease in, preload. Also, in our hands, in hearts that were already severely compromised due to the underlying disease and surgery, this increased stiffness has had a measurable effect on cardiac performance which, finally, could be resolved only by leaving the sternotomy open.

In summary, transesophageal echocardiography offers a new approach to continuous monitoring of ventricular performance, valvular and subvalvular morphology, and hemodynamic abnormalities during anesthesia and surgery. It allows echocardiograms to be obtained from the same location throughout the entire procedure without sterilization of the probe. Its use is limited neither by the surgeon's concession to interrupt his activity nor by its use being possible only while the chest is open. The surgeon can both assess precisely the operative outcome immediately after repair, and visualize residual defects. Consequently, an incomplete correction can be revised at the time in the operating room or additional procedures performed [8]. Failures and mistakes directly related to the surgical procedure and observed before the end of the operation can induce the surgeon to continue surgery, commence drug therapy and/or mechanical support, and delay sternal closure.

References

1. Cooley DA, Wukasch DC, Leachman RD (1976) Mitral valve replacement for idiopathic hypertrophic subaortic stenosis: results in 27 patients. J Cardiovasc Surg 17:380−387
2. Dahm M, Iversen S, Schmid FX, Drexler M, Erbel R, Oelert H (1987) Intraoperative evaluation of reconstruction of the atrioventricular valves by transesophageal echocardiography. Thorac Cardiovasc Surg 35:140−142
3. Drexler M, Erbel R, Dahm M, Mohr-Kahaly S, Oelert H, Meyer J (1986) Assessment of successful valve reconstruction by intraoperative transesophageal echocardiography (TEE). Int J Card Imaging 2:21−30
4. Erbel R, Mohr-Kahaly S, Drexler M, Wittlich N, Kersting H, Iversen S, Oelert H, Meyer J (1986) Erweiterung der kardialen Notfalldiagnostik bei Ventikelseptumruptur nach akutem Myokardinfarkt mittels Farb-Doppler-Echocardiographie. Z Kardiol 75:468−472
5. Erbel R, Schweizer P, Meyer J, Krebs W, Jalhinoglu O, Effert S (1985) Sensitivity of cross-sectional echocardiography in detection of impaired global and regional left ventricular function: prospective study. Int J Cardiol 7:375
6. Goldman ME, Guarino T, Mindich P (1985) Localization of aortic dissection intimal flap by intraoperative two-dimensional echocardiography. J Am Coll Cardiol 6:1155−1159
7. Gussenhoven EJ, van Hewerden LA, Roeland J, Ligtvoet KM, Bos E, Witsenburg M (1987) Intraoperative two-dimensional echocardiography in congenital heart disease. J Am Coll Cardiol 9:565−572
8. Kyo S, Takamoto S, Matsumura M, Asano H, Yokote Y, Motoyama T, Omoto R (1987) Immediate and early postoperative evaluation of results of cardiac surgery by transesophageal two-dimensional Doppler echocardiography. Circulation 76:113−121
9. Matsumoto M, Oka J, Strom J, Frishman W, Kadish A, Becker RM, Frater RWM, Sonnenblick EH (1980) Application of transesophageal echocardiography to continuous intraoperative monitoring of left ventricular performance. Am J Cardiol 46:95−105
10. McIntosh CL, Maron BJ (1988) Current operative treatment of obstructive hypertonic cardiomyopathy. Circulation 78:487−495
11. Schippers OA, Gussenhaven WJ, van Herwerden LA, Taams MA, Roeland J, Bom N, Bos E (1988) The role of intraoperative two-dimensional echocardiography in the assessment of thoracic aorta pathology. Thorac Cardiovasc Surg 36:208−213
12. Van Herwerden LA, Gussenhaven WJ, Roeland J, Bos E, Ligtvoet CM, Haalebos MM, Mochtar B, et al. (1986) Intraoperative epicardial two-dimensional echocardiography. Eur Heart J 7:386−395
13. Wilkins GT, Weyman AE, Abascal VM, Block PC, Palacios JF (1988) Percutaneous balloon dilatation of the mitral valve: an analysis of echocardiographic variables related to outcome and the mechanism of dilatation. Br Heart J 60:299−308

Practicability of Transesophageal Echocardiography in Conscious Patients

W. G. DANIEL, A. MÜGGE, C. ESCHENBRUCH, and P. R. LICHTLEN

Introduction

Since the initial description by Frazin et al. in 1976 [1], and in particular since the incorporation of phased array technology into transducers mounted at the tip of a modified gastroscope [2], transesophageal echocardiography (TEE) has been increasingly used in clinical cardiology − at least in Europe and Japan. In the United States and elsewhere, however, this technique became accepted only slowly over the years; this was due not only to the slight discomfort for the patient associated with a TEE examination but predominantly to safety considerations concerning the introduction and manipulation of the esophageal transducer under optically not controlled conditions in patients with more or less severe heart diseases.

Only a few studies have been published in the literature analyzing practicability and risks of TEE in larger series of patients [3−5]. This report describes our experience with the use of TEE in the first 1900 consecutive patients examined in our laboratory and stored in a data bank.

Patients

Between January 1984 and February 1989, 1900 patients (1105 men, 795 women) aged between 13 and 87 years underwent a TEE examination in our clinic. In the same time period, a total of approximately 18500 transthoracic echocardiographic studies were performed in the division of cardiology resulting in a ratio between conventional precordial and TEE examinations of about 10.3%. 1328 patients (84.7%) underwent one TEE examination, 221 patients (14.1%) were studied twice or three times, and in 17 patients (1.2%), TEE studies were repeated between four and nine times.

At the time of the TEE examination, 1764 patients (92.8%) were conscious; 136 patients (7.2%) were studied under mechanical ventilation. 1088 patients (57.3%) were inpatients and 812 (42.7%) were outpatients who left the clinic immediately after the TEE examination. In 171 cases (9.0%), TEE examinations were performed in an intensive care unit; the remaining 1729 patients (91%) were studied in the echocardiography laboratory or on a regular ward.

Transesophageal Echocardiography
Edited by R. Erbel et al.
© Springer-Verlag Berlin Heidelberg 1989

Table 1. Predominant clinical reasons for TEE in 1900 consecutive patients

Suspected clinical diagnosis	Patients	
	(*n*)	(%)
Prosthetic valve malfunction	543	28.6
Intra-/extracardiac tumors/thrombi	496	26.1
Endocarditis	403	21.2
Aortic dissection	184	9.7
Valvular lesions	125	6.6
Others	149	7.8
Total	1900	100.0

The predominant indications for the TEE examinations are listed in Table 1. In 607 patients (31.9%), TEE was carried out in the early or late period after open heart surgery.

Methods

All TEE examinations were performed following a conventional transthoracic echocardiographic study. The TEE approach was added only in cases in which there was a clear clinical indication insufficiently clarified by the precordial technique. Prior to TEE, all conscious patients fasted for at least 4 h, gave verbal informed consent, and were carefully questioned concerning any kind of esophageal disease. In cases with potential esophageal disorders, we insisted on a regular esophagoscopy prior to TEE. In patients with known advanced esophageal varices, an esophageal tumor, or stenosis or diverticulum, and in patients who had undergone thoracic radiation therapy, TEE was considered as contraindicated. In contrast, anticoagulation was not regarded as an impediment.

Except for patients under mechanical ventilation, all studies were performed after application of local pharyngeal anesthesia (1% lidocaine spray). Additional mild sedating intravenous premedication (e.g., 5 mg diazepam) was only given in cases with suspected acute aortic dissection (in order to prevent an inappropriate blood pressure increase) and in a few patients with a markedly elevated anxiety level.

We used two types of TEE transducer: (1) a Diasonics Echoscope (Diasonics Cardio/Imaging Inc., Salt Lake City) (3.5-MHz phased array transducer, 32 elements, sector angle 84°; (2) a Hewlett-Packard 21362 A instrument (Hewlett-Packard Co., Medical Products Group, Andover, MA) (5.0-MHz phased array transducer, 64 elements, sector angle 90°). The transducers were mounted at the tip of a modified gastroscope (distal tip diameters 15.1 mm and 16.0 mm, respectively). Neither instrument had an incorporated optical channel. Following each TEE examination the probe was carefully cleaned with luke-warm soapy water and incubated in a commercially available disinfectant solution.

The TEE probe was usually inserted with the patient in left lateral decubitus position after removal of any dentures and with the neck slightly flexed towards the chest; a bite guard was placed after probe insertion. Particular care was taken that during transducer insertion as well as during the whole examination the hand control wheels for angulation of the probe tip remained in an unlocked position. During the course of the TEE examination it was sometimes necessary to change the body position of the patient (right lateral, straight back, sitting, etc.) in order to improve the visualization of particular cardiac structures. A routine TEE study was usually completed within 5−10 min. During the examination all patients were under continuous ECG monitoring; an intravenous line was placed only in rare exceptions (advanced atrioventricular block or for contrast material injection). After the examination patients were told to not eat or drink until the pharyngeal anesthetic effect has disappeared.

TEE examinations were performed by physicians only; five of eight physicians involved in TEE in our laboratory were trained in regular gastroscopy.

Results

Failure of Probe Insertion

In 23 of the 1900 consecutive patients (1.2%), we were not able to insert the transducer. All 23 patients were conscious and had had no sedating premedication. In all cases, the reason for probe insertion failure was a lack of cooperation from the patient or inexperience of the operator. In some of these cases, TEE examinations were repeated without difficulty after additional premedication or by a more experienced operator.

Interruption of TEE Examination Prior to Completion

In 17 patients (0.9%), the TEE study had to be interrupted prior to completion (Table 2). In the majority of cases (58.8%), this was due to the fact that the patient could not tolerate the TEE probe long enough. Two patients developed a short selft-terminating ventricular tachycardia during manipulation of the probe, one patient developed a transient atrial fibrillation, and in one case interruption was necessary due to bronchospasm which resolved immediately after withdrawl of the TEE probe. Three other patients reacted with vomiting since they had apparently not fasted long enough prior to TEE. To the best of our knowledge, no patient showed any significant late side effects after the TEE procedure.

Table 2. Reasons for interruption of a TEE examination prior to completion in 17 of 1900 patients (0.89%)

Reason	Patients	
	(*n*)	(%)
Intolerance of TEE probe	10	58.5
Vomiting	3	17.6
Ventricular tachycardia	2	11.8
Atrial fibrillation	1	5.9
Bronchospasm	1	5.9
Total	17	100.0

Improvement of Diagnostic Information by TEE

In 1028 of the 1900 patients (54.1%), the TEE examination added "important diagnostic information" to what was known from the precordial echocardiographic study. In this context, "important diagnostic information" was defined as findings which were essential for the further therapeutic handling of a particular patient.

Discussion

Our data indicate that in the hands of physicians who are familiar with gastroscopic techniques, a TEE examination can be performed rapidly and with an acceptably low risk. This is in good agreement with the reports of other groups [3, 4]. In addition, the procedure — although associated with some minor discomfort to the patient — is usually tolerated without problems even when a sedating premedication (which may increase the risk of aspiration and cardiovascular complications [6, 7]) is not used.

Some additional complications caused by TEE have been published in the literature: transient second- and third-degree atrioventricular block in one patient each [3, 8]; an attack of asthma (one patient) [8]; severe arterial hypoxemia in two cases with congenital heart disease and right-to-left shunts [3]; and in two patients, unilateral vocal cord paralysis. The last two patients were studied during neurosurgery under general anesthesia with extreme neck flexion and the head in an upright position; in these two instances the echoscope remained within the esophagus during the whole surgical procedure [9].

In a still ongoing cooperative multicenter study initiated by our laboratory, the results of TEE from 15 European centers were analyzed. Up to now, the data from more than 10000 TEE examinations have been collected. There was one death closely related to a TEE study. A patient with chest pain underwent TEE for exclusion of an acute aortic dissection. During the procedure, severe hematemesis, which stopped again after a short time, caused the interruption of TEE. Thereafter, the patient underwent diagnostic gastroscopy, which showed an esophageal tumor and resulted in repeated severe bleeding, and finally to death. Autopsy revealed a lung carcinoma which had infiltrated the esophagus.

In summary, in recent years TEE has been shown to provide essential diagnostic information in a variety of cardiac diseases, as outlined in the chapters of this book. The decision to perform a TEE examination should be made carefully and contraindications such as esophageal tumors, stenoses, diverticula, advanced varices, and previous chest radiation therapy should be kept in mind. However, when a TEE examination has to be performed to improve the diagnostic information and to avoid other more invasive techniques, the procedure is usually well tolerated and the associated risks are in the range of those associated with regular gastroscopies [6, 7].

References

1. Frazin L, Talano JV, Stephanides L, Loeb HS, Kopel L, Gunnar RM (1976) Esophageal echocardiography. Circulation 54:102−108
2. Schlüter M, Langenstein BA, Polster J, Kremer P, Souquet J, Engel S, Hanrath P (1982) Transoesophageal cross-sectional echocardiography with a phased array transducer system. Technique and initial clinical results. Br Heart J 48:67−72
3. Geibel A, Kasper W, Behroz A, Przewolka U, Meinertz T, Just H (1988) Risk of transesophageal echocardiography in awake patients with cardiac disease. Am J Cardiol 62:337−339
4. Engberding R, Hasfeld I, Chiladakis I, Dohrmann A, Große-Heitmeyer W, Stoll V (1988) Transösophageale Echokardiographie: erhöhtes Untersuchungsrisiko durch Blutdruckanstieg und Herzrhythmusstörungen? Herz/Kreisl 20:233−236
5. Daniel WG, Mügge A, Schröder E, Wenzlaff P, Grote J (1988) Transesophageal echocardiography in clinical cardiology − indications, practicability and risk (abstract). Circulation 78 (Suppl II):II−297
6. Miller G (1987) Komplikationen bei der Endoskopie des oberen Gastrointestinaltraktes. Leber Magen Darm 5:299−304
7. Hart R, Hagenmüller F (1988) Komplikationen und Todesfälle in der gastroenterologischen Endoskopie. Internist 29:815−819
8. Erbel R, Boerner N, Steller D, Brunier J, Thelen M, Pfeiffer C, Mohr-Kahaly S, Iversen S, Oelert H, Meyer J (1987) Detection of aortic dissection by transoesophageal echocardiography. Br Heart J 58:45−51
9. Cucchiara RF, Nugent M, Seward JB, Messick JM (1984) Air embolism in upright neurosurgical patients: detection and localization by two-dimensional transesophageal echocardiography. Anesthesiology 60:353−355

Subject Index

**J. B. Seward, A. J. Tajik, W. D. Edwards,
D. J. Hagler,** Mayo Clinic, Rochester

Two-Dimensional Echocardiographic Atlas

Volume 1

Congenital Heart Disease

1987. XIV, 598 pp. 517 figs. in 1820 parts.
Hardcover ISBN 3-540-96473-8

This is the first volume in a comprehensive three-volume tomographic atlas. It presents congenital cardiac defects imaged by twodimensional echocardiographic techniques. Directed towards the novice as well as the expert in this area of specialization, the atlas explores the diagnosis of various types of congenital heart disease from the common to the complex, using non-invasive tomographic imaging. High quality photographic reproductions constitute a major appeal of this important work, along with anatomic tomographic correlation. Both the beginner and the experienced clinician will find this an invaluable and essential reference on the topic of congenital heart disease.

Springer-Verlag Berlin
Heidelberg New York London
Paris Tokyo Hong Kong

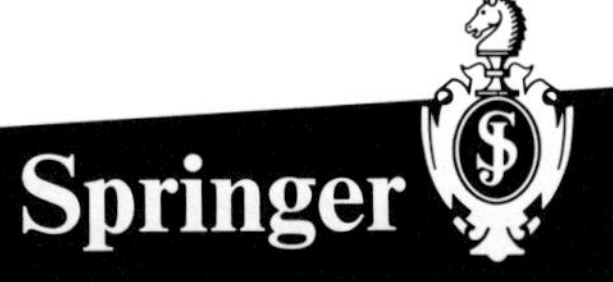

D. A. Redel, Bonn

Color Blood Flow Imaging of the Heart

1988. VII, 130 pp. 214 figs. Hardcover
ISBN 3-540-16521-5

This book looks at the newly developed technique of color blood flow imaging (CBFI) – a noninvasive ultrasonic method which will change essentially the diagnostic procedures in cardiology in the years to come. Additionally, CBFI yields new insights into physiological and pathophysiological mechanisms of the cardiovascular system which cannot be investigated with any other method. The reader will be introduced to this fascinating method by typical findings of CBFI in all common types of heart disease. The diagnostic possibilities of CBFI are shown by the presentation of high-quality color pictures which have been taken directly from the screen without video play-back; these are integrated into the text and extensively explained in the legends. The reader will also be confronted with normal findings as well as with artefacts of the method. After having studied this book he should be familiar with CBFI and be able to perform investigations by himself. This book presents typical findings of CBFI in all forms of commonly encountered heart disease to an extent not available in any other publication.

Springer-Verlag Berlin
Heidelberg New York London
Paris Tokyo Hong Kong

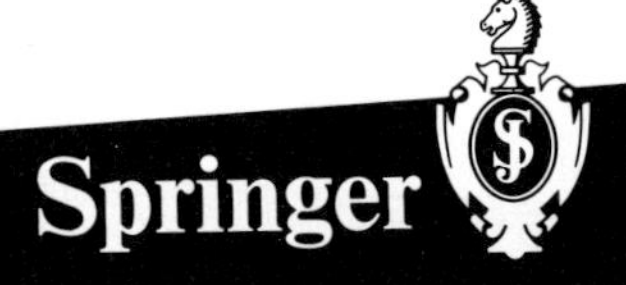